MBL Lectures in Biology
Volume 6

BLOOD CELLS OF MARINE INVERTEBRATES
Experimental Systems in Cell Biology and Comparative Physiology

MBL LECTURES IN BIOLOGY

Volume 1
The Origins of Life and Evolution
Harlyn O. Halvorson and K.E. Van Holde, *Editors*

Volume 2
Time, Space, and Pattern in Embryonic Development
William R. Jeffery and Rudolph A. Raff, *Editors*

Volume 3
Microbial Mats: Stromatolites
Yehuda Cohen, Richard W. Castenholz, and Harlyn O. Halvorson, *Editors*

Volume 4
Energetics and Transport in Aquatic Plants
John A. Raven

Volume 5
The Visual System
Alan Fein and Joseph S. Levine, *Editors*

Volume 6
Blood Cells of Marine Invertebrates: Experimental Systems in Cell Biology and Comparative Physiology
William D. Cohen, *Editor*

BLOOD CELLS OF MARINE INVERTEBRATES
Experimental Systems in Cell Biology and Comparative Physiology

Editor
William D. Cohen
Department of Biological Sciences
Hunter College of the City University of New York
New York, New York

ALAN R. LISS, INC. • NEW YORK

Address all Inquiries to the Publisher
Alan R. Liss, Inc., 41 East 11th Street, New York, NY 10003

Printed in the United States of America.

Library of Congress Cataloging in Publication Data
Main entry under title:

Blood cells of marine invertebrates.

Bibliography: p.
Includes index.
1. Marine invertebrates—Physiology. 2. Marine invertebrates—Cytology. 3. Blood cells. I. Cohen, William D.
QL364.B59 1985 592'.0116 84-26174
ISBN 0-8451-2205-3

Contents

Contributors

Peter B. Armstrong [77,251] Department of Zoology, University of California–Davis, Davis, CA 95616 and the Marine Biological Laboratory, Woods Hole, MA 02543

William D. Cohen [ix,3,251] Department of Biological Sciences, Hunter College of the City University of New York, New York, NY 10021 and the Marine Biological Laboratory, Woods Hole, MA 02543

Kenneth T. Edds [53,251] Department of Anatomical Sciences, State University at Buffalo, School of Medicine, Buffalo, NY 14214 and the Marine Biological Laboratory, Woods Hole, MA 02543

Paul R. Gross [xv] Marine Biological Laboratory, Woods Hole, MA 02543

Jack Levin [145,251] Departments of Laboratory Medicine and Medicine, University of California School of Medicine, San Francisco, CA 94143 and the Marine Biological Laboratory, Woods Hole, MA 02543

Timothy K. Maugel [167] Department of Zoology, University of Maryland, College Park, MD 20742 and the Marine Biological Laboratory, Woods Hole, MA 02543

Ronald Nagel [227] Division of Hematology, Albert Einstein College of Medicine, Bronx, NY 10461 and the Marine Biological Laboratory, Woods Hole, MA 02543

Iris Nemhauser [3,251] Department of Biological Sciences, Hunter College of the City University of New York, New York, NY 10021 and the Marine Biological Laboratory, Woods Hole, MA 02543; present address: Department of Hormone Research, Weizmann Institute of Science, Rehovot, Israel

Richard L. Ornberg [127,251] Laboratory of Cell Biology and Genetics, National Institute of Arthritis, Diabetes, Digestive, and Kidney Diseases, National Institutes of Health, Bethesda, MD 20205 and the Marine Biological Laboratory, Woods Hole, MA 02543

Sidney K. Pierce [167,251] Department of Zoology, University of Maryland, College Park, MD 20742 and the Marine Biological Laboratory, Woods Hole, MA 02543

Eric Schabtach [193] Biology Department, University of Oregon, Eugene, OR 97403

Nora B. Terwilliger [193,251] Oregon Institute of Marine Biology, University of Oregon, Charleston, OR 97420 and Biology Department, University of Oregon, Eugene, OR 97403

Robert C. Terwilliger [193,251] Oregon Institute of Marine Biology, University of Oregon, Charleston, OR 97420 and Biology Department, University of Oregon, Eugene, OR 97403

The number in brackets is the opening page number of the contributor's article.

Preface

The seeds for this text were planted almost 7 years ago, when a search of the MBL library for organized information on invertebrate blood cells ended in frustration. There was only Warren Andrew's 1966 *Comparative Hematology* (Grune and Stratton Inc., New York) to whet the appetite. The same need was obviously felt by others, as evidenced by the two volume work on *Invertebrate Blood Cells* which subsequently appeared (Ratcliffe and Rowley, Eds., Academic Press Inc., London, 1981). This accomplished the remarkable feat of thoroughly surveying the literature on the whole range of invertebrate Phyla and innumerable fascinating species. However, there still appeared to be a niche for a complementary text, one which would provide detailed information on selected physiological problems and a relatively small number of cell types of value to researchers at the cell and molecular levels. For practical purposes, animals readily available for study at the Marine Biological Laboratory and other marine laboratories were of particular interest.

The possibility of producing such a text arose with awareness that there was a nucleus of MBL summer investigators working on various aspects of invertebrate blood cell physiology. Many participated in an informal hematology seminar series organized at MBL by Jack Levin, and also presented work at the MBL General Meetings. These meetings of colleagues with mutual interests and the resulting exchange of ideas and information did much to make this book a reality.

Our objectives have been the following:

1) To provide an account of current research on specific physiological problems, utilizing various marine invertebrate blood cell types
2) To document the experimental value of these cell types in approaching problems of broad interest
3) To contribute to the fields of comparative physiology and hematology at the cellular and molecular levels
4) To generate research interest in marine species available at the MBL and other marine stations
5) To provide practical information on obtaining and maintaining the organisms and cells

In general, we have attempted to produce a text which is useful and stimulating to researchers at the cell and molecular levels, and which might remain so for some years beyond our current investigations. To this end the authors were encouraged not only to include their latest research findings, but to speculate, to point out areas of ignorance, and to raise questions for future research. No effort was made to cover the wide range of invertebrate blood cell types; on the contrary, the physiological problems were our primary consideration, with the same cells sometimes utilized in several different studies. Major chapter topics include cytoskeletal structure and function, cell motility, cellular morphogenesis, exocytosis, coagulation, osmotic regulation, and the molecular structure and function of intracellular respiratory pigments. Practical material on the animals and cells, sufficient to enable a researcher to initiate studies, has been gathered into the final chapter. Included are conditions for maintaining the animals, methods for obtaining, washing, and handling of the cells, and sources of the animals. Although the individual chapters do not undertake consideration of species identification or general anatomy and physiology of the animals themselves, a list of useful reference works dealing with such subjects is also provided in the final chapter.

As systems for research, the cells discussed in this volume offer the experimental advantages of populations of single cells together with the physiological relevance of *in vivo* origin and function. In general, they fall into two categories: (a) "erythrocytes," i.e., those containing respiratory pigments, and (b) "clotting cells," i.e., cells which have, as one of their major functions, a role in blood coagulation and/or sealing of wounds. Although the number of major invertebrate species represented in this text is relatively small, their phylogenetic range is broad. The cells studies include the hemoglobin-containing erythrocytes of certain Molluscs ("blood clams"), of Echiurans ("innkeeper worms"), and of Annelids (polychaete "blood worms"), the hemerythrin-containing erythrocytes of Sipunculans ("peanut worms"), and the clotting cells of certain Arthropods ("horseshoe crab" amebocytes and lobster coelomocytes) and of Echinoderms (sea urchin coelomocytes). It is hoped that the data and approaches for the cell types presented will not only be of intrinsic value but will also prove useful as a guide for work on blood cells of other invertebrate species.

I am indebted to Dr. Paul Gross, Director of the MBL, for his support of the project, to Alan Liss and Paulette Cohen of Alan R. Liss, Inc., who helped get it underway and waited patiently as it came to fruition, and to Barbara Schloss of Alan R. Liss, Inc., who was extremely helpful and steadfast in following it through to production. I wish also to thank my family, who tolerated me as I wrestled with editorial tasks, and especially my daughter Sarah, who contributed the drawings for the last chapter.

ABOUT THE AUTHORS

The MBL has had considerable influence on the lives and careers of many of the authors, and much of the work presented herein was performed there. It seemed to me particularly appropriate to record some of that while introducing the authors:

Peter B. Armstrong is Professor in the Zoology Department, University of California, Davis, CA. He has been a Summer Investigator at MBL in 1975–79 and 1982–84. His MBL origins are notable: "My association with MBL began considerably pre-utero with my father, Philip B. Armstrong, who began spending summers at MBL in 1928. He and my mother met at Woods Hole in 1931, and he continued to summer at Woods Hole until his death, bringing me along throughout my childhood. Exposure to the Woods Hole environment, including several summers of classes at the Children's School of Science, was instrumental in convincing me that biological research was amongst the highest callings to which one could respond. Formal association with MBL began with a stint as a summer helper collector (1956–58) for what was then called the Supply Department and continued with two summers as a research associate and a summer in the Invertebrate Zoology Course during which time I met my wife (1961). The cycle is continuing with recent summers spent as an Independent Investigator, accompanied by my own children."

Kenneth T. Edds is Assistant Professor in the Department of Anatomical Sciences, State University at Buffalo, Buffalo, NY. Ken took the MBL Invertebrate Zoology course as an undergraduate (1968), spent three summers in the laboratory of Dr. Robert D. Allen as a graduate student (1970–73), and eventually returned for year-round postdoctoral work with R.E. Stephens in 1974–76. Subsequently he set up his own year-round lab at the MBL and was an Assistant Scientist from 1976–79. He was a member of the MBL January Developmental Biology course faculty for eight years, serving as course Director in 1981–82, and has been a Summer Investigator since 1979.

Jack Levin is Professor of Laboratory Medicine and of Medicine in the Departments of Laboratory Medicine and Medicine, University of California School of Medicine, San Francisco, CA. Jack has been active in MBL research and teaching for twenty years. He began as Research Associate in 1963 and has been an Independent Investigator since 1965. From 1978 to 1983 he participated as a faculty member in the MBL Winter Course "Comparative Pathology of Marine Invertebrates". Jack recounts his MBL beginnings as follows: "My initial opportunity to work at MBL was provided by the late Frederik B. Bang, whose initial observations of the effects of bacteria on blood coagulation in *Limulus* provided the starting point for my work with *Limulus*. In addition, Dr. Bang provided continuous advice and inspiration to me, throughout our long and valued association."

Timothy K. Maugel is Director of the Laboratory for Ultrastructural Research, Department of Zoology, University of Maryland, College Park, MD. He has done research with co-author S.K. Pierce at MBL in the summers of 1982 and 1983, and has beaten Pierce in the Falmouth Road Race each time.

Ronald L. Nagel is Professor of Medicine and Head, Division of Hematology, at the Albert Einstein College of Medicine, Bronx, NY. A Summer

Investigator at MBL since 1976, he relates his background as follows: "My first trip to Woods Hole was in 1963, while a Fellow at the Albert Einstein College of Medicine. Irving London was the Chairman of our Department and an avid Woods Hole person, and was responsible for stimulating our interest in the place. But it was in 1976 that I became an annual devotee of the Marine Biological Laboratory, sharing, since then, a lab with Tom Borgese every summer. My general interest in marine biology, nevertheless, started in the Biological Station at Montemar, Chile (which is connected with the University of Chile) and to which I was exposed since my medical school days."

Iris Nemhauser is currently in the Department of Hormone Research, Weizmann Institute of Science, Rehovot, Israel, having previously (during the writing of this text) been a Post-doctoral Fellow in the Department of Pharmacology, College of Physicians and Surgeons, Columbia University, NY. As a Graduate Student with co-author W.D. Cohen at Hunter College, she spent the summers of 1977–80 at the MBL studying the cytoskeletal system of various blood cell types in local invertebrates.

Richard L. Ornberg is Senior Staff Fellow in the Laboratory of Cell Biology and Genetics, The National Institute of Arthritis, Diabetes, Digestive and Kidney Diseases, National Institutes of Health, Bethesda, MD. He has spent six summers at the MBL, beginning in 1976 as a Grass Foundation Fellow and continuing in 1977–1981 as a Co-Investigator with T.S. Reese.

Sidney K. Pierce is Professor in the Zoology Department, University of Maryland, College Park, MD. He has been associated with MBL continuously since 1968, when he was a student in the Ecology course. He returned as a graduate student in 1969–1970, and Summer Investigator in 1971–72. For the next five summers he served as Instructor in the Experimental Invertebrate Zoology course. He has been a Summer Investigator since 1978, and spent the winter of '83–84 on Sabbatical leave at the MBL.

Eric Schabtach is Director of the Electron Microscope Facility, Department of Biology, University of Oregon, Eugene, OR. His encounter with the MBL was limited to about 2 weeks in the winter of 1968, studying tunicates. Though brief, it has remained vivid: "I had a lab on the 2nd floor of the Supply Building with a great view, the weather was beautiful, and the solitude remarkable (the winter population at that time seemed miniscule). I enjoyed myself very much, and still remember the period fondly."

Nora Barclay Terwilliger is Research Associate at the Oregon Institute of Marine Biology, Charleston, OR, and the Biology Department, University of Oregon, Eugene, OR. Nora was a Graduate student in the MBL Physiology course in the summer of 1966, where she met Bob Terwilliger. According to Nora and Bob, "post-course research on mitotic spindle proteins with Shinya Inoué and *Limulus* hemocyanin with Ken Van Holde piqued our interest in other multisubunit protein systems as well. When we moved west to the University of Oregon's Oregon Institute of Marine Biology, our mutual research interests focused on the blood of marine species, specifically the structure and function of the respiratory proteins. It was a bonus for us that Ken Van Holde was at Oregon State University; we have had a very pleasant and rewarding collaboration with him. Writing this chapter has provided a good opportunity to combine a continued interest in blood cell morphology with our current work on invertebrate hemoglobins."

Robert C. Terwilliger is Professor of Biology in the Biology Department, University of Oregon, Eugene, OR, and Assistant Director of the Oregon Institute of Marine Biology in Charleston, OR. As noted above, he took the MBL Physiology Course as a graduate student in the summer of 1966, where he met Nora, and returned the following summer working in Henry de-Philips' and Ken Van Holde's lab.

Finally, I am Professor in the Department of Biological Sciences, Hunter College of the City University of New York, NY, where I maintain a bit of the sea in several tanks. While a graduate student at Columbia University I paid an initial brief visit to MBL in the summer of 1961. This was highlighted by a specimen collecting trip aboard the (then) Supply Department boat, arranged by dissertation sponsor Teru Hayashi. I spent the next summer in Tay's Lillie laboratory, a room not only conducive to research but also providing an excellent view of the Mess tennis court. A subsequent summer was spent in the MBL Library working on a book, and I have been a Summer Investigator at MBL since 1977. My personal relationship with the Atlantic began about 40 years ago on the beaches of Long Island, prowling the jetties which were richly endowed with invertebrates. I think it fair to say that all of the authors share a love and respect for the sea, with its diversity of creatures beyond imagination. That many of these species should turn out to be of considerable value to our work has been a wonderful bonus. It has been my privilege, and that of many of the other authors as noted above, to be able to perform much of this research at the MBL, a unique institution which maximizes the freedom of the individual to explore and to learn. We are grateful for these opportunities and are proud to be part of the *MBL Lectures in Biology* series.

W.D Cohen

Foreword

In 1888 C.O. Whitman, the founding Director of the MBL, delivered an evening lecture (in a famous series that continues to the present day) on Evolution and Epigenesis. Its purpose was primarily to administer some discipline to members of the two rapidly-diverging schools of embryology in the place: the cell lineagists, who were primarily observers and describers, and the experimental epigeneticists, who scorned mere observation as a device for getting at the underlying phenomena of development. Of course Whitman was also defending his own approach to embryology, which was descriptive and comparative morphology, but his admonitions were addressed to all:

". . .Many difficult questions are involved which can only be settled after the most exhaustive analysis of. . .structure and the most careful examination of its entire history. It is not enough to catch a fact here and there, in this or that species; the whole series of phenomena must be studied genetically, and in as many forms as possible. It often happens that we have to snatch facts as opportunity brings them within reach, regardless of their connections; but so long as they stand isolated, they are unsafe pegs to hang theories upon."

Whitman's influence was profound: he did not himself reconcile the lineagists with the epigeneticists, who managed that feat, more or less, by themselves in the course of time, but he did make comprehensiveness of approach a hallmark of biological research done at the MBL. And of course that made sense then, as it does now, because as opposed to what is common at universities, the gathering of investigators at the MBL is an unique opportunity, each year, for comprehensiveness. Thus no single investigator of blood cells, or using them simply as convenient material, could today give the time necessary to writing a comprehensive treatise on the blood cells of invertebrates generally. But in a place where (1) there is a long tradition of interest in those cells for their own sake; (2) many distinguished members of the community use them, not because they are particularly interested in blood cells but because the cells of a particular species are especially favorable material for studying some structure or process; and (3) the members of both groups can readily exchange information and communicate tricks of the trade in an informal way, it makes sense to use the agglomeration of knowledgeables for construction of that "exhaustive analysis" Whitman considered essential—and some of us do today—for the understanding of important biological phenomena.

That the present volume should appear among the MBL Lectures in Biology seems to me, therefore, particularly appropriate. Those published to date in the series have been the products of formal courses or of organized and intensive symposia. To have among them now a book generated in essence by a confluence of interest among investigators, independent of the external pressure of formal proceedings, seems to me an expression of that special kind of collegiality and intellectual cooperation that *is* the MBL, and has been the really unique feature of MBL science since the time of Whitman.

That the contents of this volume represent more than one scientist could find the time and expertise, today, to write alone will be self-evident. It is not, however, simply an assembly of disparate and superficial papers, stitched together by the organizers of a meeting and repeating what has already appeared elsewhere in journal articles. It is what its title says it is: a scholarly and practical work on the blood cells of marine invertebrates, meant to give form to a host of different research enterprises that are united primarily by the biological origin of the research material, and to provide for students and investigators who might choose in the future to use that material a practical and broadly-based survey of what is known about it.

I know that the book will be useful to marine biologists and cell biologists for a long time to come, but I believe that its interest can be broader than that. The comparative biology of circulating cells among invertebrates provides unique insights into processes whose importance transcends the special tissue of their origin: these processes are as diverse as cytoskeletal morphogenesis, osmoregulation and the regulation, at more fundamental levels, of osmoregulation itself, and the relations of structure to function in those unique cargoes of the blood cells, respiratory proteins. Discussed together, within a broad physiological and phylogenetic context, these matters do indeed approximate Whitman's ideal of exhaustive and genetic examination of a biologic phenomenon.

P.R. Gross

THE CYTOSKELETON

Blood Cells of Marine Invertebrates: Experimental Systems in Cell Biology and Comparative Physiology, pages 3–49

Chapter One
Marginal Bands and the Cytoskeleton in Blood Cells of Marine Invertebrates

William D. Cohen and Iris Nemhauser

Department of Biological Sciences, Hunter College of the City University of New York, New York, New York 10021 (W.D.C., I.N.) and the Marine Biological Laboratory, Woods Hole, Massachusetts 02543 (W.D.C., I.N.)

INTRODUCTION

The Cytoskeleton

Study of the cytoskeleton of eukaryotic cells has been a major activity in cell biology in recent years. The term "cytoskeleton" means, literally, skeleton of the cell, and it implies passive function by analogy with truly skeletal structures such as bones. This is misleading, however, for in actual usage the current concept of cytoskeleton is far broader. It includes all of the major fibrous or filamentous elements of cells: microtubules, microfilaments, and intermediate filaments. From an operational viewpoint, these are structures which remain behind in a relatively stable, insoluble state following extraction of membrane components with detergents such as Triton X-100 under appropriate conditions. The structure and arrangement of fibrous elements in the residue after such extraction tends to be faithful to that of the living cell and is thus referred to as the cytoskeleton. In this connection the term really indicates "bare-bones" or skeletal appearance rather than bone-like func-

Iris Nemhauser's present address is the Department of Hormone Research, Weizmann Institute of Science, Rehovot, Israel.

tional passivity. Major molecular components of the cytoskeleton may thus include tubulin, intermediate filament proteins, actin, and even myosin, and they may be involved in active motile and morphogenetic functions in cells [see Edds, this volume].

In addition, the cytoskeleton encompasses structures such as the cell surface-associated cytoskeleton (abbreviated here as SAC), which underlies the lipid bilayer of the plasma membrane. This has also been referred to as the "membrane skeleton" and was studied for many years simply as part of the plasma membrane, without reference to cytoskeletal function. From an experimental point of view, the SAC paradigm is the actin-spectrin network associated with the mammalian erythrocyte membrane [Hainfield and Steck, 1977; Branton et al., 1981]. This network does not contain long linear elements such as microtubules and filaments, but rather consists of a relatively thin, planar cross-linked layer composed of several kinds of molecules in repeating array. In addition to these structures, there is the (still controversial) microtrabecular system reported to link nearly all organelles and other cytoskeletal elements within one three-dimensional cellular lattice [Wolosewick and Porter, 1979]. Presumably such a system would be composed at least partly of various proteins that bind to and cross-link actin filaments (actin-binding proteins), as well as microtubule-associated proteins (MAPs) and intermediate filament-associated proteins (IFAPs).

Marginal Bands

Of the numerous cytoskeletal systems currently under investigation, the marginal band (MB) of microtubules present in nonmammalian vertebrate erythrocytes (and various other blood cell types) is one of the simplest. Such erythrocytes are flattened, generally elliptical, and nucleated, with the MBs present in the plane of flattening, lying close to but not touching the plasma membrane bilayer. MBs were originally discovered in amphibian erythrocytes by light microscopists, who recognized that they were continuous fibrous structures with a probable cytoskeletal role [Dehler, 1895; Meves, 1911]. Fawcett was the first to show that nonmammalian vertebrate erythrocyte and thrombocyte MBs were constructed of microtubules [Fawcett, 1959; Fawcett and Witebsky, 1964], and subsequently similar MBs were discovered in mammalian blood platelets by Behnke [1965] and others. MBs also occur in the immature erythrocytes of camels (the only mammalian family with elliptical erythrocytes) [Barclay, 1966; Cohen and Terwilliger, 1979] and in the primitive (yolk-sac) nucleated erythrocytes of mammalian embryos [van Deurs and Behnke, 1973]. However, MBs are not present in mammalian splenic erythroblasts [Grasso, 1966; Repasky and Eckert, 1981] or in circulating mammalian erythrocytes. It is clear that, among the vertebrates, mammals have the most atypical erythrocytes.

Marginal Bands in Invertebrate Blood Cells

Some years ago, armed with knowledge of widespread MB distribution in vertebrate blood cells, we wondered whether any invertebrate erythrocytes and/or clotting cells contained similar structures. The sparse and scattered literature on such cells yielded few unequivocal examples in our initial literature search. Thus, beginning in 1977, we spent part of several summers at the Marine Biological Laboratory surveying the blood cells of local invertebrates for the presence of MBs. The task had been facilitated by recent advances in understanding the conditions for assembly of tubulin into microtubules in vitro, initially demonstrated by Weisenberg [1972]. We were able to lyse cells directly in detergent (Triton X-100) under microtubule-stabilizing conditions and examine the cytoskeletons in phase contrast for the presence of MBs [Cohen et al., 1977]. To our great delight, we found that the waters of Cape Cod offered a wonderful smorgasbord of readily available invertebrates with MB-containing blood cells. These included hemerythrin-bearing erythrocytes of the "peanut worm" *Phascolopsis gouldii* (formerly known as *Phascolosoma* and *Golfingia;* phylum Sipuncula), hemoglobin-containing erythrocytes of the "blood clams" *Anadara ovalis* and *Anadara transversa* (phylum Mollusca), amebocytes of the "horseshoe crab" *Limulus polyphemus* (Arthropoda-Xiphosura), and hemocytes of the lobster *Homarus americanus* and of the marine crabs *Libinia emarginata* and *Cancer borealis* (Arthropoda-Crustacea). Subsequent literature searches revealed well-documented MBs in hemocytes of the cockroach *Periplaneta americana* (Arthropoda-Insecta) [Baerwald and Boush, 1970], hemoglobin-containing erythrocytes of the sea cucumber *Cucumaria miniata* (phylum Echinodermata) [Fontaine and Lambert, 1973], and hemerythrin-containing erythrocytes of the marine worm *Priapulus caudatus* (phylum Priapulida) [Mattison and Fange, 1973].

In this chapter we discuss the MB-containing erythrocytes and clotting cells of the peanut worm, blood clam, horseshoe crab, and lobster. These cells are of intrinsic interest with respect to function(s) in the animals, and they also provide a comparative perspective from which to view vertebrate blood cells. Of equal or surpassing importance, however, is their value as experimental systems for analysis of cytoskeletal structure, composition, assembly, and function.

EXPERIMENTAL STUDIES: ERYTHROCYTES

Erythrocytes of the Blood Clam *Noetia ponderosa* and Closely Related Species

Certain members of the Arcidae, known colloquially as blood clams, are unusual among the mollusks in that they possess hemoglobin-bearing erythrocytes. These animals are common, however, and have a worldwide distribution including species such as the "bloody cockle" of West Africa *(Anadara senilis)* [Yoloye, 1975] and the Sydney cockle of Australia *(A. trapezia)* [Sullivan, 1961]. Along the eastern coast of the United States one finds *Noetia ponderosa, Anadara transversa,* and *Anadara ovalis* as typical representatives. The hemoglobin in these species is of considerable interest from the standpoint of evolution and comparative biochemistry [see Nagel, this volume], and the cells are of value for work on osmotic regulation [see Pierce and Maugel, this volume]. These erythrocytes also have a fascinating cytoskeletal system, and in this chapter we will consider some of its major structural and functional features.

The living erythrocytes are flattened, nucleated, and usually elliptical in profile (Fig. 1). When removed from the animal and kept in their native fluid, they typically undergo a rapid morphological change, appearing lumpy or amorphous after 5–10 min. The significance of this change is unknown at present, but it appears to be caused by a factor in the clam "blood." It occurs

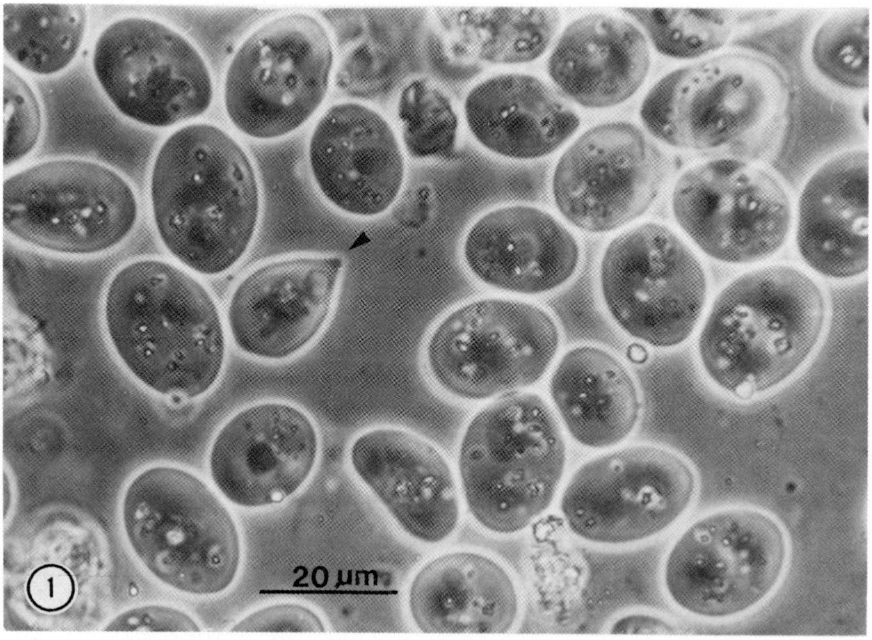

Fig. 1. Living erythrocytes of *Noetia ponderosa*, observed in phase contrast. The cells are typically flattened and elliptical, but occasionally a pointed cell (arrowhead) is present. Figures 1, 2, 4, 6, 7, 8, 10 from Nemhauser et al. [1983], reproduced from The Journal of Cell Biology 96:979–989, by copyright permission of The Rockefeller University Press.

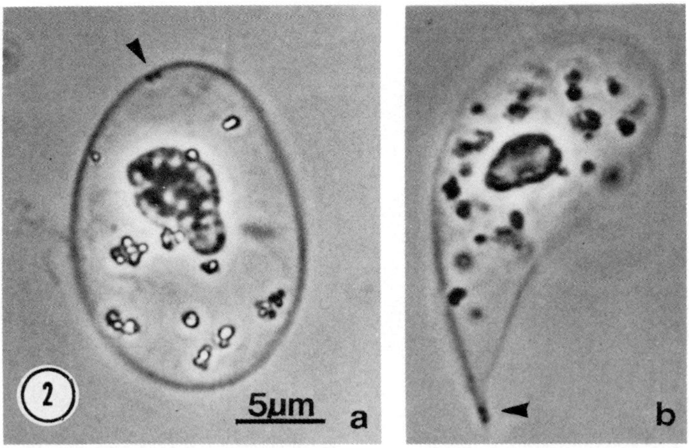

Fig. 2. a. Lysed erythrocytes ("cytoskeletons") of *N. ponderosa* (phase contrast). The phase-dense MB lies in the original plane of flattening, corresponding in size and shape to the living cell. A pair of centrioles visible as phase-dense "dots" is associated with every MB (arrowhead). b. Typical cytoskeleton of a pointed cell, in this case from animals tentatively identified as juveniles of *A. lienosa*. In this as well as the other blood clam species, pointed MBs typically have the centrioles at the tip (arrowhead).

far less frequently in *Noetia* than in the *Anadara* species, making *Noetia* more convenient to work with in experiments in which preservation of native cell morphology is important. Further information and methods for preventing this shape change are presented in the final chapter of this volume.

When living cells of normal morphology are suspended in microtubule-stabilizing medium containing the nonionic detergent Triton X-100 (typical medium = 0.4% w/v Triton, 100 mM PIPES buffer, 1 mM $MgCl_2$, 5 mM EGTA, + protease inhibitors, pH 6.8), they are rapidly cleared of hemoglobin and other soluble components. The MB, previously invisible, is now readily apparent at the periphery of the resulting "cytoskeleton," with size and shape corresponding to that of the original cell (Fig. 2). The MBs of these cells have a striking structural feature: A pair of centrioles is physically associated with each MB, usually at one end of the ellipse [Cohen and Nemhauser, 1980]. These centrioles are easily visible as a pair of dense dots in phase contrast under oil immersion (Fig. 2a). They are usually adjacent but have been found separated by up to 1.3 μm in some cytoskeletons. Both MB and centrioles bind anti-tubulin, as shown by indirect immunofluorescence (Fig. 3). The morphological correspondence between cell and MB holds even in pointed (i.e., teardrop-shaped) erythrocytes which are occa-

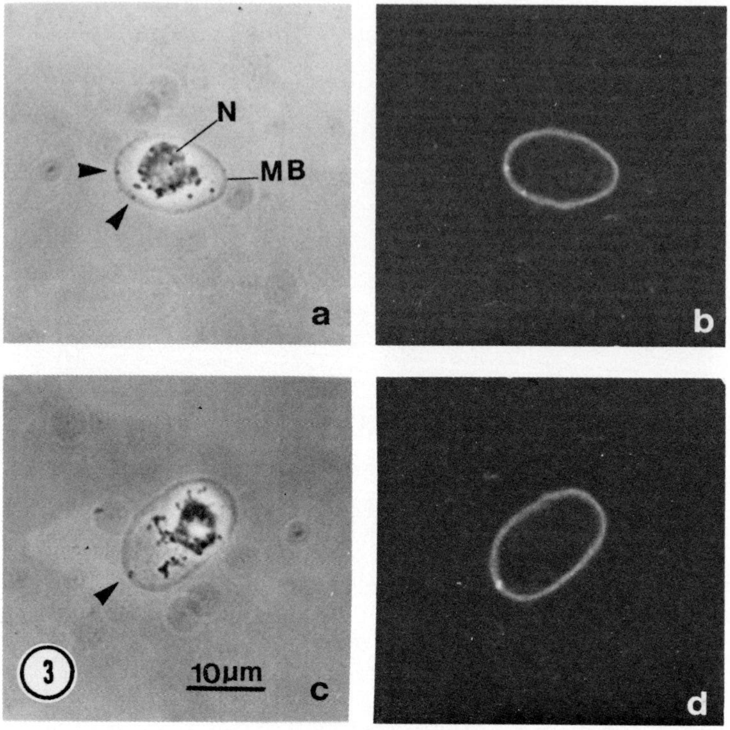

Fig. 3. Cytoskeletons of *A. transversa* examined by means of anti-tubulin immunofluorescence (indirect method). a,b and c,d are phase/fluorescence pairs. Both MB and centrioles (arrowheads) bind anti-tubulin. In this case centriolar fluorescence exceeds that of the MB, but MB fluorescence often masks the centrioles. Centrioles are usually close together as in panels c and d but are occasionally separated as in panels a and b. N, nucleus.

sionally observed (Fig. 1). Pointed MBs are present with corresponding frequency in cytoskeleton preparations, with the centrioles invariably located at the apex. In one of the species that we have examined, tentatively identified as *A. lienosa* (juveniles), pointed cells and cytoskeletons were consistently present in large numbers (Fig. 2b). We do not know whether the pointed erythrocytes are an abnormality, a stage of cellular morphogenesis, or a normal, functional variant cell type. Identification of the erythropoietic organ(s) in these species would be a first step in answering this question.

If glutaraldehyde is included in the Triton-containing lytic medium, simultaneous lysis and fixation for thin sectioning can be achieved. The cell surface-associated cytoskeleton (SAC) is observed enclosing the MB, nucleus, and remains of other organelles. When the MB is present in cross section, the SAC is always tightly apposed to it, giving the impression that it is "stretched" or held in an extended state by the MB (Fig. 4a). At higher magnifications, cross-bridges are often seen between adjacent MB microtubules (Fig. 4a, inset, and 4b). The centrioles have typical 9-triplet ultrastructure (Fig. 4c). Marginal band microtubules appear to be in contact with the centriolar surfaces rather than the ends of the triplets, and some centrioles are clearly at right angles to each other and to the MB (Fig. 4d).

General cytoskeletal features are evident in whole mounts stained with uranyl acetate and observed in the transmission electron microscope (TEM) (Fig. 5). The MB circumscribes the cytoskeleton, and the densely staining centrioles are usually readily apparent. The SAC collapses onto the grid and is visible as a network covering and enclosing the MB, within which the nucleus and remnants of other organelles are suspended. Whole mounts are of value because the cytoskeletons are derived from cells that are naturally flat, and therefore the depth of material through which one must look is within a useful range.

Since the site of erythropoiesis in "blood clams" is unknown [Sullivan, 1961], we have not been able to determine whether the centrioles, presumably remaining from the last mitotic division, participate in MB biogenesis during cell differentiation. However, the MB is cold-labile in the species we have studied, disassembling in about 1 hr at 0°C and reassembling in about the same time upon rewarming to more physiological temperatures (for clams!). This permits study of the reassembly sequence [Nemhauser et al., 1983]. The centrioles are present in the cytoskeleton at 0°C, but MB microtubules are absent (Fig. 6). Within minutes of the onset of rewarming, microtubules are observed radiating from the centrioles (Fig. 7a,b), and the cytoskeleton subsequently takes on a pointed appearance (Fig. 8a,b,c,d). Ultimately a normal-looking MB reforms, although it is sometimes thinner than in non-cooled controls. The centrioles are associated with the reassembling MB at all stages, and even in late stages it is evident that they are functioning as organizing centers (Fig. 8e,f). Our proposal for the MB reassembly sequence is illustrated in Figure 9.

In recent experiments utilizing the microtubule-stabilizing agent taxol [Schiff et al., 1979; Schiff and Horwitz, 1980], the participation of centrioles in MB reassembly in these cells has been further documented [Joseph-Silverstein and Cohen, 1983a]. When taxol is added to cells lacking MBs at 0°C, MBs slowly reassemble even without rewarming, and this unusual reassembly at 0°C is also initiated at the centrioles.

In addition to providing a means for demonstrating centriole function in MB formation, the low temperature lability of the blood clam erythrocyte MB is very useful for studies of cytoskeleton composition and function. As

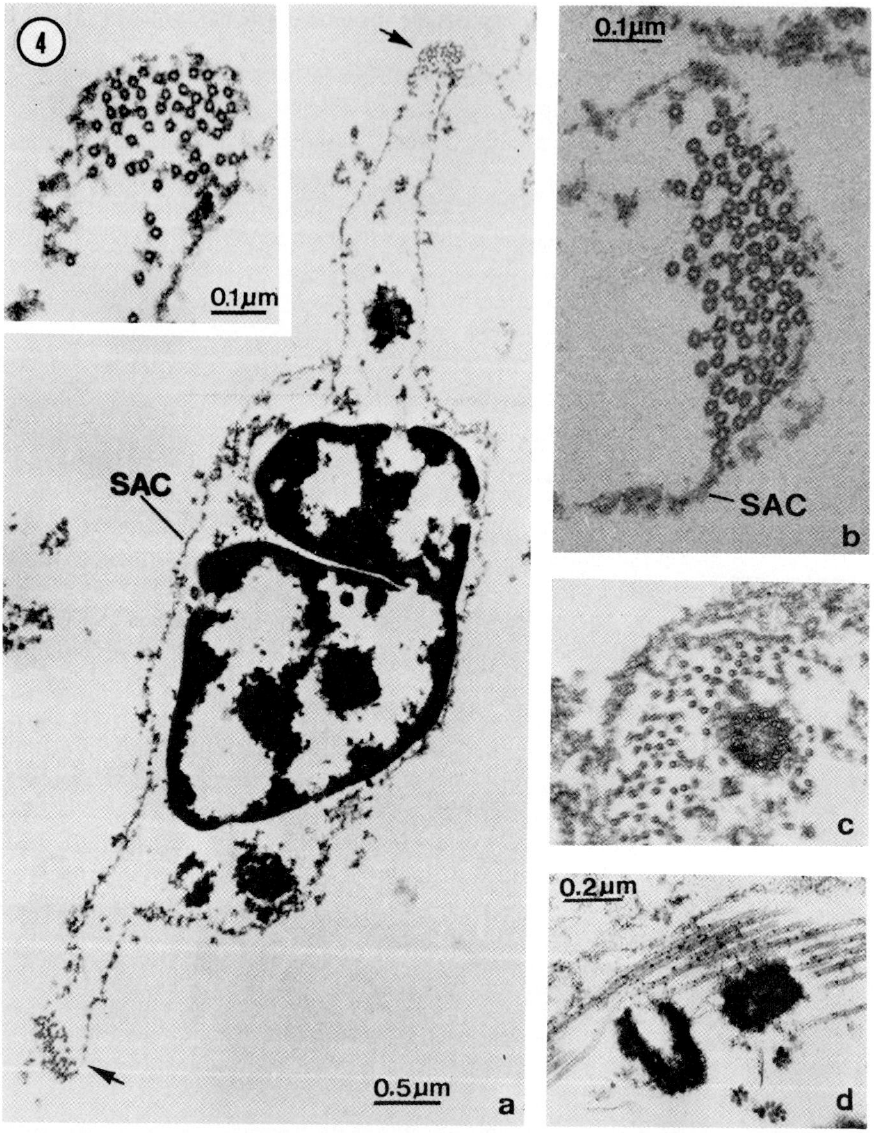

Fig. 4. Cytoskeletal structure as seen in thin section (transmission electron microscopy) after simultaneous lysis and fixation of blood clam erythrocytes. a. Entire cytoskeleton, with the MB in cross section at the extremities (arrows). The MB is in contact with the cell surface-associated cytoskeleton (SAC), which encloses it and all other components. The MB appears to press against the SAC, keeping it extended and maintaining flattened morphology as in the living cell. *Inset:* Higher-magnification view of MB at upper arrow. About 50 microtubules are present, some connected by bridges. b. Cross section through a thicker MB (~85 microtubules), in which many bridges are visible. c. MB-associated centrioles exhibit classical 9-triplet ultrastructure. d. In some cases at least, one member of a centriole pair is aligned perpendicular to the MB, and the two centrioles are arranged orthogonally. Magnification in c as in d. All are *N. ponderosa* except c, which is *A. transversa.* Figures 4c and 5 from Cohen and Nemhauser [1980], reproduced from The Journal of Cell Biology 86:286–291 by copyright permission of the Rockefeller University Press.

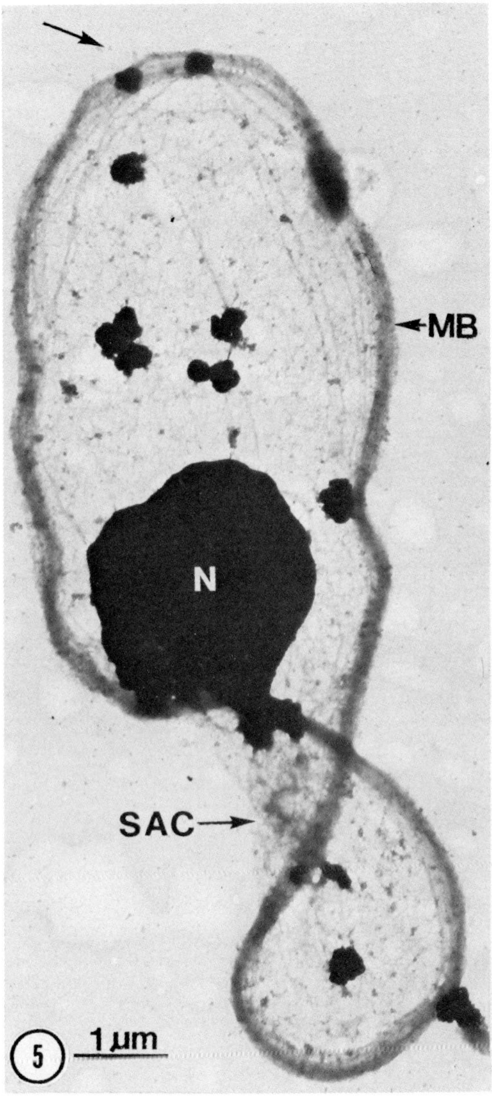

Fig. 5. Whole mount of *A. transversa* erythrocyte cytoskeleton (glutaraldehyde fixation, uranyl acetate staining, TEM). The MB is twisted into a figure-8 (an artifact of preparation), with the heavily stained centrioles readily visible (arrow). The SAC collapses onto the grid, appearing as a rough network within which the nucleus (N) and all other structures are trapped.

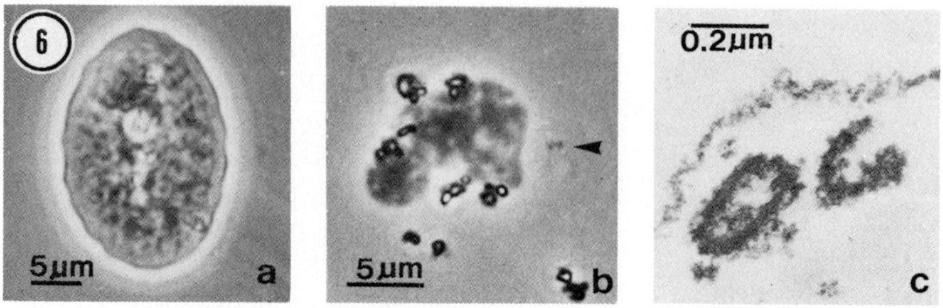

Fig. 6. *N. ponderosa* erythrocytes at 0°C. a. Intact erythrocyte; general flattened, elliptical morphology is maintained. b. Lysed cell; MB has disassembled, but centrioles (arrowhead) remain. c. Part of a lyse-fixed cytoskeleton with pair of centrioles adjacent to the SAC. a,b, Phase contrast; c, TEM.

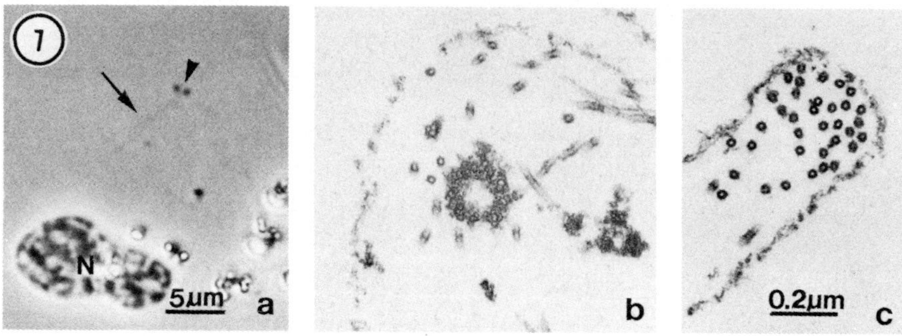

Fig. 7. *N. ponderosa* erythrocyte cytoskeletons prepared from cells during rewarming at 25°C after MB disassembly at 0°C. a. Two-minute rewarming; centrioles are visible (arrowhead) and fibers (arrow) are already observed emanating from centriolar region (compare with Fig. 6b). Phase contrast. b. Two-minute rewarming, TEM thin section; microtubules are present in vicinity of centrioles, but are not observed elsewhere in the cytoskeletons. c. A nascent MB after 15 min rewarming, already maintaining the SAC in extended form (compare with Fig. 4a). Thin section, TEM. Magnification in b as in c.

seen in thin section, cytoskeletons at 0°C have lost the MB but retain the SAC (Fig. 10). The SAC loses its normal shape in the absence of the MB, however. When cytoskeletons are prepared from room temperature cells and analyzed by SDS-PAGE, the major components are tubulin and two proteins that co-migrate with human erythrocyte α-spectrin and actin (Fig. 11). Comparison with cytoskeletons prepared from cells at 0°C, in which MBs have

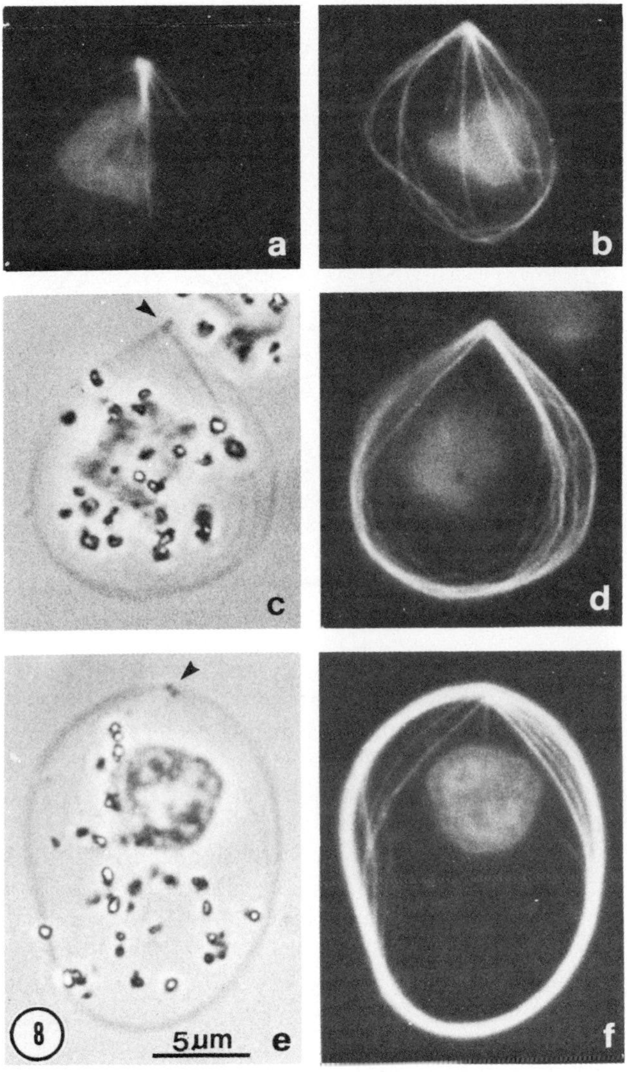

Fig. 8. Function of centrioles as organizing centers during MB reassembly in *N. ponderosa* erythrocytes (18°C). a,b. Indirect anti-tubulin immunofluorescence of cytoskeletons prepared from cells rewarmed 5 min (a) and 10 min (b). MB microtubules initiate and grow from centriolar points. c,d and e,f are phase contrast/immunofluorescence pairs, 20-min and 45-min rewarming, respectively. At 20 min many MBs are continuous but still pointed, with centrioles at apex (arrowhead) as shown. At 45 min the MB is no longer pointed, but microtubules still radiate from the centrioles (arrowhead), joining the MB at a distance.

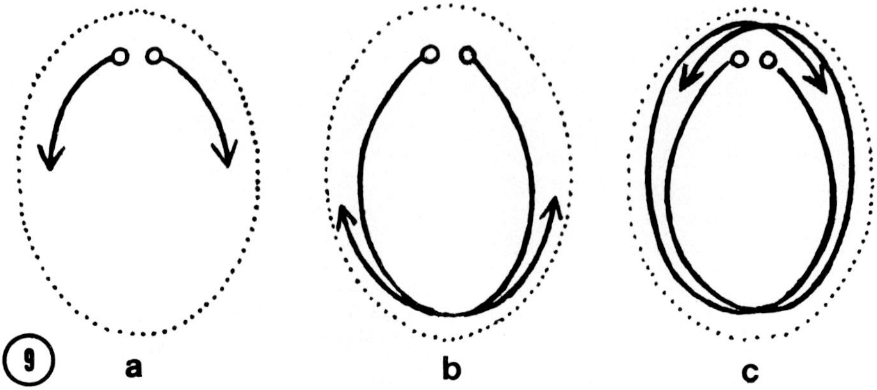

Fig. 9. Model for MB reassembly in blood clam erythrocytes. a. Microtubules initiate at centrioles and grow in diverging directions towards distal end of cell. b. Pointed stage in which a continuous MB is formed when microtubules of one polarity pass those of opposite polarity at distal end of cell. c. Microtubules continue growing and pass each other proximally, between the SAC and the centrioles. This would close the ellipse and result in attentuation of MB points.

disassembled, shows that most of the tubulin is lost but the α-spectrin and actin correlates remain. Thus proteins analogous to human α-spectrin and actin are probably present in the SAC of this molluscan erythrocyte, although further experiments are required for their characterization and localization.

An understanding of MB assembly and function requires knowledge not only of MB tubulin but also of quantitatively minor proteins associated with it. Such microtubule-associated proteins would be expected to function in cross-bridging MB microtubules to form the bundle (Fig. 4b) and perhaps in linking the outer MB microtubules to the SAC. The ability to disassemble the MB at 0°C and reassemble it upon rewarming provides an approach to identifying such components. In recent work [Joseph-Silverstein and Cohen, 1983b] two minor proteins (~80K, ~105K) have been observed to temperature-cycle with the *Noetia* MB in addition to tubulin (Fig. 11, arrowheads). That these are not simply cold-labile proteins which happen to co-cycle can be demonstrated through use of taxol and the tubulin polymerization inhibitors colchicine and nocodazole. The ~80K and ~105K proteins remain present in cytoskeletons prepared from cells containing taxol-stabilized MBs at 0°C, and they are not present in cytoskeletons prepared from cells at room temperature in which MB reassembly has been inhibited by either colchicine or nocodazole. These two proteins thus exhibit co-assembly/disassembly with the MB, and are tentatively identified as MB MAPs. It will be of considerable

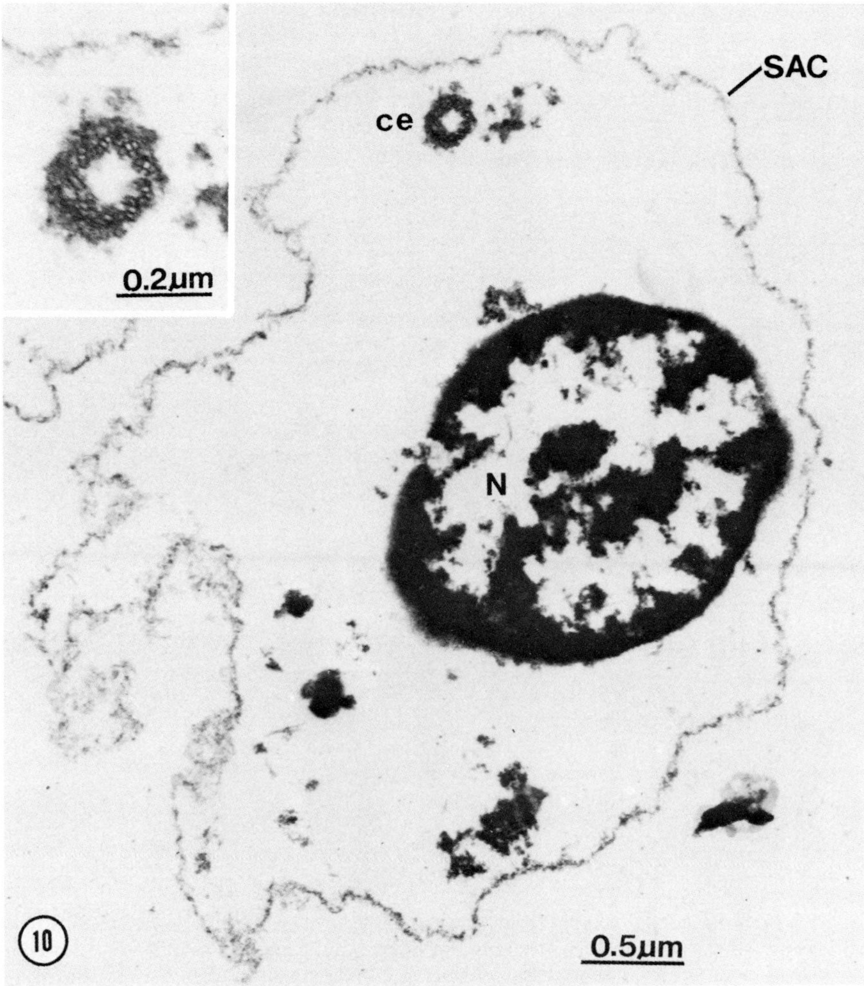

Fig. 10. Cytoskeleton of *N. ponderosa* erythrocyte after incubation of cells at 0°C. Note lack of MB or any microtubules, as well as the shapeless SAC. A centriole (ce) with closely adherent electron-dense material is present, shown at higher magnification in the inset. Simultaneous lysis/fixation, TEM.

interest to localize these proteins by independent means at the ultrastructural level and to test for their presence in MBs of other species and cell types.

The availability of erythrocytes with and without MBs at 0°C (taxol stabilization vs. no taxol) and at room temperature (colchicine and nocoda-

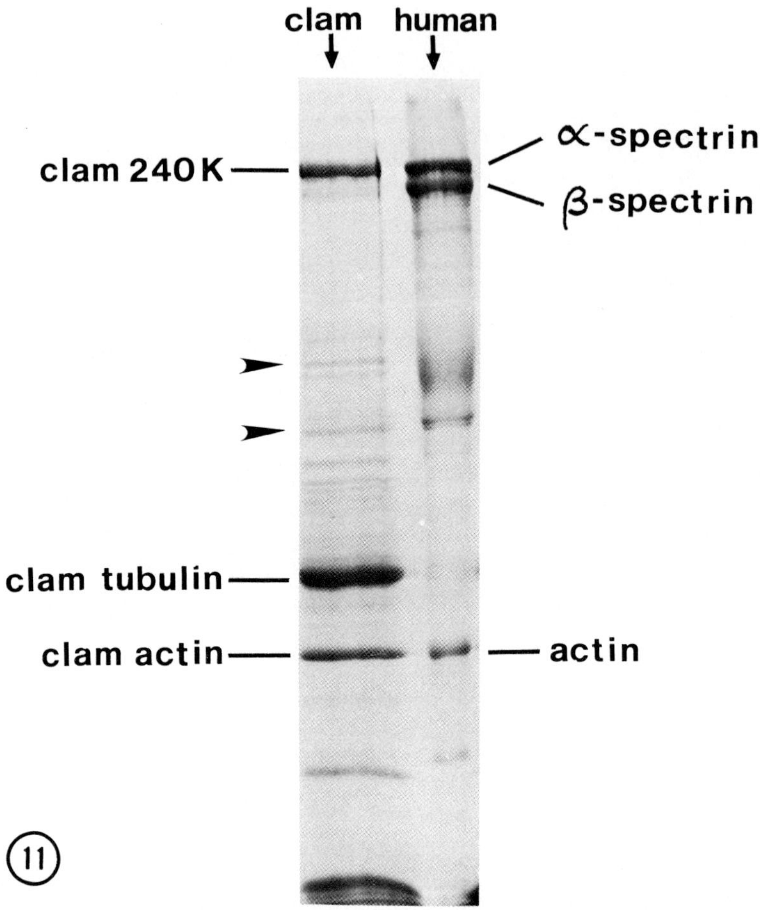

Fig. 11. SDS-polyacrylamide gel electrophoresis of *N. ponderosa* erythrocyte cytoskeletons (left lane). Human erythrocyte standards are shown for comparison (right lane). Major components of the clam erythrocyte cytoskeleton co-migrate with human α-spectrin (clam 240K) and actin. Clam tubulin co-migrates with mammalian tubulin standards (not shown). The arrowheads point to two proteins that show co-assembly/disassembly with MB tubulin in living cells and which may be MB microtubule-associated proteins. Courtesy of J. Joseph-Silverstein.

zole inhibition of reassembly vs. no inhibitors) has permitted a more direct examination of MB function than previously possible. The initial observation, made by J. Joseph-Silverstein, was that some of the cells lacking MBs appeared to have buckled or folded during preparation. When intentionally subjected to mechanical stress by fluxing through glass capillary tubes, most cells with MBs remained flattened and elliptical (98%), whereas many of those without MBs became deformed (up to 45%) (Fig. 12). This supports the view that the blood clam erythrocyte MB plays a continuing role in cell shape maintenance, resisting shape change and/or effecting the rapid recovery of erythrocyte shape following deformation in vivo [Joseph-Silverstein and Cohen, 1983a,b]. The observations on these invertebrate erythrocytes have reopened questions about MB function in the vertebrates, providing the impetus for recent studies with dogfish erythrocytes, which are discussed in the last section of this chapter.

The blood clam erythrocyte provides a relatively simple model system for studying the genesis and spatial control of a microtubule bundle. It is a "poor man's mitotic spindle" with respect to centriole function and in vivo disassembly/reassembly. As such it should be of considerable value for future work.

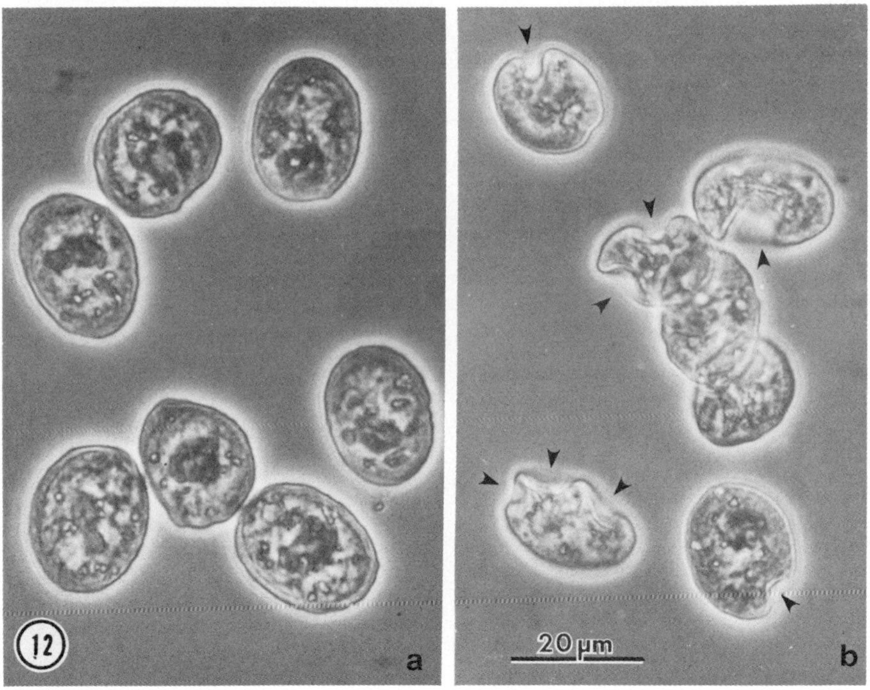

Fig. 12. Effect of mechanical stress (fluxing through capillary tubes) on blood clam erythrocytes *(N. ponderosa)* that contain MBs (a) or lack MBs (b). Nearly all cells containing MBs are normal in shape, whereas many without MBs are deformed (arrowheads). In this case, a cell suspension was divided and taxol added to half. After 3 hr at 0°C, MBs had disassembled in cells without taxol but were still present in cells with taxol. Similar results are obtained using cells with and without MBs at room temperature, in which MB reassembly was inhibited in half the population by colchicine or nocodazole. Courtesy of J. Joseph-Silverstein.

Erythrocytes of the Peanut Worm, *Phascolopsis gouldii*

Phascolopsis gouldii (formerly known as *Golfingia* and *Phascolosoma*) is a common marine Sipunculan that inhabits estuarine mud flats along the eastern coast of the United States. Much of the body volume is occupied by coelomic fluid, in which erythrocytes are suspended. The erythrocytes are nucleated, highly flattened, and generally elliptical, with the long axis in the 20- to 30-μm range (Fig. 13). They contain hemerythrin, a respiratory protein unique to cells of certain invertebrates [see Terwilliger, Terwilliger, and Schabtach, this volume, for detailed discussion of hemerythrin properties and distribution].

When these cells are suspended in microtubule-stabilizing medium containing Triton X-100, they are rapidly cleared of hemerythrin and other soluble components [Nemhauser et al., 1980]. The MB is just visible as a phase-dense line delimiting the resulting cytoskeleton, with circumference approximating that of the original cell (Fig. 14). It is considerably thinner than in the blood clams and is difficult to see in phase contrast. In untwisted cytoskeletons the MBs are elliptical, corresponding to cell shape. However,

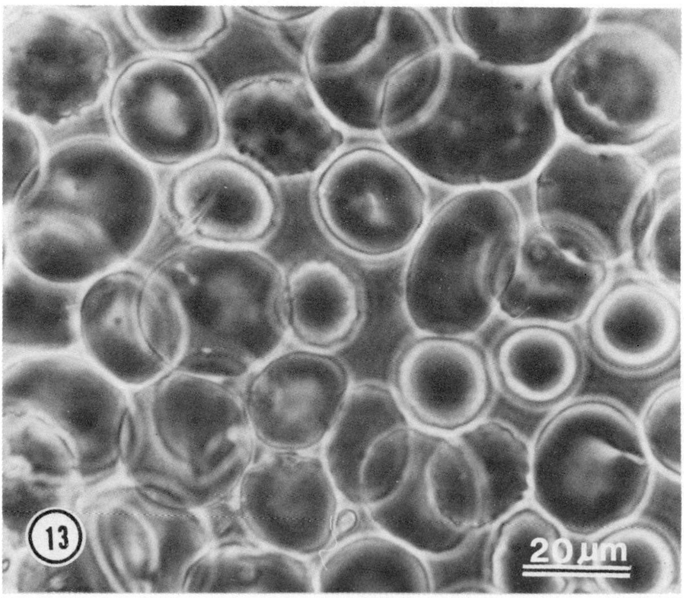

Fig. 13. Living erythrocytes of the Sipunculan worm *Phascolopsis gouldii*. The native cells are flattened and usually elliptical, with considerable size variation; some in this field have become spherical because of contact with glass slide. Phase contrast. Figures 13, 14, 16, 20, 21 from Nemhauser et al. [1980], with permission of Academic Press.

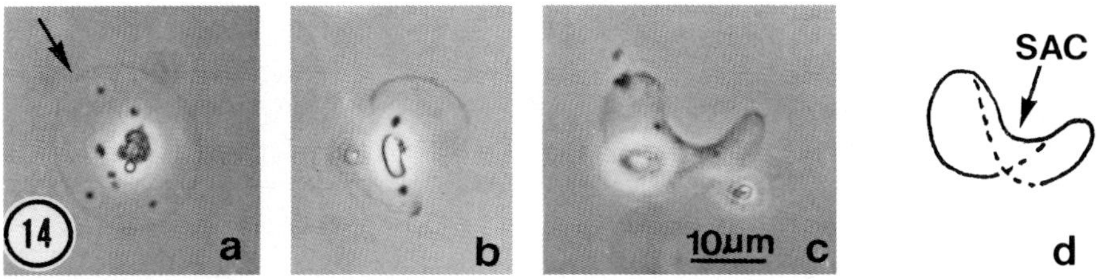

Fig. 14. Cytoskeletons produced by Triton lysis of *P. gouldii* erythrocytes (phase contrast). a. A flat cytoskeleton, with typically thin MB barely visible (arrow). The large dense central object is the nucleus. b,c. Cytoskeletons as more commonly observed, in which the MB is twisted into a figure-8 shape. Because of such twisting, it is possible to capture only parts of the MB in one optical section, as shown. d. Drawing of the saddle-shaped cytoskeleton in c, with dotted lines indicating out-of-focus MB sections. Figure-8 MB twisting generates a saddle-shaped SAC, and is a tell-tale sign that MBs are present in cases such as this, in which the MB itself is difficult to see in phase contrast.

the MBs are usually in a figure-8 configuration (an artifact of cell lysis), giving the cytoskeleton a three-dimensional "saddle" shape and permitting one to visualize the cell surface-associated cytoskeleton (SAC). In phase contrast the SAC has the appearance of a transparent surface layer, within which the nucleus and other remaining organelles are trapped or suspended (Fig. 14). As in the blood clam erythrocytes, the SAC is more readily visualized in thin sections of cytoskeletons; when obliquely sectioned it appears as a fuzzy layer of material in contact with the MB (Fig. 15a).

As observed by indirect immunofluorescence, anti-tubulin antibody is specifically bound by the MB (Fig. 15b), showing that there are few, if any, microtubules elsewhere. The thinness of the MB in these cells is verified by counts of microtubules in thin sections of intact cells or cells simultaneously lysed and fixed (TEM). The MB typically contains 7–8 microtubules, with a range of 2–13 in different cells. In intact cells the microtubules are often not as tightly bundled as one would predict from the phase contrast image or as observed in lyse-fixed cells (Fig. 16). The reason for this is not known at present, but fixation artifact is a possibility. As observed in situ the MB microtubules lie adjacent to but not in direct contact with the plasma membrane bilayer. Our explanation for this is that the SAC, though not differentially stained, is located between the MB and the bilayer.

Are centrioles associated with these MBs? The twisting of most cytoskeletons upon lysis obscures parts of many MBs. However, careful phase-contrast (oil immersion) examination of MBs that can be followed for their entire circumference reveals paired phase-dense "dots" in many but not all

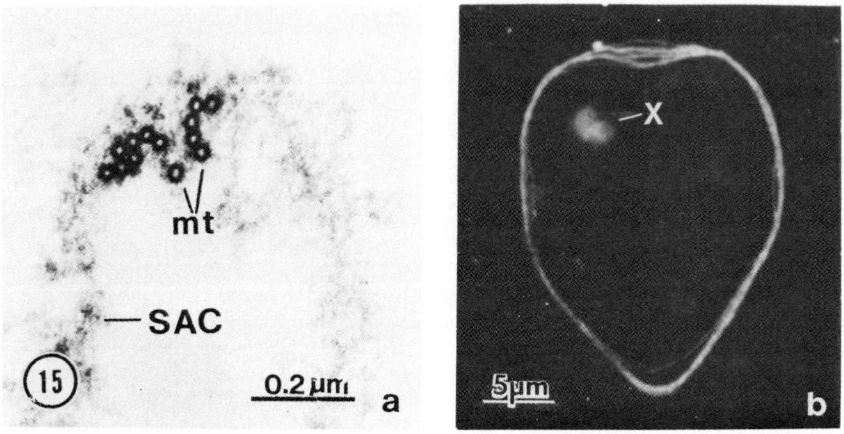

Fig. 15. Microtubular structure of the *P. gouldii* MB. a. Thin section of lyse-fixed cell (TEM) showing 13 microtubules (mt) closely associated with the SAC. The latter appears as a fuzzy layer, more diffuse where obliquely sectioned. b. Indirect immunofluorescence of whole cytoskeleton using anti-tubulin. Ready visibility of MB fluorescence makes this a method of choice for the initial detection of such thin MBs. In addition to the MB, consistent specific binding to a patch of material (×) was observed in most cells. Its nature and significance are unknown.

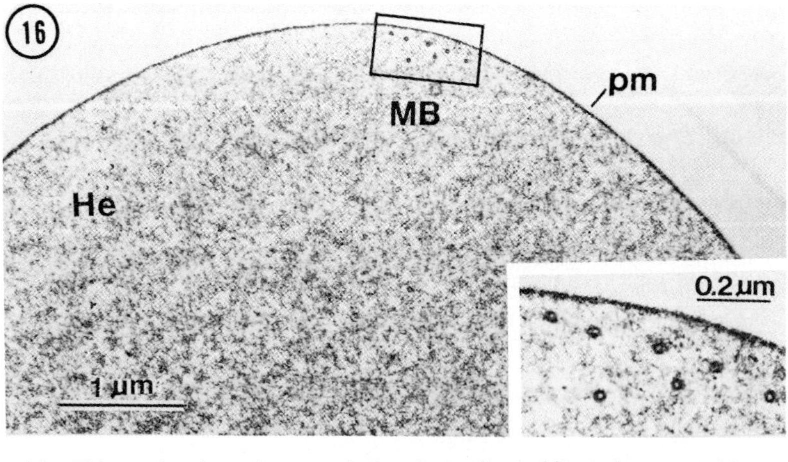

Fig. 16. Thin section through one end of an intact *P. gouldii* erythrocyte, with seven MB microtubules near the cell surface. pm = plasma membrane; He = hemerythrin. In the inset it can be seen that the MB microtubules do not contact the plasma membrane bilayer directly.

cases. Whenever they have been seen, the two "dots" are aligned at an angle to the MB, with only one member of the pair in contact with it (Fig. 17). Although we think it highly likely that these are centrioles, their identity requires verification in thin section.

If the cells are lysed with Triton in the presence of very high ATP concentrations (nonphysiological levels, up to 25 mM), the cytoskeletons become unstable with time. Initially, the SAC appears to solubilize and MBs are liberated. When whole mounts are examined at high magnifications (TEM), individual microtubules can be traced around the entire circumference in some of these very thin MBs, with few free ends visible (Fig. 18). The MB of the *Phascolopsis* erythrocyte thus appears to be constructed of only a few very long, multiply wound microtubules (or possibly only one, since breakage might have occurred). Very high ATP concentrations also liberate MBs from vertebrate erythrocyte cytoskeletons [Cohen, 1978b]; while the mechanism is unknown, the effect is useful as a means of partially dissecting the cytoskeleton.

Although not directly related to our cytoskeleton theme, certain other features of *P. gouldii* erythrocytes of interest with respect to cell function are visible in thin sections. Most prominent are membrane-bound electron-dense masses of material in the cytoplasm (Fig. 19a). As shown by energy-dispersive X-ray microanalysis, this material contains high concentrations of iron (Fig. 19b,c). Similar dense material containing ferritin has been observed previously in "vacuoles" of Sipunculan erythrocytes [Dybas, 1981]. Tangen-

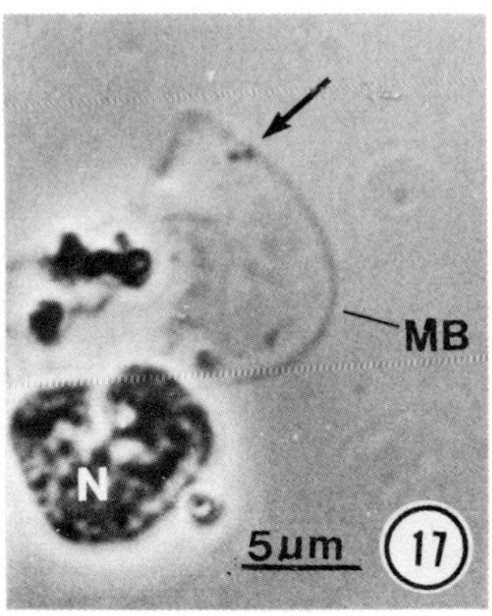

Fig. 17. Possible centriole pair (arrow) associated with the *P. gouldii* erythrocyte MB, as seen in phase contrast under oil immersion. Many but not all MBs of this species exhibit such a pair of dense dots, only one of which seems to be in contact with the MB. The MB of this particular cytoskeleton is twisted, such that only part of it is in focus. N = nucleus.

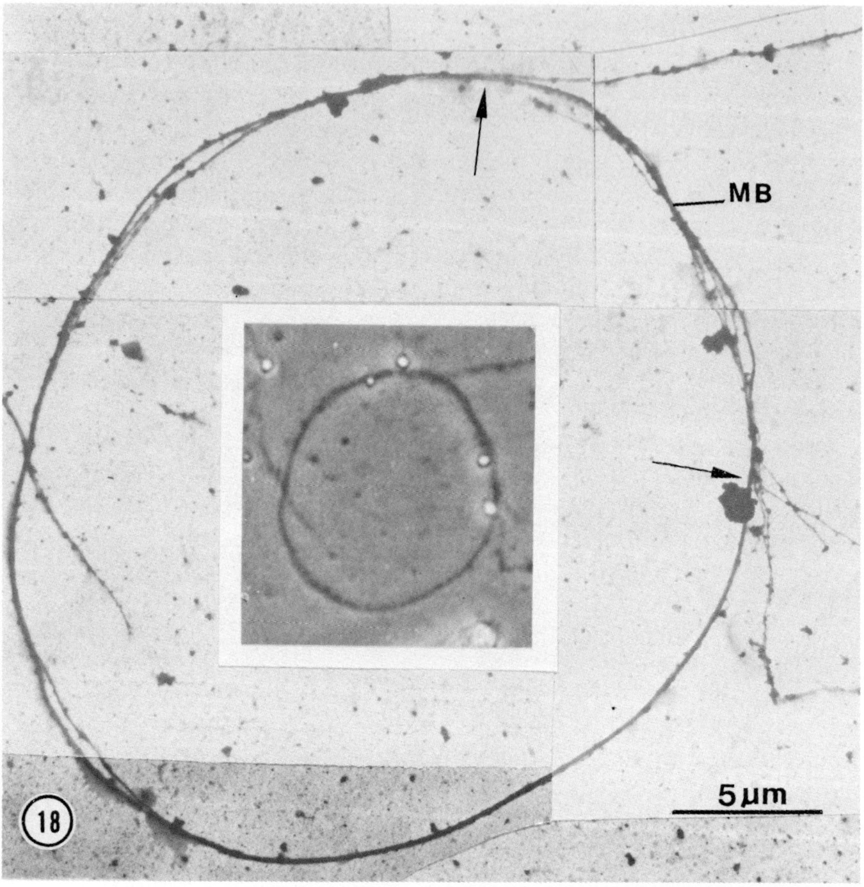

Fig. 18. Montage of a *P. gouldii* MB liberated from the SAC by use of a high concentration of ATP (uranyl acetate staining, TEM). When examined at higher magnifications, individual microtubules can be traced around the entire circumference. Microtubules "fray" off the MB surface at two points (arrows), and relatively few free microtubule ends are visible. Inset: the same isolated MB as seen in phase contrast on the grid prior to TEM examination.

tial sections through the plasma membrane of these cells show numerous electron-dense granules that also exhibit high iron content (Fig. 19d); presumably they function in iron metabolism associated with hemerythrin synthesis.

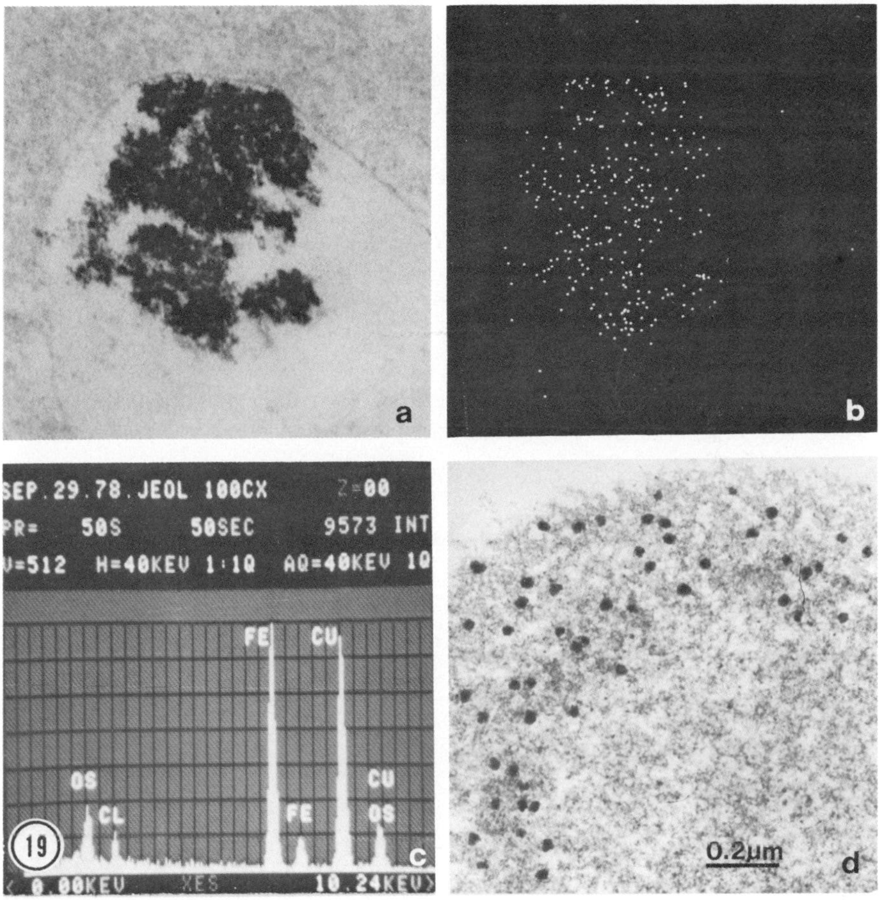

Fig. 19. a. Membrane-bound electron-dense material in the cytoplasm of an intact *P. gouldii* erythrocyte. b. Energy-dispersive x-ray microanalysis showing the presence of iron in this section, localized to the dense material. c. Spectrum containing an iron peak. d. Electron-dense granules associated with the tangentially sectioned plasma membrane were found to contain iron by the same method. Magnification in a and b as in d.

EXPERIMENTAL STUDIES: CLOTTING CELLS

Amebocytes of the Horseshoe Crab *Limulus polyphemus*

The clotting cells or "amebocytes" of *Limulus* are of great value as experimental material, both because one can easily obtain essentially pure populations in large quantities and because they exhibit a variety of interesting properties. These properties are thoroughly documented elsewhere [see chapters by Armstrong, by Levin, and by Ornberg, this volume]. Like clotting cells in general, *Limulus* amebocytes undergo very rapid morphological changes when removed from the animal unless precautions are taken to prevent activation [see final chapter]. We have examined the amebocyte cytoskeleton prior to activation, i.e., when the cells still have their native flattened and generally oval shape [Nemhauser et al., 1980]. This morphology (Fig. 20a; also Figure 1 in Armstrong, this volume) is similar to that of vertebrate erythrocytes and thrombocytes (unactivated), which initially suggested to us that MBs might be present. MBs cannot be seen in the living cells in phase contrast or with Nomarski differential interference optics [Armstrong, 1977]. This is due at least partly to the presence of numerous refractile granules, which contain all of the clotting factors [Murer et al., 1975]. After lysis of the cells with Triton X-100 under conditions similar to

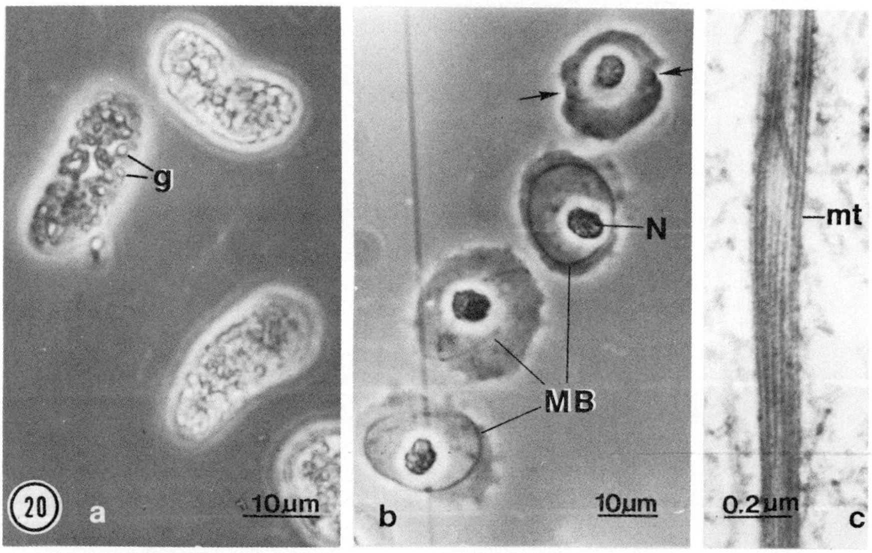

Fig. 20. a. Living amebocytes of *Limulus polyphemus* treated with 2 mM propranolol at low temperature to inhibit activation and shape transformation. Under these conditions the cells remain flattened and ovoid, but are not quite the normal native shape, which is smoothly elliptical (see Fig. 1 in chapter by Armstrong, this volume). Refractile granules (g) pack the cytoplasm of the living cells. b. Cells lysed with Triton immediately upon removal from the animal (no other treatment). MBs are visible at the periphery of the cytoplasmic remnant of every cell. In fortuitous cases the MB is observed to constrict this remnant (arrows). Granules are no longer visible, presumably having been lysed. Nuclei (N) retain integrity. c. Thin section through a pellet of lysed amebocytes, showing tightly bundled MB microtubules (mt) in longitudinal section.

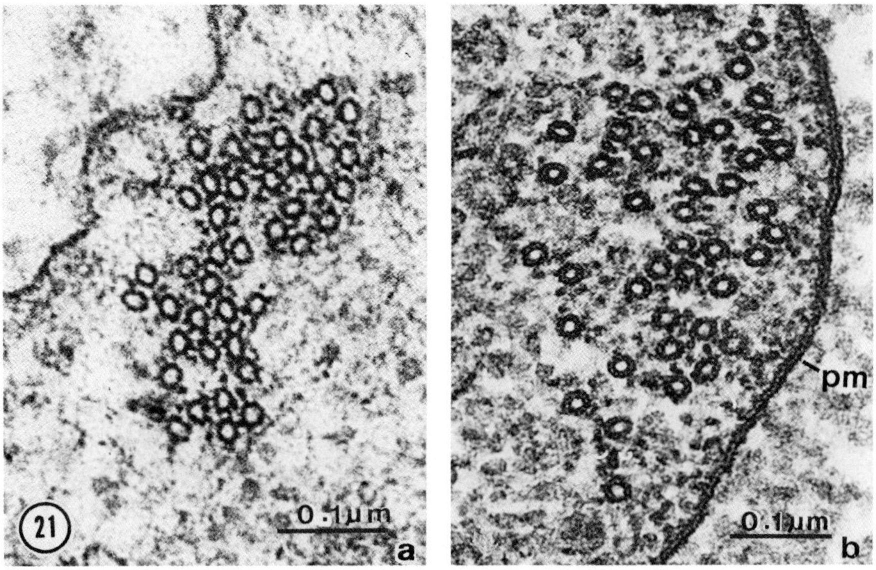

Fig. 21. The MB of the *L. polyphemus* amebocyte as seen in thin sections of quick-frozen,, freeze-substituted cells. a. Cross-bridges link many of the microtubules. b. The microtubules do not directly contact the bilayer of the plasma membrane (pm), but are separated from it by at least one microtubule diameter. This suggests the presence of a cortical cytoskeletal layer (SAC).

those used for erythrocytes, these granules are no longer visible. The cytoplasmic residue appears as a relatively homogeneous mass, within which the nucleus and the MB are now readily apparent in phase contrast (Fig. 20b). Electron microscopy of thin sections through pellets of lysed cells confirms the presence of MB microtubules (Fig. 20c). In situ features are visible in quick-frozen and freeze-substituted amebocytes, as observed originally by R. Ornberg (Fig. 21). The number of MB microtubules in cross sections in such preparations is variable, ranging from 12 to 47, and averaging about 32. Many of them are linked by cross-bridges (Fig. 21a). The microtubules do not contact the plasma membrane bilayer directly, but appear to be separated from it by a material-filled space at least 500 Å thick (Fig. 21b). We believe that this is a continuous specialized cortical layer, constituted at least in part by the SAC of the amebocyte.

Clotting Cells of the Lobster *Homarus americanus*

As an experimental animal, the American lobster *Homarus* offers routine commercial availability and ease of laboratory maintenance. Although cytological studies of its hemocytes have been conducted by several laboratories, there is still uncertainty regarding the number of cell types present. This is attributable in part to classification of cell types on different bases by different workers [Toney, 1958; Hearing and Vernick, 1967; Cornick and Stewart, 1978], and in part to complexity engendered by morphological changes after removal of cells from the animal. Our studies [Cohen et al., 1983] support the view that clotting cells, originally identified as such and named "explosive refractile granulocytes" by Toney [1958], constitute the majority of "hemocytes" within lobster "hemolymph." Toney described these cells as being round or oval immediately after removal from the animal. Subsequently there occurred extensive morphological changes, with cells spreading very thinly and large granules at their surface disintegrating so as to produce

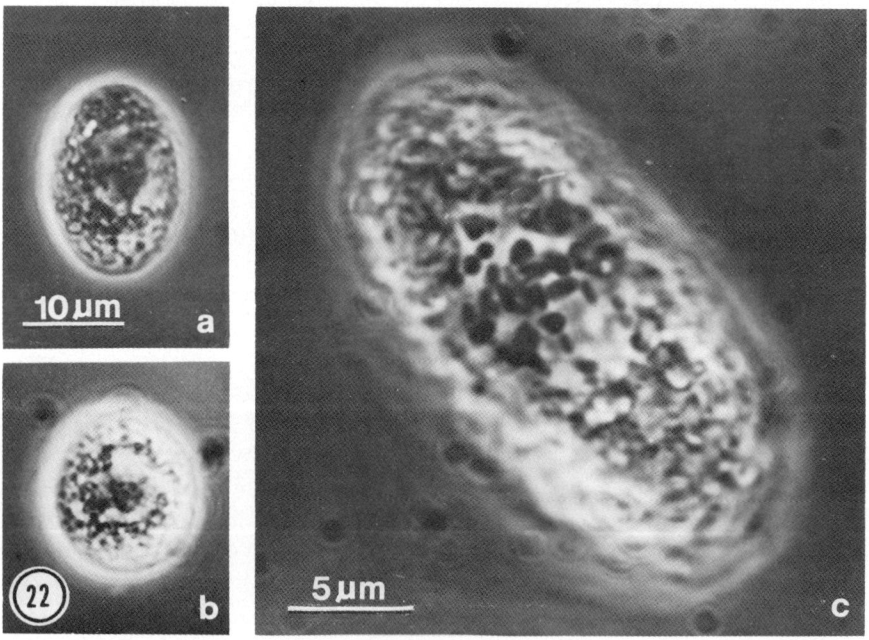

Fig. 22. Hemocytes of the American lobster, *Homarus americanus,* fixed immediately upon removal from the animal (Crustacean Ringer's solution containing 1% glutaraldehyde). The majority of cells are flattened and ellipsoidal, as in panel a, or are slight distortions of this shape. A smaller percentage are discoidal, as in panel b, or have points at one or both ends. Cytoplasmic granules, numerous in most cells, are readily examined microscopically in the thin cytoplasmic layer above or below the nucleus (c). Cells such as these are identifiable as the clotting cells described by Toney [1958]. Magnification in b same as in a. Figures 22–27 from Cohen et al [1983], with permission of the Marine Biological Laboratory.

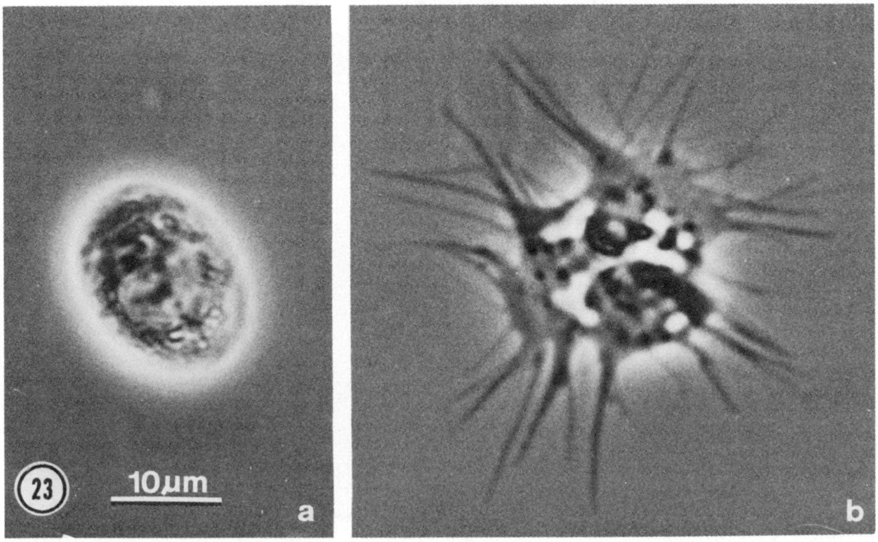

Fig. 23. Morphological transformation of *H. americanus* clotting cell in contact with glass slide. a. One minute after removal from animal the cell is still flattened and elliptical. b. Same cell, at same magnification, 9 min later. The cell has sent out numerous filopodia and is spread very thinly against the surface.

an "explosive" or "bubbling" effect. It is apparent that this phenomenon is exocytosis [see Ornberg, this volume].

The clotting cells of *Homarus* are similar to those of *Limulus* in size (15–20 μm, long axis), appearance, and general behavior, but show somewhat greater morphological variation on a basic flattened elliptical theme. They contain cytoplasmic granules of various sizes (Fig. 22). These granules are probably not identical in content to those of *Limulus,* however. In *Limulus* amebocytes, all of the clotting factors, including clottable protein, are believed to be present in the cytoplasmic granules [Murer et al., 1975; see also Levin, this volume], whereas in *Homarus*, a "fibrinogen" has been reported to be a normal component of hemolymph plasma [Stewart et al., 1966]. Upon removal from the animal, the initially flattened lobster blood cells undergo dramatic shape changes, sending out filopodia and spreading thinly on substrata (Fig. 23).

Immediate dilution of fresh hemolymph into microtubule-stabilizing medium containing Triton X-100 causes the cells to lyse before the morphological transformations associated with clotting can occur. This procedure nevertheless produces "clots" of lysed cells in which nuclei are prominent (Fig. 24). Granules are no longer visible, presumably having lysed and contributed their contents to formation of the mass. Careful examination

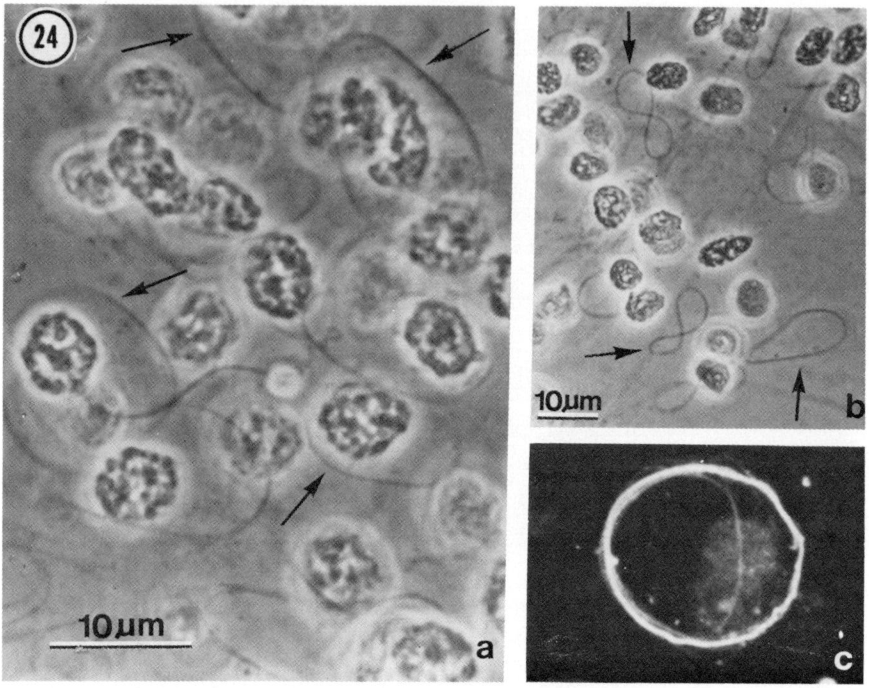

Fig. 24. *H. americanus* hemocytes lysed immediately, before the onset of morphological transformation. A "clot" consisting of cytoskeletons in a matrix results (a), in which there is nearly a 1:1 correspondence between nuclei and MBs (arrows) as determined by careful focusing. MBs can be separated from nuclei by squashing the "clot" (b, arrows). c. MB visualized by indirect anti-tubulin immunofluorescence. Magnification for c as in a.

under phase contrast shows that each nucleus has a circumscribing MB. The MBs are particularly obvious in squashes of the "clot," with many of them separating from nuclei and twisting into figure-8 forms (Fig. 24b). Thin sections of intact flat-embedded cells show that the MB lies in the plane of flattening, exhibiting classical cross sections at opposite extremities of the cell (Fig. 25). As in the case of *Limulus* amebocytes, MB microtubules do not contact the plasma membrane bilayer directly (Fig. 25b).

What happens to the MB when the cells undergo morphological transformation? When well-spread cells are lysed by perfusion, no MBs are visible (Fig. 26). As revealed by anti-tubulin immunofluorescence, MBs are still recognizable as such after 5 min spreading, although many have a grossly twisted appearance. Subsequently they become highly disorganized and ultimately disappear (Fig. 27). Morphological transformation is thus accom-

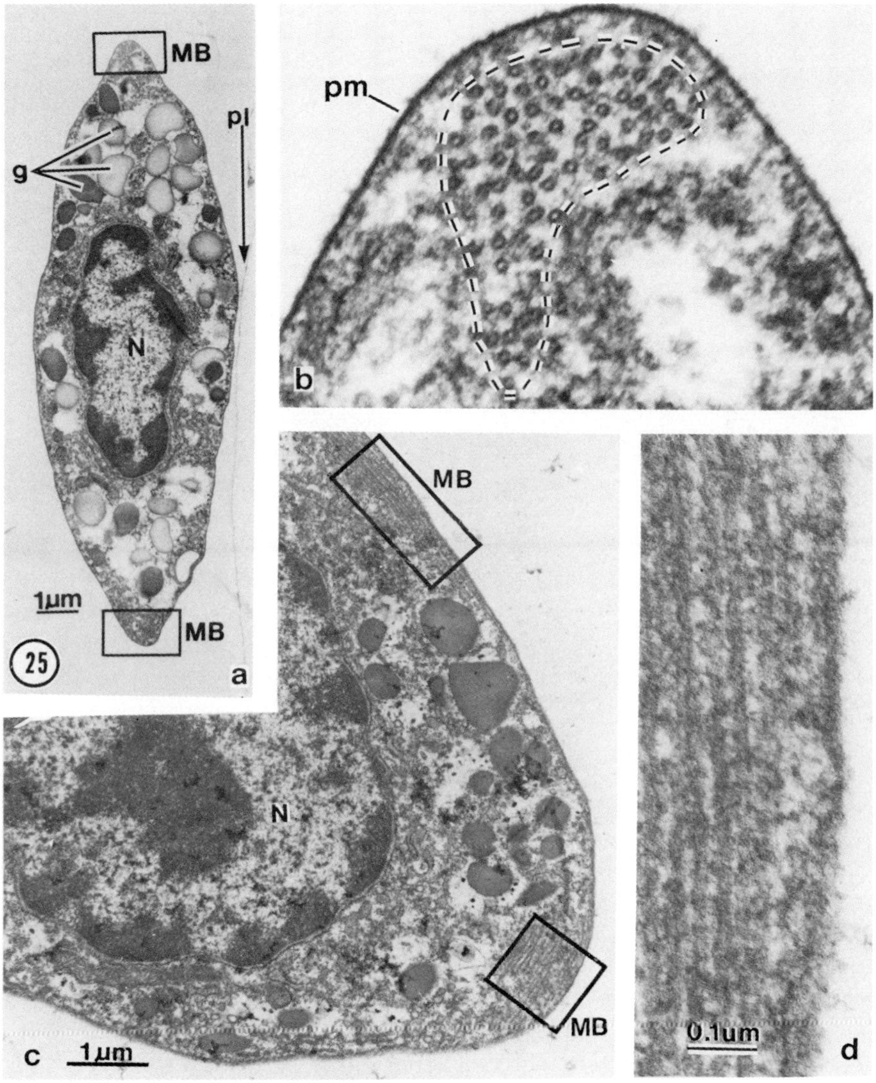

Fig. 25. Intact clotting cells of *H. americanus*, oriented for sectioning either perpendicular to (a) or parallel to (c) the plane of flattening. a. Cell lies flat against polylysine-coated substratum (pl), with nucleus (N) and numerous granules (g) visible. MB microtubules appear in cross section at opposite ends of the section (rectangles), shown at higher magnification within dotted line in (b). As in *Limulus* (Fig. 21), MB microtubules do not contact the plasma membrane bilayer (pm) directly. In sections through the plane of flattening (c) MB microtubules appear in longitudinal view at the cell periphery (rectangles). Part of the area in the upper rectangle is shown at higher magnification in d. Magnification of b as in d.

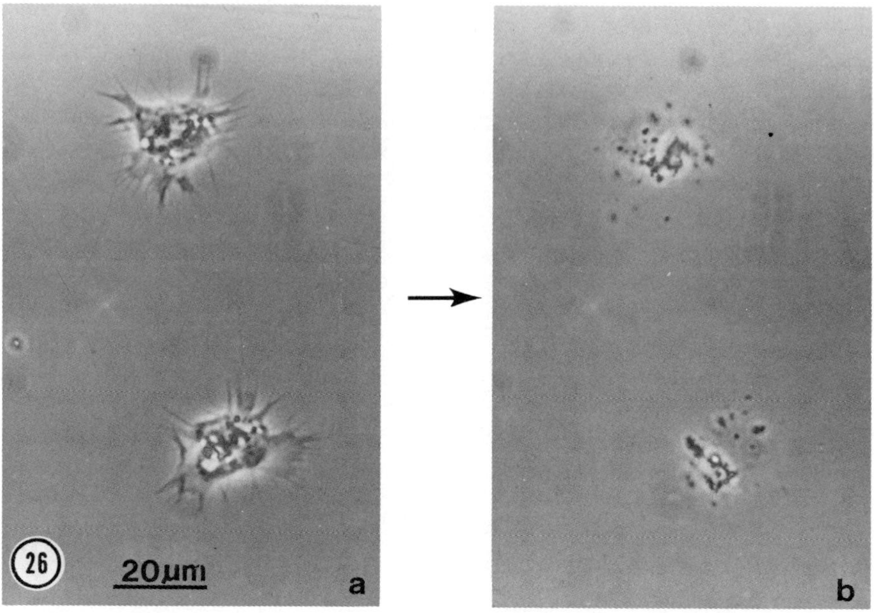

Fig. 26. a. Hemocytes of *H. americanus* allowed to spread on glass substratum for 12 min. Lysis by perfusion with Triton in microtubule-stabilizing medium shows that the spread cells do not contain MBs (b).

panied by MB disorganization, but we do not know whether MB disorganization is a causal or controlling step that permits transformation, or simply one of many simultaneous changes triggered by clotting cell activation.

Do clotting cells similar to those of *Homarus* occur in other crustacea? Do they contain MBs? Using the lytic technique, we have found obvious MBs in blood cells of the marine crabs *Libinia emarginata* (spider crab) and *Cancer borealis* ("Jonah" rock crab), and less obvious MBs appear to be present in several other marine crustaceans, including *Cancer irroratus* ("rock" crab), *Ovalipes ocellatus* (calico or "lady" crab), and *Emerita talpoida* ("sandbug" or mole crab). "Explosive refractile granulocytes" were also described by Toney [1958] as being the major cell type in the blood of the crayfish *(Cambarus bartoni)* and the blue crab *(Callinectes sapidus),* but the lytic technique has not revealed MBs in blood samples of a crayfish (probably *Cambarus*) or of the blue crab. This result must be treated cautiously, however. Using the lytic technique alone on cells such as these, it is more difficult to establish the absence of MBs than their presence. The clotting cells of some species may be activated so quickly by removal from the animal that we have already lost the MBs by the time of lysis. In addition, MBs could be destabilized rapidly upon cell lysis by endogenous proteases or other factors, or they might not be readily visible in phase contrast because of thinness or for other optical reasons. Therefore, although MB-containing cells are certainly present in some crustacea, a reliable judgment cannot yet

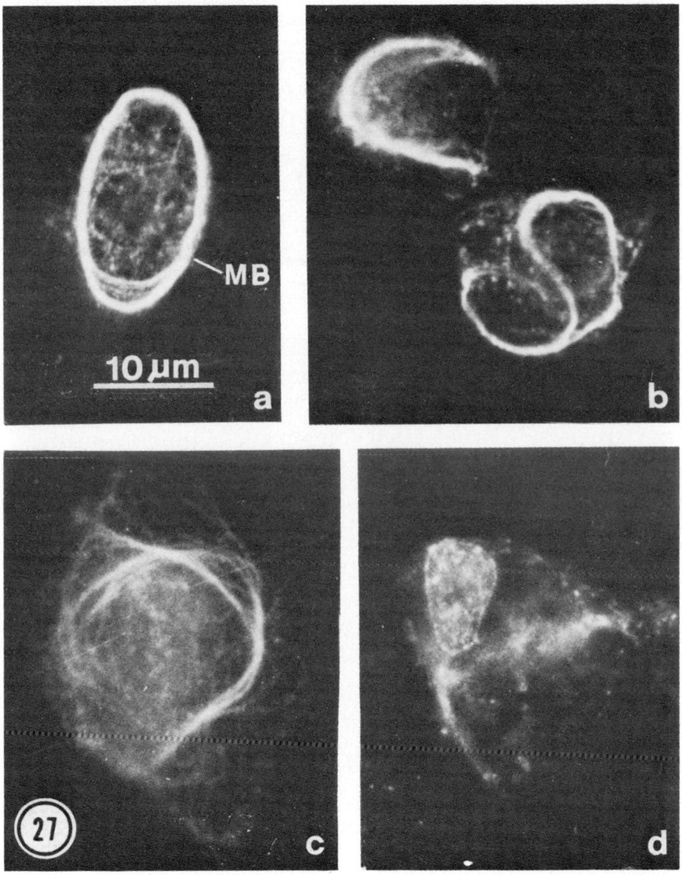

Fig. 27. Changes in the MB during spreading of *H. americanus* hemocytes as visualized by indirect anti-tubulin immunofluorescence. a,b. After 5 min spreading, some MBs are still nearly intact. The majority have begun to twist and splay apart, however, as shown in panel b. After 10 min, microtubule bundles are present, but MBs are no longer recognizable as such (c). After 20 min spreading, MBs and most microtubules have disappeared, though some background fluorescence is present (d).

be made concerning the universality of their distribution or their restriction to clotting cells.

DISCUSSION

Phylogenetic Distribution of the MB System

The marginal band was probably the first "cytoskeletal" structure discovered and considered as such by light microscopists [Dehler, 1895; Meves, 1911; Dustin, 1978]. It is a distinctive feature that is common to a variety of cell types in phylogenetically distant species. The first well-documented report of MBs in invertebrates appears to be that of Baerwold and Bousch [1970] on cockroach "hemocytes" (leukocytes of undetermined function). The presence of MBs has also been reported in erythrocytes of several species of sea cucumber [Fontaine and Lambert, 1973; Fontaine and Hall, 1981], and in the hemerythrin-containing erythrocytes of *Priapulus caudatus* (phylum Priapulidae, unsegmented marine worms) [Mattison and Fange, 1973]. These and additional references are listed in Table I, which summarizes the phylogenetic distribution of MBs according to cell type and species. As can be seen in Table I, MBs are present in cells containing hemoglobin (most erythrocytes) or hemerythrin (certain invertebrate erythrocytes) and in cells with no respiratory proteins (platelets, thrombocytes, invertebrate clotting cells). They are present in cells that contain nuclei (nonmammalian vertebrate erythrocytes and thrombocytes; invertebrate erythrocytes and clotting cells) and in cells that lack nuclei (*Batrachoseps* erythrocytes, platelets). Their occurrence spans at least seven phyla and a remarkable diversity of species (Table I). What do these cells have in common? MBs are a normal component only of cells that exist as individuals in a fluid tissue of a multicellular animal. All of these cells, as far as is known, have flattened elliptical or discoid morphology. MBs are therefore thought to function universally in cellular morphogenesis and in the adaptation of cells to existence in a fluid, flowing environment. These functions are discussed in more detail below.

Continuous circumferential bundles of microtubules do occur in some cases in cells of non-fluid tissues, but these are sufficiently distinct to preclude application of the term "marginal band." For example, there is the preprophase band in plant cells, a transient structure that, unlike the MB, is composed of relatively short overlapping microtubule segments [Hardham and Gunning, 1978]. A microtubule system perhaps more closely resembling the MB occurs at nodes of Ranvier [Gray and Westrum, 1979], and recently Gray et al. [1982] and others have shown that circumferential microtubule coils resembling MBs can form in synaptosomes under certain conditions.

TABLE I. Phylogenetic Distribution of the Marginal Band System

Phylum, species[a], and common name	Cell types[b]	Cell morphology[c]	References
SIPUNCULA			
Phascolopsis gouldii (peanut worm)	Erythrocyte (He)	F, C or E, N	Nemhauser et al. [1980]
PRIAPULIDA			
Priapulus caudatus (priapulid worm)	Erythrocyte (He)	F, C, N	Mattison and Fange [1973]
ANNELIDA			
Travisia japonica (a polychaete)	Erythrocyte	F, E, N	Ochi [1969, 1980]
MOLLUSCA			
Anadara transversa (blood clam)	Erythrocyte	F, C or E, N	Cohen and Nemhauser [1980]
ARTHROPODA			
Xiphosura			
Limulus polyphemus (horseshoe crab)	Clotting cell (amebocyte)	F, E, N	Nemhauser et al. [1980]
Crustacea			
Homarus americanus (American lobster)	Clotting cell	F, E, N	Cohen et al. [1983]
Cancer borealis (rock crab)	Hemocyte	F, E, N	Cohen et al. [1977]
Insecta			
Periplaneta americana (cockroach)	Hemocyte	F, ?, N	Baerwold and Boush [1970]
ECHINODERMATA			
Cucumaria miniata (sea cucumber)	Erythrocyte	F, E, N	Fontaine and Lambert [1973]
CHORDATA (Vertebrate Classes)			
Agnatha			
Eptatretus stoutii (Pacific hagfish)	Erythrocyte	F, E, N	Sekhon and Maxwell [1970]
Chondrichthyes			
Mustelus canis (smooth dogfish)	Erythrocyte	F, E, N	Cohen et al. [1982a]
Osteichthyes			
Opsanus tau (toadfish)	Erythrocyte, Thrombocyte	F, E, N	Fawcett and Witebsky [1964]
Carrasius auratus (goldfish)	Erythrocyte	F, E, N	Weinreb and Weinreb [1965]
Amphibia			
Rana pipiens (leopard frog)	Erythrocyte	F, E, N	Maser and Philpott [1964]
Batrachoseps attenuata (slender salamander)	Erythrocyte	F, E, A	Cohen [1982]
Reptilia			
Dipsosaurus dorsalis (desert iguana)	Erythrocyte	F, E, N	Maser and Philpott [1964]

(continued)

TABLE I. Phylogenetic Distribution of the Marginal Band System (continued)

Phylum, species[a], and common name	Cell types[b]	Cell morphology[c]	References
Aves			
Gallus domesticus (chicken)	Erythrocyte, Thrombocyte	F, E, N	Behnke [1970a], Edmonds [1968]
Mammalia			
Homo sapiens (human)	Platelet	F, C or E, A	Behnke [1965]
Homo sapiens (human)	Erythrocyte (primitive)	F, E?, N	van Deurs and Behnke [1973]
Lepus (rabbit)	Erythroblast (fetal liver)	?, ?, N	Grasso [1966]
Camelus dromedarius (camel)	Erythrocyte (immature)	F, E, A	Cohen and Terwilliger [1979]
Llama glama (llama)	Erythoblast (bone marrow)	F, E, A	Goniakowska-Witalinska and Witalinski [1977]

[a]Only well-documented cases are listed; where there are many possible examples, representative species are given.
[b]Erythrocyte = hemoglobin-containing red cell; erythrocyte (He) = hemerythrin-containing cell; hemocyte = nonerythroid cell of undetermined function; thrombocyte = nonmammalian vertebrate clotting cell. Thrombocytes were originally described in toadfish as containing "endoplasmic rings" of microtubules [Fawcett and Witebsky, 1964] deeper within the cytoplasm than erythrocyte MBs. Subsequent work on other species (e.g., see Edmonds [1968] and Behnke [1970]) shows their similarity to erythrocyte MBs.
[c]F = flattened, C = circular, E = elliptical, N = nucleated, A = anucleate, ? = data lacking.
Modified from Nemhauser et al. [1980] with permission of Academic Press.

Synaptosomes are membrane vesicles produced from neurons by fractionation procedures, so these coils are not naturally occurring structures. They may well prove to be an excellent model system for studying MB formation and function, however.

MB Function

What function or functions do MBs serve? How is MB function achieved? The literature on MB function is principally that of the vertebrates. In platelets, the native flattened discoid or slightly elliptical shape is lost upon MB disassembly at low temperature, and the platelet becomes spherical. When the MB reassembles upon rewarming, most platelets regain their flattened shape [Behnke, 1967]. In contrast, in those nonmammalian vertebrate erythrocytes that have cold-labile MBs (chicken, dogfish),[1] the flat-

[1]Not all MBs are cold-labile, e.g., those of *Rana catesbiana* [Behnke, 1970a] and *Xenopus laevis* [Gambino et al., 1982].

tened, elliptical erythrocyte shape is retained at 0°C even though MBs have disassembled [Barrett and Dawson, 1974; Behnke, 1970a; Cohen et al., 1982a]. In addition, in certain species (chicken, trout) the number of microtubules diminishes as the cell matures, suggesting at least some loss of function [Barrett and Dawson, 1974; Yamamoto and Iuchi, 1975]. Reversion of chicken erythrocyte shape to a sphere upon MB disassembly occurs only in immature bone marrow cells, and flattening of cells during differentiation is concomitant with MB biogenesis [Barrett and Scheinberg, 1972; Small and Davies, 1972; Goniakowska-Witalinska and Witalinski, 1977]. On the basis of such observations, there is general agreement that MBs function universally in cellular morphogenesis, bringing about the conversion of spherical or amorphous cells to a flattened, elliptical or discoid shape. Such a shape is presumed to be of adaptive value for flow conditions [Fischer, 1978] and for metabolic exchange. Some investigators have concluded that the erythrocyte MB is not required for continued shape "maintenance" in mature cells of at least some species [Behnke, 1970a; Barrett and Dawson, 1974]. This conclusion would seem to be valid for any erythrocyte that does not lose native shape when its MB is experimentally disassembled, including the blood clam erythrocyte (Fig. 6). However, as discussed above, our laboratory has recently obtained evidence that the MBs of blood clam erythrocytes serve to stabilize normal shape against external deforming forces. This is compatible with the observations of several earlier investigators suggesting that MBs play some continuing role in mature cells. Fawcett and Witebsky [1964], for example, noted that MBs in stained preparations of amphibian *(Amphiuma)* erythrocytes sometimes exhibited loops indicative of the flexibility required for a shape maintenance role. Goniakowska-Witalinska and Witalinski [1976] reported a correlation between cell size and MB microtubule number in different vertebrate species, suggestive of a mechanical role. How are these various observations to be reconciled?

The literature really encompasses two kinds of cell shape "maintenance": a) maintenance of the differentiated state, and b) maintenance of shape in the face of external deforming forces. Thus, in erythrocytes with cold-labile MBs (chicken, dogfish, blood clam), the MB is needed to attain the differentiated shape (flattened disc or ellipse) but not to maintain it. However, the latter conclusion is valid only for the static experimental conditions of microscopic examination. It says little about MB function under dynamic conditions, i.e. the second kind of maintenance referred to above, to which observations on MB flexibility and thickness in mature erythrocytes apply. Behnke [1970b] alluded to this distinction, stating that "although the marginal bundle may not maintain cell shape, there is suggestive evidence that the bundle will resist changes in shape." Based on the work with blood clam erythrocytes, we have tested MBs of vertebrate erythrocytes (dogfish) for such a continuing maintenance role by comparing the responses of cells with and without MBs to mechanical stress [Joseph-Silverstein and Cohen, 1984]. The results are similar: Significantly more of the dogfish erythrocytes that lack MBs are found to be deformed. In addition, those containing MBs maintain elliptical shape in hyperosmotic media, whereas many of those without MBs do not. Continuing MB function in "type b" maintenance of mature cell shape is therefore indicated for erythrocytes in general.

By what mechanism could the MB achieve such a function? In our current general model for the cytoskeletal system of all MB-containing cells, the MB is in contact with the cytoplasmic face of the SAC. We believe that the MB acts as a flexible frame supporting the SAC and other membrane components attached to it, and that tension within the SAC is applied across this frame (Fig. 28). Flexibility permits the MB to be deformed by external forces, as would be required during passage of cells through small vessels or during other surface contacts. Upon removal of those forces the MB rapidly springs back to equilibrium shape because of redistribution of strain within it. Is there any evidence of strain within MBs? Isolated MBs tend to circularize,

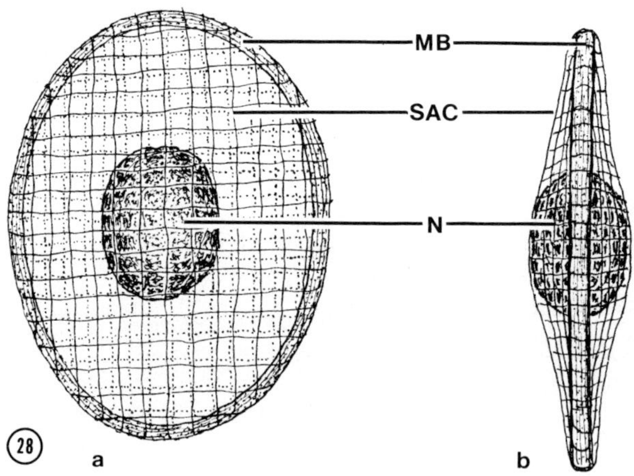

Fig. 28. A model of the nucleated erythrocyte cytoskeleton, illustrating the relationship between the MB and the cell surface-associated cytoskeleton (SAC). a. Face view. b. Edge view. The SAC completely encloses the MB and is in contact with it. In cells with a relatively thick nucleus there will be a central bulge (biconvexity in edge view, as in b). The SAC is thought to be under tension, which is applied across the MB acting as a frame. Bending strain within the MB would account for its return to equilibrium morphology after deformation by external forces. For simplicity, other possible cytoskeletal elements, such as intermediate filaments, are omitted.

suggesting equalization of strain [Bertolini and Monaco, 1976; Cohen, 1978a]. In addition, microtubule bundles that strip away from the MB surface during protease-induced disorganization straighten as they do so, and completely transsected MBs tend to open outward into a much more linear configuration [Cohen, 1978a]. Both are indicative of release of strain, i.e., the curved MB microtubules "prefer" to be straight.

What evidence indicates that the MB is in contact with a SAC in all cell types in which MBs are present? In the vertebrate and invertebrate erythrocytes, direct contact between MB and SÁC is seen in thin sections of cytoskeletons (as in Fig. 4). Such contact has not yet been visualized directly in thin sections of intact cells because cytoplasmic homogeneity and electron density (especially due to hemoglobin) mask the SAC. However, MB microtubules are never observed directly touching the lipid bilayer of erythrocyte plasma membranes, and the same is true for clotting cells (for example, Figs. 21 and 25; *Limulus,* lobster) and for mammalian platelets [Behnke, 1970a; White, 1971]. In addition, an actin-containing cytoskeletal layer external to the MB has recently been observed by electron microscopy of whole cytoskeletons prepared from unstimulated platelets [Boyles et al., 1983]. Cytoplasmic granules such as those of *Homarus* and *Limulus* clotting cells are also separated from the bilayer by a space [Ornberg and Reese, 1981; Cohen et al., 1983], and passage of the granule through a cortical layer in the *Limulus* amebocyte is believed to be a critical event in exocytosis [see Ornberg, this volume].

MB Structure and Biogenesis

The biogenesis of MBs, like that of any microtubule system, encompasses general problems of spatial and temporal control of tubulin assembly. Since the literature on these general subjects is enormous, we will consider only selected aspects restricted principally to MBs.

Microtubule-associated proteins (such as the high-molecular-weight brain MAPs) promote and can be critical for microtubule assembly under certain conditions [Murphy and Borisy, 1975; Sloboda et al., 1976]. Some MAPs appear to be widely distributed among species and tissues, while others are restricted to certain organelles and cell types [Solomon et al., 1979; Zieve and Solomon, 1982; Duerr et al., 1981]. Specific MAP functions have been difficult to assign in any system, but the relative simplicity of the MB suggests that it may ultimately prove useful for this purpose. As noted earlier, one such function is the cross-bridging of microtubules into arrays, which occurs in many systems [Dustin, 1978]. Cross-bridges are observed in thin sectioned MBs of *Noetia* erythrocytes and *Limulus* amebocytes (Figs. 4b and 21a), as well as vertebrate MBs [Cohen et al., 1982a; Behnke, 1967].

Bridging proteins have not been identified or characterized in MBs or in most other microtubule systems, but both dynein and MAP-2 have been shown to bridge microtubules in vitro [Haimo et al., 1979; Kim et al., 1979].

The literature on MB MAPs and other possible non-tubulin MB components is currently in a complex state. Platelet microtubule protein preparations obtained by temperature-cycling contain high-molecular-weight components similar to brain MAPs 1 and 2 [Castle and Crawford, 1977]. However, it has not been demonstrated directly that these are actually associated with the platelet MB in situ. The MBs of chicken and amphibian *(Bufo marinus)* erythrocytes appear to contain a protein analogous to brain MAP 2, as determined by anti–MAP 2 immunofluorescence [Sloboda and Dickersin, 1980]. Although its molecular weight is higher than that of brain MAP 2, making identification uncertain, gold-labelled anti-MAP 2 has been localized to cross-bridges between microtubules of amphibian MBs [Centonze et al, 1984]. MBs isolated from amphibian *(Triturus cristatus)* erythrocytes are reported to contain 14 components, including actin, myosin, and 90K glycoprotein, as well as tubulin [Monaco et al., 1982]. However, the published gel pattern contains proteins similar to those of the dogfish or chicken erythrocyte SAC, the most prominent of which are the high-molecular-weight triplet (> 200,000) in the spectrin range, and actin [Bartelt et al., 1982]. This raises some doubt about whether MBs were truly isolated. MBs isolated from dogfish erythrocytes do not contain high-molecular-weight MAPs, actin, or myosin [Cohen et al, 1982a]. After one disassembly/reassembly cycle of MB-derived tubulin, the only major associated proteins are in the Mr 30,000 range [Cohen et al., 1982b]. In addition, microtubule protein extracted from chicken erythrocytes and purified by temperature-cycling does not contain high-molecular-weight MAPs or other proteins, but rather components in the tau molecular weight range [Murphy and Wallis, 1983b]. However, although these last-cited studies are in agreement with respect to absence of high-molecular-weight MAPs, they do not rule out the possibility of proteolytic degradation of MAPs during cell lysis and/or MB isolation. Protease (elastase) was used to remove the SAC during isolation of MBs from dogfish erythrocytes [Cohen et al., 1982a], and endogenous proteases which degrade membrane proteins rapidly after cell lysis have been observed in chicken erythrocytes [Jackson, 1975] and could be present in erythrocytes of other species as well.

Further studies are required before these apparently conflicting data can be resolved. While the diversity of potential MB MAPs may be disconcerting, it is not necessarily indicative of faulty data. MBs of different cell types may contain different MAPs related to specific functions. For example, MAPs of clotting cells and mammalian platelets may be specialized to permit rapid splaying and reorganization of MB microtubules during morphological changes associated with clotting. Considerable work on MB MAP identification obviously remains to be done—in particular attempting to minimize the possibility of in vitro artifact. The approach that we have taken in recent work with the blood clam MB is promising in this regard, with potential MAPs identified on the basis of co-assembly with the MB in living cells [Joseph-Silverstein and Cohen, 1983a,b]. Such an approach has been taken previously by others in different systems [Solomon et al., 1979; Duerr et al., 1981].

Although the problem of MB structure was defined by Fawcett and Witebsky in their original paper [1964], the data on MB microtubule numbers and lengths are still incomplete. Platelet MB microtubules traverse the platelet circumference at least several times, and it is possible that the entire platelet MB is a single coiled microtubule [Behnke and Zelander, 1967; Nachmias et al., 1977; Nachmias, 1980]. Current work in our laboratory on experimentally disorganized goldfish erythrocyte MBs reveals at least some microtubules to be longer than required for one complete circumferential turn (DeFour and Ginsburg, 1983, unpublished). The isolated *Phascolopsis* erythrocyte MB similarly contains very long microtubules with few free ends visible (Fig. 18). This is consistent with recent work on chicken erythrocyte tubulin indicating that it has an unusual β-subunit which may be responsible for assembly of microtubules of great length [Murphy and Wallis, 1983a]. It is highly unlikely that any MB consists of relatively short overlapping microtubule segments such as occur in the plant cell cortex [Hardham and Gunning, 1978].

As in other systems, relatively little is known about spatial and temporal control of MB microtubule assembly and polarity in vivo. To our knowledge, the blood clam erythrocyte is the only cell type in which a microtubule organizing center (MTOC) involved in MB assembly has been identified. Recent work confirms the presence of MB-associated centrioles in three Japanese species of blood clams (*Barbatia virescens, Arca boucardi,* and *Pseudogrammatodon dalli* [Ochi and Cohen, 1984]), and we assume that they are a universal feature of all such species. Sea cucumber erythrocytes also contain centrioles that are regularly associated with the MB [Fontaine and Lambert, 1973], and we have observed what appear to be centriole pairs associated with at least some of the *Phascolopsis* erythrocyte MBs (Fig. 17). However, studies have not yet been conducted on centriole function in these cells. In nonmammalian vertebrate erythrocytes, centrioles are not regularly observed on or near MBs, although they have been found adjacent to the nucleus in amphibian erythrocytes [Euteneuer et al., 1982; Gambino et al., 1982]. In chicken erythrocytes, centriole-containing MTOCs are not present during MB reassembly [Miller and Solomon, 1984]. We have not found MB-associated centrioles in our phase contrast surveys of invertebrate clotting cell cytoskeletons, though centrioles have been observed close to the nucleus in *Limulus* amebocytes [Dumont et al., 1966]. In mammals, numerous centrioles are present in megakaryocytes [Behnke, 1969], but their number is about 100 times lower than required for a 1:1 correspondence with platelets produced by these cells, and centrioles are rarely found in mature platelets [Behnke, 1970b; White, 1971]. Therefore, if centrioles have *any* role in platelet MB biogenesis, it would have to be indirect, such as one involving distribution of pericentriolar material. MTOC activity has been localized to pericentriolar material in several systems (for example, see Gould and Borisy [1977]), and this also appears to be the case for the MTOC of blood clam erythrocytes [Nemhauser et al, 1983]. However, little is known about its composition and mechanism of action.

Both theoretical and experimental analysis indicates that the "+" or net assembly ends of microtubules are distal to centriole-containing MTOCs [Heidemann and McIntosh, 1980; Bergen et al., 1980; Kirschner, 1980]. Our model for MB formation in the blood clam erythrocytes (Fig. 9) thus predicts that this MB is constructed of microtubules of opposite polarity. In contrast, the platelet MB is expected to have uniform microtuble polarity, assuming that it is a single coiled microtubule. Initial results using the tubulin hook addition technique [Heidemann and McIntosh, 1980] indicate that vertebrate erythrocyte MBs of a given species sometimes contain microtubules of uniform polarity and sometimes of opposite polarity. The authors [Euteneuer et al., 1982] have raised the provocative possibility that the mechanism of MB biogenesis permits such variability within a given species, implying that the particular mode of MB construction may not be important to its function. This would be consistent with the existence of a variety of mechanisms for generating MBs (centrioles vs. no centrioles, etc.) and with a universal functional mechanism that is independent of microtubule polarity, such as that based upon MB strain as discussed above.

Other mechanisms may be at work in the spatial control of MB assembly. Since blood clam erythrocytes and other erythrocytes with cold-labile MBs remain flattened and elliptical at 0°C and during rewarming, the MB must reassemble in its original location in the existing plane of flattening. Otherwise, intermediate stages of cell shape would be observed as a new plane of flattening was being established. One possibility is that the centrioles, when present, remain in their original location and initiate microtubules in a specific plane. Another plausible explanation is that there exists some kind of "track" along the SAC in the plane of flattening. In fact microtubule "tracks" have recently been observed in replicas of the inner surface of the chicken erythrocyte membrane [Granger and Lazarides, 1982]. It is not yet clear whether they are present in erythrocytes lacking MBs or whether they are produced by pressure of MB microtubules against the SAC during fixation. If real, such tracks could function to guide and stabilize reassembling MB microtubules and might contain MAPs or other components that link the outer MB microtubules to the SAC. In recent work, Swan and Solomon [1984] have depleted chicken erythrocytes of microtubules at 0°C, and incubated their cytoskeletons with calf-brain tubulin. Most microtubules reassembled in curved bundles at the cytoskeleton periphery, with close similarity to the original MB, providing functional evidence of such "tracks."

Our understanding of the possible role of centrioles and of other mechanisms involved in MB biogenesis would benefit greatly from further detailed structural studies of hematopoietic tissue. Unfortunately, information is currently lacking on the site(s) of erythropoiesis in marine invertebrates.

ADDITIONAL COMPARATIVE ASPECTS AND PROBLEMS FOR FUTURE WORK

Cell Size Vs. Microtubule Number: Comparison of cytoskeletal structure and behavior in erythrocytes and clotting cells of invertebrates and vertebrates reveals certain additional features of interest. As noted previously, there is a general correlation between microtubule number and cell size in erythrocytes of diverse nonmammalian vertebrate species [Goniakowska-Witalinska and Witalinski, 1976]. This correlation presumably has some mechanical significance associated with MB function in maintaining erythrocyte shape in response to deformation. The relationship does not hold for the invertebrate erythrocyte MBs, however. Blood clam erythrocytes are smaller than those of *Phascolopsis,* yet the latter have extremely thin MBs (2–13 microtubules counted), whereas the former have thick ones (20–40 microtubules). The *Phascolopsis* MBs have far fewer microtubules than would be predicted on the basis of the vertebrate data. This suggests that the invertebrate erythrocyte cytoskeletal systems have more wide-ranging properties commensurate with great differences in interphylum physiology. *Phascolopsis gouldii,* for example, is a well-known osmoconformer, and its erythrocytes may be specially adapted to survive a wide range of osmolarities in vivo.

Although a relationship between cell size and MB microtubule number does not appear to hold across invertebrate Phyla, Ochi [1980] has observed a positive correlation between cell size and MB microtubule number in erythrocytes of the polychaete *Travisia japonica.* Animals of higher body weight have larger erythrocytes and greater numbers of MB microtubules (counted in cross section) than those of lower body weight. This is an interesting case of cytoskeletal regulation within cells of a single species.

MB Disorganization During Clotting Cell Activation: MBs or "endoplasmic rings" of microtubules are present in mammalian platelets, nonmammalian vertebrate thrombocytes, and at least some invertebrate (Arthropod) clotting cells (Table I). In human platelets, MB internalization and partial disorganization are among the first signs of activation [White, 1971]. Anti-tubulin immunofluorescence reveals spiral ring forms suggestive of MB splaying, and at later stages, when the platelet MB is no longer recognizable as such, microtubules are still present [Debus et al., 1981]. Anti-tubulin immunofluorescence shows that MB disorganization also accompanies morphological changes during spreading of lobster hemocytes (Fig. 27). The MB twists and splays apart in activated cells, and the microtubules ultimately disappear. This suggests that a process of complete cellular self-destruction may be involved in the lobster clotting mechanism [Cohen et al., 1983]. It would be of interest to determine whether the MBs of other invertebrate clotting cells and of nonmammalian vertebrate thrombocytes suffer a similar fate. At least the first step, MB disorganization, does occur: After initiation of clotting, *Limulus* amebocytes show a much more random and internalized arrangement of microtubules [Dumont et al., 1966] than that which we have observed in MBs of unactivated cells.

SAC Components: While our emphasis in this chapter has been on MBs, the SAC is obviously a cytoskeletal component of major intrinsic interest. How does the molecular composition of the SAC in mammalian erythrocytes compare with that of nonmammalian erythrocytes and of non-erythroid cells? Actin appears to be a ubiquitous SAC component, and is particularly evident in erythrocytes. The function served by spectrin as the major network-forming and actin-binding SAC component in the mammalian erythrocyte is apparently served by fodrin (also referred to by various workers as "brain spectrin" or "non-erythroid spectrin") in most non-erythroid cells [Levine and Willard, 1981; Glenney and Glenney, 1983]. Mammalian brain fodrin has subunits of Mr 240,000 and 235,000, compared with 240,000 and 220,000 for mammalian spectrin. The higher-molecular-weight fodrin subunit (α-fodrin) binds calmodulin in a calcium-dependent manner as shown by the "gel overlay" technique [Glenney et al., 1982; Carlin et al., 1983]. Similar calmodulin binding is displayed by the co-migrating subunit of *nonmammalian* vertebrate erythrocyte "spectrin" [Bartelt et al., 1982; Glenney et al., 1982; Palfrey et al., 1982], and antibody to this subunit reacts with the SAC of a wide range of cell types [Repasky et al., 1982]. Mammalian erythrocyte spectrin is different, however; it does not bind calmodulin under the same conditions [Andreason et al., 1981; Bartelt et al., 1982]. In addition, antibody to mammalian erythrocyte spectrin generally does not cross-react well with the "spectrin" of nonmammalian vertebrate erythrocytes, whereas anti-fodrin shows strong cross-reactivity. In these respects the

SAC proteins referred to as "spectrin" in the literature on nonmammalian vertebrate erythrocytes appear to be more closely related to fodrin of nonerythroid cells than to mammalian erythrocyte spectrin [Bartelt et al., 1984].

The blood clam erythrocyte cytoskeleton contains a major protein component that co-migrates on gels with α-spectrin of mammalian erythrocytes (Fig. 11) and with α-fodrin. Contrary to our expectations, however, preliminary experiments indicate that it does not bind calmodulin via the "gel-overlay" assay (Bartelt and Cohen, 1981, unpublished observation). This, together with the absence of a stoichiometric lower-molecular-weight subunit analogous to β-spectrin or to β-fodrin, suggests that SAC construction and properties in the blood clam erythrocyte differ in certain respects from that of both mammalian and nonmammalian vertebrate erythrocytes. The presence of "spectrin" has also been reported for erythrocytes of the marine polychaete *Terebella lapidaria* on the basis of antibody binding [Pinder et al., 1978], but a stoichiometric doublet corresponding to that of vertebrate spectrin or to fodrin was not observed on gels. Obviously, much remains to be learned about the SAC in invertebrate erythrocytes. If fodrin or spectrin subunit analogs are shown to be present, then there may also be functional analogs of ankyrin and band 4.1, respectively, involved in linking the mammalian erythrocyte SAC to the bilayer and in binding actin [Branton et al., 1981; Cohen, 1983].

The SAC of mammalian platelets, and of clotting cells such as nonmammalian vertebrate thrombocytes and *Limulus* amebocytes, is presumed to differ considerably from that of erythrocytes. It must remain highly responsive to signals which trigger the rapid changes in cell morphology that accompany clotting [see chapters by Armstrong and by Levin, this volume]. Little is known about SAC components and properties in invertebrate clotting cells, but tools such as antibodies to potentially relevant molecules like spectrin and fodrin are now at hand to make progress in this area [see Edds, this volume].

MB-SAC Interaction: The MB-SAC interaction proposed for erythrocytes and clotting cells may be but a specialized case in which the microtubule component of the system is unusually obvious. Smaller groups of microtubules or even individual microtubules could similarly interact with the SAC to generate a variety of cell shapes in different cell types. An interesting case in point is the erythrocyte of the holothurian (sea cucumber) *Eupentacta quinquesemita* [Fontaine and Hall, 1981]. This cell is reported to undergo a transition from immature spheroid to flattened ellipse and then back to a sphere on maturation. The flattened elliptical cells contain MBs, but the spherical ones are described as containing microtubules distributed like "meridians of longitude." The authors suggest that this arrangement constitutes a spherical frame, over which SAC tension is symmetrically distributed. Similarly, a model involving a strained MB "frame" and tension in the overlying SAC "fabric" might be generalized to apply to morphogenesis and shape maintenance in single-celled organisms, in which complex arrays of microtubules underlie specialized cortical layers.

In seeking to understand the role of MBs, one must consider them as part of a more complex system involving not only the SAC but possibly other kinds of cytoskeletal elements. In chicken erythrocytes, for example, there are intermediate filaments that span the cytoplasmic space between nucleus and SAC and also connect one SAC cytoplasmic face to the other [Granger and Lazarides, 1982]. The function of intermediate filaments in erythrocytes and their possible mechanical interaction (direct or indirect) with the MB are unknown. However, their presence, as well as that of the MB and SAC, indicates that nucleated erythrocytes are a good model system for obtaining data relevant to cytoskeletal function in eukaryotic cells in general.

It is important to remember that MBs are not a universal feature of blood cells. Typical mammalian erythrocytes lack them, for example, and the behavior of mammalian erythrocytes in flow is considerably different from that of nonmammalian vertebrate erythrocytes [Fischer, 1978]. Electron microscopy and the lytic technique with Triton have failed to reveal MBs in some invertebrate erythrocytes as well, such as those of *Glycera dibranchiata* [see Pierce and Maugel, this volume] and of *Themiste dyscrita* [see Terwilliger et al., this volume]. Thus there may be more to learn about MB and cell function by comparing the properties of cells in which MBs are or are not naturally present, correlating their cytoskeletal structure and behavior with the specific physiological conditions under which they normally function.

ACKNOWLEDGMENTS

We are indebted to the staff of the MBL Department of Marine Resources, particularly to John and Francis Valois and to the late Lewis Lawday, for their efforts in obtaining and identifying the animals. We thank Jacquelyn Joseph-Silverstein (Hunter College), Dr. Diana Bartelt (Rutgers University), and Dr. Osamu Ochi (Ehime University), for making unpublished material available, Dr. Roger Sloboda (Dartmouth College) for reviewing part of the manuscript, and Dr. A.R. Fontaine (University of Victoria) for a helpful personal communication. W.D.C. also wishes to thank Dr. Nobu Sawada and Dr. Osamu Ochi (Ehime University) for their hospitality and use of their laboratory facilities while collaborating on a brief study of marine invertebrate blood cells in Japan. Much of the research discussed in this chapter was supported by PSC-CUNY grants 13313 and 13567, by National Institutes of Health grant HL 20902, and by National Science Foundation grant PCM-8107195.

REFERENCES

Andreasen TJ, Keller CH, LaPorte DC, Edelman AM, Storm DR (1981): Preparation of azidocalmodulin: A photoaffinity label for calmodulin-binding proteins. Proc Natl Acad Sci USA 78:2782–2785.

Armstrong PB (1977): Interaction of the motile blood cells of the horseshoe crab, *Limulus*. Studies on contact paralysis of pseudopodial activity and cellular overlapping *in vitro*. Exp Cell Res 107:127–138.

Baerwald RJ, Boush GM (1970): Fine structure of the hemocytes of *Periplaneta americana* (orthoptera: Blattidae) with particular reference to marginal bundles. J Ultrastruct Res 31:151–161.

Barclay NE (1966): Marginal bands in duck and camel erythrocytes. Anat Rec 154:313.

Barrett LA, Dawson RP (1974): Avian erythrocyte development: Microtubules and the formation of disc shape. Dev Biol 36:72–81.

Barrett LA, Scheinberg SL (1972): The development of avian red cell shape. J Exp Zool 182:1–14.

Bartelt DC, Carlin RK, Scheele GA, Cohen WD (1984): Similarities between the Mr 245,000 calmodulin-binding protein of the dogfish erythrocyte cytoskeleton and α-fodrin. Arch Biochem Biophys 230:13–20.

Bartelt DC, Carlin RK, Scheele GA, Cohen WD (1984): Similarities between the Mr 245,000 calmodulin-binding protein of the dogfish erythrocyte cytoskeleton and α-fodrin. Arch Biochem Biophys 230 (in press).

Behnke O (1965): Further studies on microtubules. A marginal bundle in human and rat thrombocytes. J Ultrastruct Res 13:469–477.

Behnke O (1967): Incomplete microtubules observed in mammalian blood platelets during microtubule polymerization. J Cell Biol 34:697–701.

Behnke O (1969): An electron microscope study of the rat megakaryocyte. II. Some aspects of platelet release and microtubules. J Ultrastruct Res 26:111–129.

Behnke O (1970a): A comparative study of microtubules of disc-shaped blood cells. J Ultrastruct Res 31:61–75.

Behnke O (1970b): Microtubules in disk-shaped blood cells. Int Rev Exp Pathol 9:1–92.

Behnke O, Zelander T (1967): Filamentous substructure of microtubules of the marginal bundle of mammalian blood platelets. J Ultrastruct Res 19:147–165.

Bergen LG, Kuriama R, Borisy GG (1980): Polarity of microtubules nucleated by centrosomes and chromosomes of Chinese hamster ovary cells in vitro. J Cell Biol 84:151–159.

Bertolini B, Monaco G (1976): The microtubule marginal bundle of the newt erythrocyte. Observations on the isolated band. J Ultrastruct Res 54:57–67.

Boyles J, Fox JEB, Phillips DR (1983): The filamentous cytoskeleton of the discoid platelet. J Cell Biol 97:274a.

Branton P, Cohen CM, Tyler J (1981): Interaction of cytoskeletal proteins on the human erythrocyte membrane. Cell 24:24–32.

Carlin RK, Bartelt DC, Siekevitz P (1983): Identification of the high molecular weight calmodulin-binding protein of postsynaptic densities as fodrin. J Cell Biol 96:443–448.

Castle AG, Crawford N (1977): The isolation and characterisation of platelet microtubule proteins. Biochim Biophys Acta 494:76–91.

Centonze VE, Ruben GC, Sloboda RD (1984): Immunogold labeled microtubules and cross-bridges in freeze-dried replicas of *Bufo marinus* erythrocyte cytoskeletons. J Cell Biol 99:197a.

Cohen CM (1983): The molecular organization of the red cell membrane skeleton. Semin Hematol 20:141–158.

Cohen WD (1978a): Observations on the marginal band system of nucleated erythrocytes. J Cell Biol 78:260–273.

Cohen WD (1978b): Lability of the marginal band system in vitro. J Cell Biol 7:309a.

Cohen WD (1982): The cytomorphic system of anucleate non-mammalian erythrocytes. Protoplasma 113:23–32.

Cohen WD, Nemhauser I (1980): Association of centrioles with the marginal band of a molluscan erythrocyte. J Cell Biol 86:286–291.

Cohen WD, Terwilliger NB (1979): Marginal bands in camel erythrocytes. J Cell Sci 36:97–107.

Cohen WD, Nemhauser I, Jaeger R (1977): Rapid visualization of the marginal band system in blood cells of marine species. Biol Bull 153:420.

Cohen WD, Bartelt D, Jaeger R, Langford G, Nemhauser I (1982a): The cytoskeletal system of nucleated erythrocytes. I. Composition and function of major elements. J Cell Biol 93:828–838.

Cohen WD, Langford GM, Sloboda RD (1982b): Temperature-induced disassembly of isolated marginal bands and reassembly of marginal band tubulin. Biol Bull 163:356.

Cohen WD, Nemhauser I, Cohen MF (1983): Marginal bands of lobster blood cells: Disappearance associated with changes in cell morphology. Biol Bull 164:50–61.

Cornick JW, Stewart JE (1978): Lobster *(Homarus americanus)* hemocytes: Classification, differential counts, and associated agglutinin activity. J Invert Pathol 31:194–203.

Debus E, Weber K, Osborn M (1981): The cytoskeleton of blood platelets viewed by immunofluorescence microscopy. Eur J Cell Biol 24:45–52.

Dehler A (1895): Beitrag zur Kenntnis de feineran Baues der roten blutkorperchen beim huhnerembryo. Arch Mikrosk Anat Entwicklungsmech 46:414–430.

Duerr A, Pallas D, Solomon F (1981): Molecular analysis of cytoplasmic microtubules in situ: Identification of both widespread and specific proteins. Cell 24:203–211.

Dumont JN, Anderson E, Winner G (1966): Some cytologic characteristics of the hemocytes of *Limulus* during clotting. J Morphol 119:181–207.

Dustin P (1978): "Microtubules." New York: Springer-Verlag.

Dybas L (1981): Sipunculans and Echiuroids. In Ratcliffe NA, Rowley AF, eds (1981): "Invertebrate Blood Cells." London: Academic Press, Vol 1.

Edmonds RH (1968): Electron microscope studies on the hemostatic process in bird embryos. 1. The initial plug. J Ultrastruct Res 24:295–310.

Euteneuer U, Ris HR, Borisy GG (1982): Polarity of marginal band microtubules in bullfrog erythrocytes. J Cell Biol 95:346a.

Fawcett DW (1959): Electron microscopic observations on the marginal band of nucleated erythrocytes. Anat Rec 133:379.

Fawcett DW, Witebsky F (1964): Observations on the ultrastructure of nucleated erythrocytes and thrombocytes with particular reference to the structural basis of their discoidal shape. Z Zellforsch 62:785–806.

Fischer TM (1978): A comparison of the flow behavior of disc shaped versus elliptic red blood cells (RBC). Blood Cells 4:453–461.

Fontaine AR, Hall BD (1981): The haemocyte of the holothurian *Eupentacta quinquesemita:* Ultrastructure and maturation. Can J Zool 59:1884–1891.

Fontaine AR, Lambert P (1973): The fine structure of the haemocyte of the holothurian *Cucumaria miniata* (Brandt). Can J Zool 51:323–332.

Gambino J, Gavin RH, Eckhardt RA (1982): The depolymerization of non-steady state cytoplasmic microtubules of *Xenopus laevis* erythrocyte cytoskeletons by Ca++ activated cytoplasmic factors. J Cell Biol 95:354a.

Glenny JR, Glenny P (1983): Fodrin is the general spectrin-like protein found in most cells whereas spectrin and the TW protein have a restricted distribution. Cell 34:503–512.

Glenny JR, Glenny P, Weber K (1982): Erythroid spectrin, brain fodrin, and intestinal brush border proteins (TW-260/240) are related molecules containing a common calmodulin-binding subunit bound to a variant cell type-specific subunit. Proc Natl Acad Sci USA 79:4002–4005.

Goniakowska-Witalinska L, Witalinski W (1976): Evidence for a correlation between the number of marginal band microtubules and the size of vertebrate erythrocytes. J Cell Sci 22:397–401.

Goniakowska-Witalinska L, Witalinski W (1977): Occurrence of microtubules during erythropoiesis in llama, *Llama glama.* J Zool (Lond) 181:309–313.

Gould PR, Borisy GG (1977): The pericentriolar material in Chinese hamster cells nucleates microtubule formation. J Cell Biol 73:601–615.

Granger BL, Lazarides E (1982): Structural associations of synemin and vimentin filaments in avian erythrocytes revealed by immunoelectron microscopy. Cell 30:263–275.

Grasso JA (1966): Cytoplasmic microtubules in mammalian erythropoietic cells. Anat Rec 156:397–414.

Gray EG, Westrum LE (1979): Marginal bundles of axoplasmic microtubules at nodes of Ranvier within muscle. Cell Tissue Res 199:281–288.

Gray EG, Burgoyne RD, Westrum LE, Cumming RB, Barron J (1982): The enigma of microtubule coils in rat synaptosomes. Proc R Soc B 216:385–396.

Haimo LT, Telzer BR, Rosenbaum JL (1979): Dynein binds to and cross-bridges cytoplasmic microtubules. Proc Natl Acad Sci USA 76:5759–5763.

Hainfield JF, Steck TL (1977): The sub-membrane reticulum of the human erythrocyte: A scanning electron microscope study. J Supramol Struct 6:301–311.

Hardham AR, Gunning BES (1978): Structure of cortical microtubule arrays in plant cells. J Cell Biol 77:14–34.

Hearing V, Vernick SH (1967): Fine structure of the blood cells of the lobster, *Homarus americanus.* Chesapeake Sci 8:170–186.

Heidemann SR, McIntosh JR (1980): Visualization of the structural polarity of microtubules. Nature 286:517–519.

Jackson RC (1975): The exterior surface of the chicken erythrocyte. J Biol Chem 250:617–622.

Joseph-Silverstein J, Cohen WD (1983a): Taxol-induced stabilization and reassembly of functional marginal bands in erythrocytes at 0°C. J Cell Biol 97:212a.

Joseph-Silverstein J, Cohen WD (1983b): Composition and function of the cytoskeleton in "blood clam" erythrocytes. Biol Bull 165:492.

Joseph-Silverstein J, Cohen WD (1984): The cytoskeletal system of nucleated erythrocytes. III. Marginal band function in mature cells. J Cell Biol 98:2118–2125.

Kim H, Binder LI, Rosenbaum JL (1979): The periodic association of MAP2 with brain microtubules *in vitro.* J Cell Biol 80:266–276.

Kirschner MW (1980): Implications of treadmilling for the stability and polarity of actin and tubulin polymers in vivo. J Cell Biol 86:330–334.

Levine J, Willard M (1981): Fodrin: Axonally transported polypeptides associated with the internal periphery of many cells. J Cell Biol 90:631–643.

Maser MD, Philpott CW (1964): Marginal bands in nucleated erythrocytes. Anat Rec 150:365–382.

Mattison A, Fange R (1973): Ultrastructure of erythrocytes and leucocytes of *Priapulus caudatus* (De Lamarck) (Priapulida). J Morphol 140:367–380.

Meves F (1911): Gesammelte Studien an den roten Blutkorperchen der Amphibien. Arch Mikrosk Anat Entwicklungsmech 77:465–540.

Miller M, Solomon F (1984): Kinetics and intermediates of marginal band reformation: Evidence for peripheral determinants of microtubule organization. J Cell Biol 99:70s–75s.

Monaco G, Salustri A, Bertolini B (1982): Observations on the molecular components stabilizing the microtubular system of the marginal band in the newt erythrocyte. J Cell Sci 58:149–163.

Murer EH, Levin J, Holme R (1975): Isolation and studies of the granule of the amebocytes of *Limulus polyphemus,* the horseshoe crab. J Cell Physiol 86:533–542.

Murphy DB, Borisy GG (1975): Association of high molecular weight proteins with microtubules and their role in microtubule assembly *in vitro.* Proc Natl Acad Sci USA 72:2696–2700.

Murphy DB, Wallis KT (1983a): Brain and erythrocyte microtubules from chicken contain different β-tubulin polypeptides. J Biol Chem 258:7870–7875.

Murphy DB, Wallis KT (1983b): Isolation of microtubule protein from chicken erythrocytes and determination of the critical concentration for tubulin polymerization *in vitro* and *in vivo.* J Biol Chem 258:8357–8364.

Nachmias VT (1980): Cytoskeleton of human platelets at rest and after spreading. J Cell Biol 86:795–802.

Nachmias VT, Sullender J, Asch A (1977): Shape and cytoplasmic filaments in control and lidocaine-treated human platelets. Blood 50:39–53.

Nemhauser I, Ornberg R, Cohen WD (1980): Marginal bands in blood cells of invertebrates. J Ultrastruct Res 70:308–317.

Nemhauser I, Joseph-Silverstein J, Cohen WD (1983): Centrioles as microtubule-organizing centers for marginal bands of molluscan erythrocytes. J Cell Biol 96:979–989.

Ochi O (1969): Blood pigments and erythrocytes found in some marine annelida. Mem Ehime Univ Sci Ser B (Biol) VI:23–131.

Ochi O (1980): Personal communication in 1984 of unpublished data obtained 1979–80 at Ehime University, Matsuyama, Japan.

Ochi O, Cohen WD (1984): Unpublished observations, Ehime University, Matsuyama, Japan.

Ornberg RL, Reese TS (1981): Beginning of exocytosis captured by rapid-freezing of *Limulus* amebocytes. J Cell Biol 90:40–54.

Palfrey HC, Schiebler W, Greenbard P (1982): A major calmodulin-binding protein common to various vertebrate tissues. Proc Natl Acad Sci USA 79:3780–3784.

Pinder JC, Phethean J, Gratzer WB (1978): Spectrin in primitive erythrocytes. FEBS Lett 92:278–282.

Repasky EA, Eckert BS (1981): Microtubules in mammalian erythroblasts. Are marginal bands present? Anat Embryol 162:419–424.

Repasky EA, Granger BL, Lazarides E (1982): Widespread occurrence of avian spectrin in non-erythroid cells. Cell 29:821–833.

Schiff PB, Horwitz SB (1980): Taxol stabilizes microtubules in mouse fibroblast cells. Proc Natl Acad Sci USA 77:1561–1565.

Schiff PB, Fant J, Horwitz SB (1979): Promotion of microtubule assembly *in vitro* by taxol. Nature 277:665–667.

Sekhon SS, Maxwell DS (1970): Fine structure of developing hagfish erythrocytes with particular reference to the cytoplasmic organelles. J Morphol 131:211–236.

Sloboda RD, Dickersin K (1980): Structure and composition of the cytoskeleton of nucleated erythrocytes. 1. The presence of microtubule-associated protein 2 in the marginal band. J Cell Biol 87:170–179.

Sloboda RD, Dentler WL, Rosenbaum JL (1976): Microtubule-associated proteins and the stimulation of tubulin assembly *in vitro.* Biochemistry 15:4497–4505.

Small JV, Davies HG (1972): Erythropoiesis in the yolk sac of the early chick embryo: An electron microscope and microspectrophotometric study. Tissue Cell 4:341–378.

Solomon F, Magendantz M, Salzman A (1979): Identification with cellular microtubules of one of the co-assembling microtubule-associated proteins. Cell 18:431–438.

Stewart JE, Dingle JR, Odense PH (1966): Constituents of the hemolymph of the lobster *Homarus americanus* Milne Edwards. Can J Biochem 44:1447–1459.

Sullivan GE (1961): Functional morphology, microanatomy, and histology of the "Sydney cockle," *Anadara trapezia* (Deshayes) (Lamellibranchia: Arcidae). Aust J Zool 9:219–257.

Swan JA, Solomon F (1984): Reformation of the marginal band of avian erythrocytes in vitro using calf-brain tubulin: Peripheral determinants of microtubule form. J Cell Biol, in press.

Toney ME, Jr (1958): Morphology of the blood cells of some Crustacea. Growth 22:35–50.

van Deurs B, Benhke O (1973): The microtubule marginal band of mammalian red blood cells. Z Anat Entwicklungsgesch 143:43–47.

Weinreb EL, Weinreb S (1965): Studies on the fine structure of teleost blood cells. II. Microtubular elements of erythrocyte marginal band. Z Zellforsch Mikrosk Anat 68:830–836.

Weisenberg RC (1972): Microtubule formation *in vitro* in solutions containing low calcium concentrations. Science 177:1104–1105.

White JG (1971): Platelet morphology. In Johnson SA (ed): "The Circulating Platelet." New York: Academic Press.

Wolosewick JJ, Porter KR (1979): Microtrabecular lattice of the cytoplasmic ground substance. Artifact or reality? J Cell Biol 82:114–139.

Yamamoto M, Iuchi I (1975): Electron microscope study of erythrocytes in developing rainbow trout, *Salmo gairdneri irrideus,* with particular reference to changes in the cell line. J Exp Zool 191:407–426.

Yoloye V (1975): The habits and functional anatomy of the West African bloody cockle, *Anadara senilis* (L.). Proc Malacol Soc Land 41:277–299.

Zieve G, Solomon F (1982): Proteins specifically associated with the microtubules of the mammalian mitotic spindle. Cell 28:233–242.

CELLULAR MORPHOGENESIS

Blood Cells of Marine Invertebrates: Experimental Systems in Cell Biology and Comparative Physiology, pages 53–74

Chapter Two
Morphological and Cytoskeletal Transformation in Sea Urchin Coelomocytes

Kenneth T. Edds

Department of Anatomical Sciences, State University at Buffalo, School of Medicine, Buffalo, New York 14214, and the Marine Biological Laboratory, Woods Hole, Massachusetts 02543

INTRODUCTION

Sea urchin coelomocytes were first described in the latter part of the 19th century by Geddes [1880] and Cuenot [1891]. Since then there has been periodic interest in them as a model system for investigations of phenomena ranging from invertebrate immune responses to cellular morphogenesis. Several good descriptive studies have appeared on these remarkable cells, and for a complete review of the earlier literature and background material the reader is referred to the following articles concerning general aspects of the biology of coelomocytes: Endean [1966], Ratcliffe and Rowley [1979], and Smith [1981]. The present article will describe the use of the petaloid/filopodial coelomocytes (amebocytes) as a model system for investigations into mechanisms of cell shape changes at the light microscope and ultrastructural levels as well as molecular mechanisms involved during the differentiation of cell shape.

The petaloid/filopodial coelomocytes to be discussed have been termed leukocytes, phagocytic leukocytes, bladder/filopodial amebocytes, or transitional amoebocytes by various authors (see Smith [1981] for a summary of cell types and their synonyms) and all of the terms have validity in that they each describe some aspect of the motility, form, or function of these cells. The coelomocytes normally reside in the coelomic cavity of the sea urchin and are a first line of defense against injury and, presumably, disease. For example, should the outermost epithelial covering of the sea urchin's test receive physical injury during especially vigorous wave action in nature or because of rough handling, the petaloid coelomocytes will migrate via ameboid motion to the site of injury and will help to form a clot of coelomic cells there. In forming the clot the petaloid cells change shape, i.e., become filopodial, and they link up with other similarly configured cells as well as with an extracellular matrix of unknown composition. Other coelomic cell types participate in the clotting mechanism as well, but the physical basis of the clot is largely due to the filopodial cells and the enmeshed extracellular matrix material. The composition of the matrix material and the nature of its formation are uncharacterized but can be demonstrated by staining coelomic fluid that has been allowed to clot in vitro with toluidine blue (Edds, unpublished observations). If there has been extensive tissue damage at the site of injury, the area of the clot grows considerably, sometimes covering several square centimeters on the animal's surface, and it turns dark red. The redness is due to the en masse migration of another coelomocyte type, a red-spherule-containing ameboid cell, into the clot. The spherules contain a napthoquinone-based pigment termed echinochrome. The function of the pigment is not fully understood, although there are some reports that when released from the cell it acts as an algicide [Vevers, 1966] and it therefore may act as a disinfectant at the site of injury. The petaloid/filopodial cells, in addition to helping form the clot, will phagocytose tissue debris resulting from the injury or elsewhere in the animal for that matter [Cuenot, 1891; Kindred, 1921; Johnson, 1969; Chien et al, 1970]. The fact that one cell type, the petaloid/filopodial coelomocyte, can assume such a diversity of forms and functions gives some insight into the reasons why they are a good model system for studying cellular morphogenesis, for example. On the basis of work from my laboratory, I will discuss 1) the phenomenology of the morphological transformation from petaloid to filopodial forms, 2) the dynamic relationship between the cell's ultrastructure and it's gross morphology, 3) which cytoplasmic linear elements are involved in the changes in shape, and 4) the presence, identity, and possible function(s) of proteins that are associated with the cytoskeleton and/or plasma membrane and are involved in the transition from one coelomocyte morphology to the other.

PETALOID/FILOPODIAL TRANSFORMATION—PHENOMENOLOGY

The petaloid cells have been described as bladder or vacuolated cells but the term petaloid is perhaps most descriptive of their morphology. Whether they are in suspension in the coelomic cavity or in isotonic buffer in vitro they assume a variety of configurations all of which resemble one another, but just as no two snowflakes are the same I suspect that no two petaloid coelomocytes have the same configuration of their petals. In this sense the petaloid cells are polymorphic. For example, Figures 1 and 2 are stereophotographs of two petaloid cells that had just settled onto a glass slide at the time of fixation and were then prepared for scanning electron microscopy (SEM). They demonstrate the remarkable beauty and diversity of form observed in these cells (see also Edds [1980a]). When these cells are separated from their coelomic fluid, washed in an isotonic buffer, and allowed to settle onto a glass slide, they display one of three forms of motility. They 1) retain their petaloid morphology with the petals undergoing a series of continuous ruffling-like motions but without producing any translocation of the cell across the substratum; 2) flatten into a nonmotile, more or less two-dimensional disk morphology, or 3) spontaneously transform to the filopodial form. The transformation to the filopodial form sometimes occurs en masse when the cells are collected and are probably stimulated by the "injury" induced when Aristotle's lantern is removed to access the coelomic fluid (see last chapter in this volume). Remarkably, upon standing as a suspension in an isotonic salt solution (0.5 M NaC1, 20 mM Tris-HC1, pH 7.5), the filopodial cells will revert to their petaloid morphology within 1 hr or less at room temperature. Thus even though the coelomocytes may not be in the shape you wish at the beginning, simply allowing them to overcome the trauma of collection will result in petaloid cells. This reversibility can be exploited for studies of cytoskeletal dynamics, as will be discussed later.

The transition to the filopodial form begins with the appearance of small protrusions (microspikes) on the periphery of the petals (Fig. 3). These can be induced with hypotonic shock or appear spontaneously when the cells begin to transform following settling and attachment to a substrate. They appear very rapidly, within seconds, after exposure to hypotonic solutions (see below). Regardless of what elicits their formation each petal forming these protrusions need not be in contact with the substratum to form filopodia, i.e., it is not a contact-mediated or -initiated phenomenon. In fact, cells form filopodia faster if they are not in contact with a surface but rather are in suspension.

The microspikes grow into filopodia in a biphasic manner by two distinct mechanisms that overlap in time and space. The first mechanism involves a reorganization of the microfilaments that make up the cytoskeleton; individual filaments become aggregated into bundles. This is followed by a centripetal retraction of the membrane and cytoplasm between the microspikes away from the periphery of the petals. The filopodia are thus left as fingerlike extensions of the cytoplasm. By this method there is no overall increase in the diameter of the cell; the distal tips of the newly formed filopodia represent the edge of the original petals. The second phase involves an active extension of the microspikes by a molecular mechanism that is as yet uncharacterized but in which there is sure to be a reordering and/or growth of the axial elements (actin filaments) contained within and supporting the filopodia. This

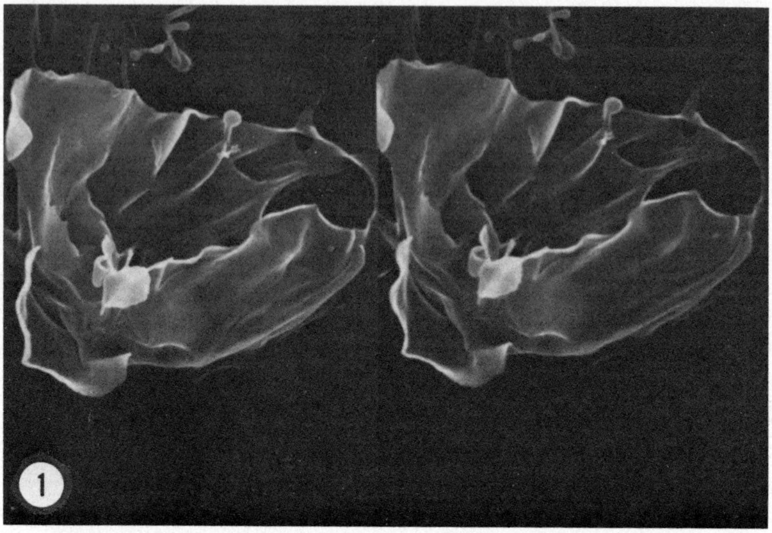

Fig. 1. Each petaloid coelomocyte is constantly changing shape and when fixed for microscopy they provide a kaleidoscope of shapes to marvel over. Their three-dimensional nature is best appreciated with stereo pairs of cells prepared for SEM as shown here and in Figures 2 and 4. The petals are thin veils of cytoplasm much like lamellipodia described in other cell types, e.g., the growth cone of outgrowing neurites. The petals undergo billowing undulations in time, and when viewed speeded up by time-lapse video techniques, they present an impressive view of this facet of their motile abilities (see Edds [1984] for a videodisk presentation of this motility). Readers are urged to use stereo viewers to fully appreciate the three-dimensional nature of these cells. These cells average 25–30 μm in diameter in vivo. ×3,600.

type of rapid extension may be mechanistically similar to that which occurs in some echinoderm sperm acrosome processes [Tilney et al., 1973]. In the acrosome reaction of the sperm of the sea cucumber *Thyone*, for example, there is an explosive burst of actin filament polymerization producing an acrosomal process that rapidly elongates several microns into the surrounding media. A similar mechanism, i.e., actin polymerization, may be acting in this second mode of coelomocyte filopodial formation as well. In addition, one often observes the active extension of filopodia without the cytoskeletal reorganization/membrane retraction phase, from sheets of coelomocyte cytoplasm (lamellipodia) that are in contact with the substrate and spread over the surface of the glass. The active protrusion of filopodia in coelomocytes is quite fast in relation to other motile phenomena, the extension proceeding at approximately 1 μm/sec and resulting in a significant increase in the cell's diameter [Edds, 1980a; Edds et al., 1983].

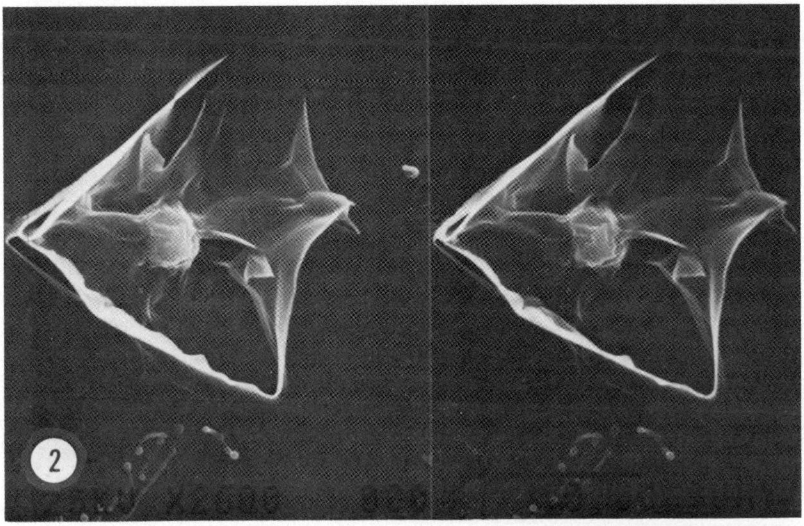

Fig. 2. A petaloid cell that displays another variation on the petaloid theme. In addition to being able to form cellular protrusions (filopodia) these cells can also phagocytically engulf bacteria [Johnson, 1969]. ×2,600.

The transformation of the whole cell to the filopodial form is complete within 5 min when elicited en masse in suspension. The process generally proceeds more slowly when the cells are in contact with the substrate and, in fact, may not reach completion at all in cells that are attached. Those cells not becoming completely filopodial remain in some intermediate morphology and have been alluded to in earlier works as transitional cells. The reasons for this difference in the degree of transformation are not understood but they appear to be related to the cell's propensity to spread rather than become filopodial when in contact with a glass slide. When cells are completely transformed, the filopodia can be 40 μm long, although half that length is more normal. In some cells all of the petals are transformed into filopodia, each petal becoming anywhere from 6 to 20 or more filopodia (Fig. 4). On the other hand, there are many cells that never become fully filopodial but rather stop somewhere in the transition. Any of these transition forms are fully capable of continuing on or reverting to the petaloid morphology.

Physiological stimuli that induce the transformation are presumed to be related to factors released from tissues, but they are largely uninvestigated. For in vitro purposes one can elicit the transformation to the filopodial form by diluting the salt buffer in which the cells are suspended from 0.5 M NaC1,

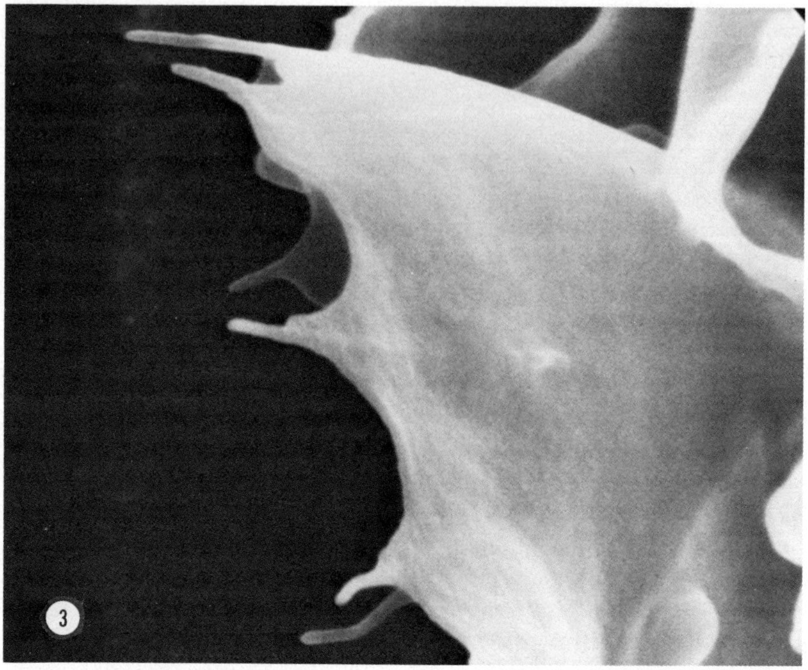

Fig. 3. The first stages of transformation to the filopodial form become evident at the periphery of the petals, where small protrusions or microspikes form and later extend into full-length filopodia. This high-power scanning electron micrograph shows several microspikes forming. ×15,500.

0.02 M Tris-HC1, pH 7.5 to 0.3 M NaC1, 0.02 M Tris-HC1, pH 7.5 [Edds, 1977a]. The osmotic stress thus induced is enough to trigger the cells and causes them to transform in synchrony. The stress is not severe enough to lyse them, and in time the cells will revert to their petaloid morphology while still immersed in the diluted buffer. They can be diluted still further and a second transformation response can be elicited, but repeated exposure to osmotic stress will eventually damage the cells irreversibly. A more efficient method is to elicit the change in shape by addition of a tissue factor [Edds, 1977c] to a suspension of cells in isotonic buffer. There are several components in this crude extract, but the active component appears to be greater than 100,000 daltons in size, is heat-stable, and is not lost during dialysis. There is a recent report of the calcium ionophore A 23187 being used in the presence of calcium-containing buffers, to elicit the morphological transformation in cells of a closely related sea urchin [Henson, personal communication; Hyatt, et al., 1984]. It is not clear what the tissue factor, hypotonic

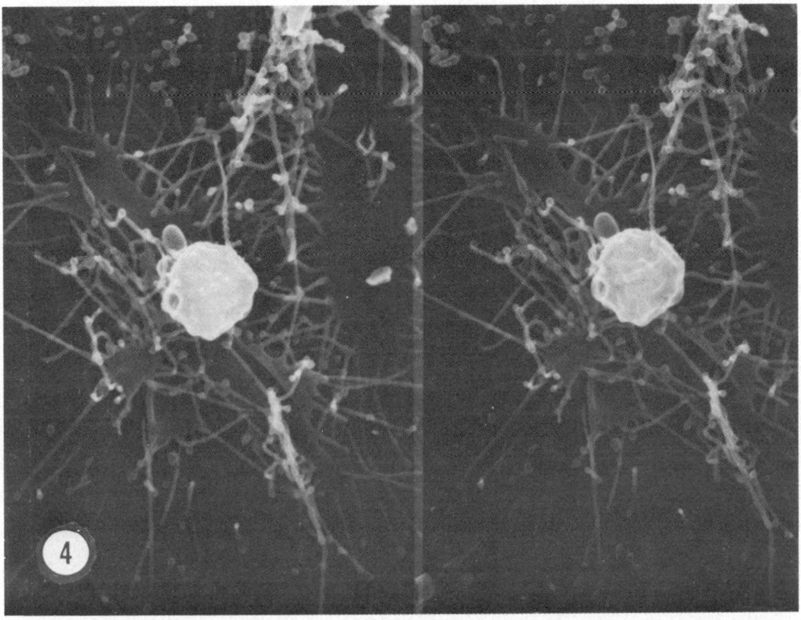

Fig. 4. As the transformation proceeds, each petal is transformed into several filopodia. Each filopodium has an actin filament bundle that acts as an axial core in helping to extend and support the structure. The filopodia can extend up to 40 μm or more into the surrounding fluid, but half that length is more usual. ×3,000.

shock, and calcium ionophore have in common that could result in the observed effect.

We have recently found (rediscovered) that if the cells are left in their coelomic fluid, even in the presence of the anticlotting agents (EGTA and Tris-HC1), they will exhibit ameboid motion and will actively translocate across the substratum. However, if purified and washed first, they lose this ability [Edds et al., 1983]. Earlier investigators did not purify the cells but observed them in the coelomic fluid and hence reported their natural motility as ameboid. The nature of the component in the coelomic fluid that is responsible for the observed whole-cell translocation is unknown but may be related to a fibronectin-like molecule or other cell-spreading factors in the coelomic fluid. Addition of bovine fibronectin to washed coelomocytes does nothing to enhance their motility, but if we add back cell-free coelomic fluid to cells that have been initially washed, there is a change in the morphology of the cells and they tend to spread and flatten to an extreme degree on the glass slide. We are currently investigating what other factors are necessary, in addition to the coelomic fluid components, for whole-cell spreading and translocation to occur.

In summary, the effect of various media and their components on the morphological transformation of these cells is to elicit one of several modes of motility. The motile mechanisms and control processes involved in each mode are currently poorly understood. It will be necessary in the future to identify the coelomic fluid components, cell surface receptors, membrane ion channels, and intracellular messengers that are involved in these processes of communication between environment and cytoskeleton and that result in the striking changes in cell shape.

RELATIONSHIP OF ULTRASTRUCTURE TO GROSS CELL MORPHOLOGY

A popular method of assessing cytoskeletal organization relative to cell shape has been to lyse immobilized cells with a mild nonionic detergent in a buffer formulated to stabilize cytoskeletal structure (see also Cohen and Nemhauser, this volume). Most membranes are dissolved by this procedure, leaving many of the cytoskeletal elements relatively untouched. This is followed by negative staining with uranyl acetate to render the cytoskeletal elements and, in many cases, the boundaries of the cell distinguishable. We can then assess the overall distribution of those linear structures within the cell that are important in forming and maintaining cell shape. A detergent-insoluble matrix of a petaloid cell produced in this manner is shown in Figure 5. Here we see that the petals that were in a three-dimensional array around the nucleus when the cell settled onto the substrate are now collapsed onto the planar surface of the electron microscope grid. The meshwork is composed largely but not exclusively of actin-containing filaments that are apparently arranged randomly, with no filament bundles present at this stage of transformation. This same meshwork arrangement and organization of the actin cytoskeleton is observed in the lamellipodial leading edge of many tissue culture cells. In fact, the cytoskeletal dynamics described here for coelomocytes can also be applied to many tissue culture cells as well [Small and Celis, 1978]. As the transformation begins, in coincidence with the appearance of microspikes at the periphery of the petals, we see the beginning of the formation of filament bundles that are to act as the axial core in supporting the filopodia. That is, actin filaments are initially gathered at the outermost aspects of the petals into small groups of filaments [Edds, 1977a]. Subsequently, the bundling of filaments continues in an inwardly directed fashion such that those portions of the bundle closest to the cell center will be formed last (Fig. 6). Recall that, as outlined earlier, the membrane and cytoplasm between the microspikes will be retracting centripetally, leaving thin fingers of cytoplasm, now supported by bundles of actin filaments,

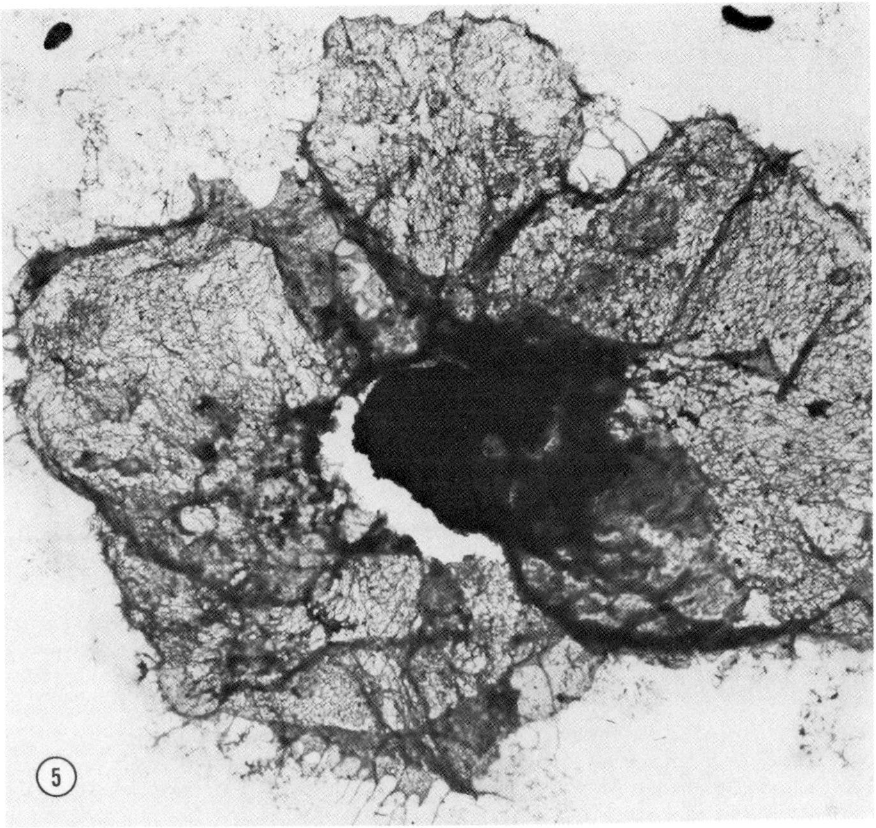

Fig. 5. When the cell membrane is solubilized with detergent, the residual detergent-insoluble cytoskeleton reveals the organization of the filamentous elements of the cytoskeleton. Here a petaloid cell was lysed and then negatively stained to visualize the actin– and microtubule-based cytoskeletal network. At this stage of transformation the cytoskeleton is an apparently random meshwork. ×3,900.

extending outward into the surrounding medium. The bundling continues until approximately 50–100 actin filaments are incorporated into each bundle. Upon completion one can see a tightly packed bundle of actin filaments that, visualized by optical diffraction techniques and to a lesser extent by visual examination of electron micrographs, contains a series of cross striations that represent the orderly distribution of a protein involved in cross-linking the filaments within the bundles [Edds, 1979; DeRosier and Edds, 1980]. This 58,000-dalton actin cross-linking protein has been termed fascin [Otto et al.,

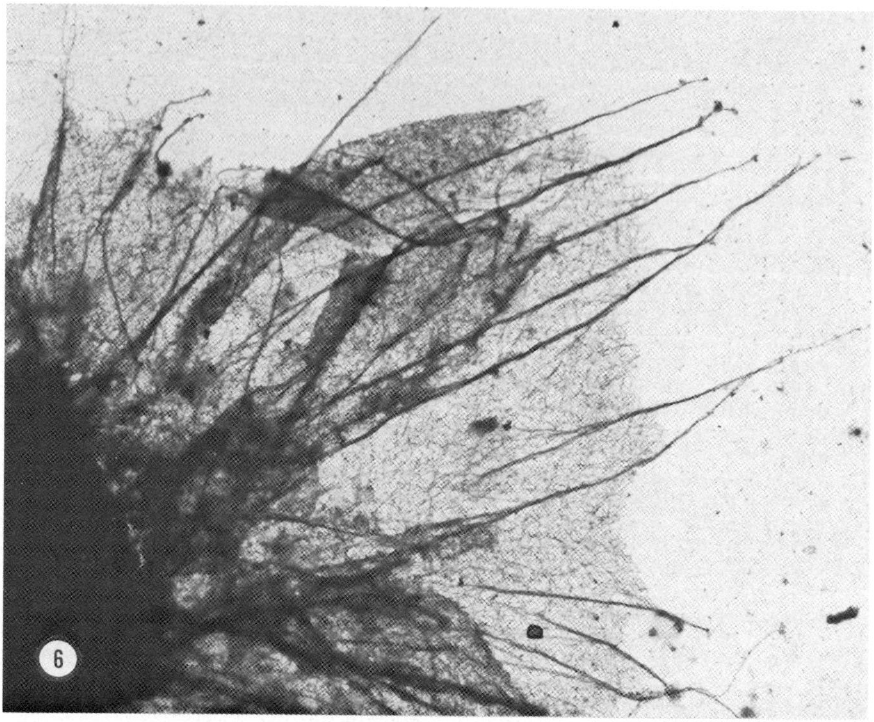

Fig. 6. A filopodial coelomocyte was prepared as described in Figure 5. Here we see the appearance of bundles of actin filaments that are the reorganized meshwork shown above. The reorganization begins at the periphery and proceeds inward. The filament bundles act to support the filopodia and, in some cases, are formed first, before the cell membrane is retracted. ×5,500.

1978] and appears to be found only in echinoderms. A summary of actin filament reorganization occurring during the initial stages of filopodial formation is diagrammed in Figure 7. The reorganization of existing filaments followed by a retraction of membrane down over the filament bundle appears to be sufficient to account for the first phase of filopodial formation discussed earlier.

From such studies on static cells, we have not been able to distinguish molecular mechanisms that may be involved in the second phase or mode (active extension) of cell protrusion activity. Although there is an increase in the amount of polymerized actin in the filopodial versus the petaloid coelomocyte morphology, it is not known whether the increased actin polymerization is contributing directly to the formation of the filopodia [Edds, 1980b; Otto et al., 1979]. An interesting correlate of the studies of cytoskeletal actin dynamics would be to test whether there is any relationship of total polymer-

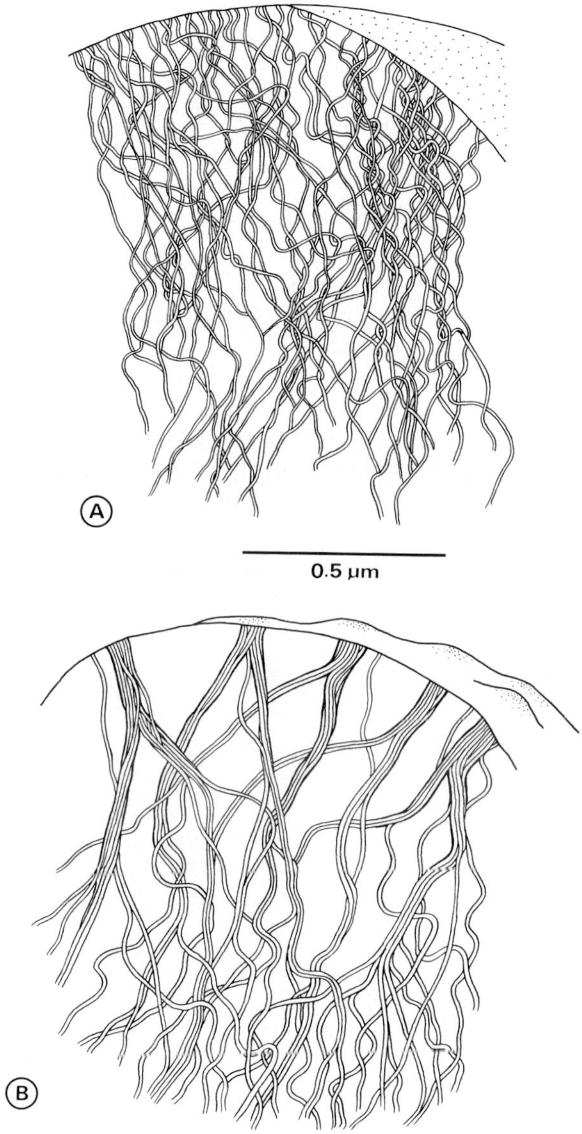

Fig. 7. The filopodia are able to form and be extended because of the rearrangements of the underlying cytoskeleton. The initial stages of that rearrangement are shown schematically in panels A and B. In the petaloid form (A) the filaments are arranged in a meshwork. There is some circumstantial evidence that the ends of those unbundled filaments are attached by a link (spectrin-like, see text) to the membrane in an end-on fashion as indicated. The polarity of the actin filaments at this stage is such that the barbed ends of the heavy meromyosin-decorated filaments are in contact with the membrane surface. As the bundles are formed (B), initially by an aggregation of the filaments at the periphery of the petals and later towards the center of the cell, that uniform polarity is maintained [Edds, 1977b].

ized actin to the forward and, later, to the reverse (filopodial to petaloid) transformation. Documentation of an increase in polymerized actin in the forward followed by a decrease in the reverse will make more tenable the notion of a polymerization-augmented reorganization of microfilaments as a means of cell extension.

Reorganization of actin-containing microfilaments occurs during the extension of microspikes both in tissue culture cells [Small et al., 1980] and in the formation of the sea urchin egg microvilli [Begg and Hyatt, 1982]. The mechanism of actin filament reorganization into bundles first described in echinoderm coelomocytes may be a universal mechanism utilized by all cell types in the formation of filopodia.

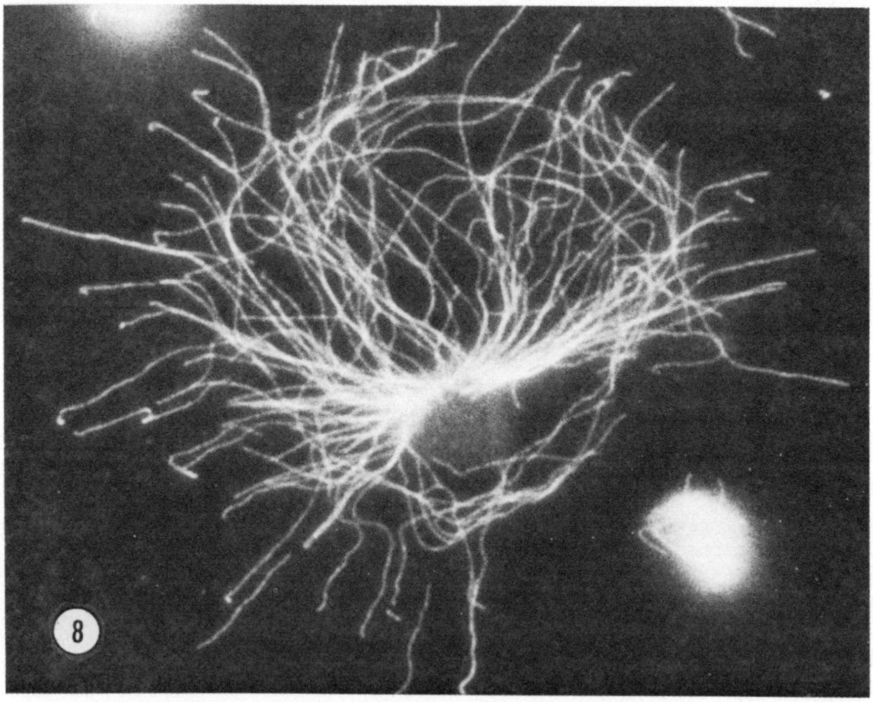

Fig. 8. Antibodies directed against the microtubule protein, tubulin, were used in conjunction with standard immunofluorescence techniques [Osborn and Weber, 1982] to assess the distribution of microtubules in the coelomocytes. These linear elements constitute a smaller portion of the cytoskeleton than does the actin and appear to emanate from a centrosomal region near the nucleus. However, the microtubules do not always extend to the cell periphery, indicating that they are not involved in production of those cellular protrusions but rather may act to stabilize them once they are formed. The tubulin antibody utilized here was the kind gift of Dr. Keigi Fujiwara. ×2,200.

Microtubules are also present in the cytoskeleton of the coelomocytes, and these 250-Å hollow tubes emanate from and are presumed to be organized by a juxtanuclear centrosomal region. Thus, they overlap with the actin filaments in the cytoskeletal meshwork (Figs. 5 and 6). I have investigated the distribution of the microtubules relative to the actin filaments in the coelomocytes using antibodies specific for tubulin and actin [Edds, 1983]. It is evident that the microtubules are not involved in producing the filopodia because they are not present in these structures as they form. However, as the whole cell becomes filopodial the microtubules can be included in some of the larger filopodia and may serve to stabilize these cellular protrusions as they do in other cell types. Their incorporation into the filopodia happens as the cytoplasm is withdrawn toward the cell center and the microtubules are necessarily included in these structures.

Another striking feature of the microtubules in these cells is their small numbers compared to what is often observed in tissue culture cells. Individual microtubules can be followed for several microns and in many cases for their entire length as they course through the cytoplasm towards the periphery of the cell (Fig. 8). The microtubules may serve to position the nucleus or other organelles within the cell in addition to helping stabilize the cellular protrusions formed by the actin filaments. Future studies will involve investigations of the dynamics of filopodial formation with regard to linear elements other than actin, i.e., actin-associated proteins and microtubules, and will be enlightening in terms of mechanisms of cell morphogenesis.

There is currently no evidence for intermediate (100-Å) filaments in the petaloid/filopodial coelomocyte cytoskeletons. There are, however, several other important cytoskeleton-associated proteins in these cells that have been investigated; these are discussed below.

CYTOSKELETON-ASSOCIATED PROTEINS

Fascin

Fascin, a 58,000-dalton actin bundling protein, was first observed in extracts of sea urchin eggs and was determined to be one of the three components necessary for the formation of a three-dimensional macromolecular complex (gel) of actin filaments that was observed upon warming of these extracts [Bryan & Kane, 1978]. Subsequently, the same protein was observed in sea urchin coelomocytes and was seen in biochemical comparisons of the two cell morphologies to increase its stoichiometric relation to actin as much as threefold in the filopodial form. That is, relative to the amount of actin in both cell morphologies, there was approximately 3 times more actin bundling protein in the cytoskeleton of the filopodial form [Edds, 1979]. This incorporation of fascin into the cytoskeleton is not surprising in view of the highly cross-linked nature of the filament bundles in the filopodia. We examined the repeating nature of the fascin-actin cross-links within filament bundles with optical diffraction methods and observed a pattern that was very similar to that observed in the gelled extracts of eggs observed by Kane and Bryan [DeRosier and Edds, 1980]. Furthermore, using an antibody directed against the egg gel-derived fascin, Otto and co-workers localized the fascin in coelomocyte filopodia as well as sea urchin egg microvilli [Otto et al., 1979; 1980]. This interesting actin cross-linking protein has apparently not been conserved in other evolutionary lines and is found in echinoderms exclusively.

Calmodulin

We have structural and biochemical evidence indicating that calmodulin is found in association with the actin cytoskeleton of coelomocytes. Using an affinity-purified antibody to calmodulin, we have observed by immunofluorescence techniques that calmodulin is associated with the general pattern of actin as seen in either negatively stained images or immunofluorescence images of anti-actin-stained coelomocytes (Figs. 6, 9). We also observe calmodulin in SDS gels of detergent-insoluble cytoskeletons and to a lesser extent with the detergent-soluble phase of those cells [Edds and Venuti-Henderson, 1982] (Figure 10). The fact that calmodulin is present in these cells does not seem surprising in retrospect, because calmodulin is now known to be ubiquitous [Means et al., 1982]. Its function(s) in the coelomocytes, however, is not fully understood. In general, we know that if coelomocytes are incubated in compounds that interact with calmodulin, such as 20 mM trifluoperazine, they are dramatically inhibited in their ability to change to the filopodial morphology [Edds and Venuti-Henderson, 1981]. Thus, it is probable that calmodulin acts as a calcium-sensitive regulator of the cytoskeletal elements and/or control mechanisms involved in the petaloid/filopodial transformation. A more precise localization and characterization of this cytoskeleton-associated protein in coelomocytes will allow a more rigorous testing of its purported function.

Spectrin

Some of the most recent work that we have been concerned with involves the presence of an α-spectrin-like protein in coelomocytes. The spectrins (alpha and beta) have for a long time been thought to be found exclusively in mammalian red blood cells. However, it is now clear that they are present in many cell types from mammals to protozoa [Glenney et al., 1982]. The function(s) of the spectrins, on the other hand, are still being sorted out in these diverse cell types. If the spectrin in nonerythroid cells acts as it does in human red blood cells, it is part of the link between the actin cytoskeleton and the plasma membrane. If true, this is very exciting, because cell biolo-

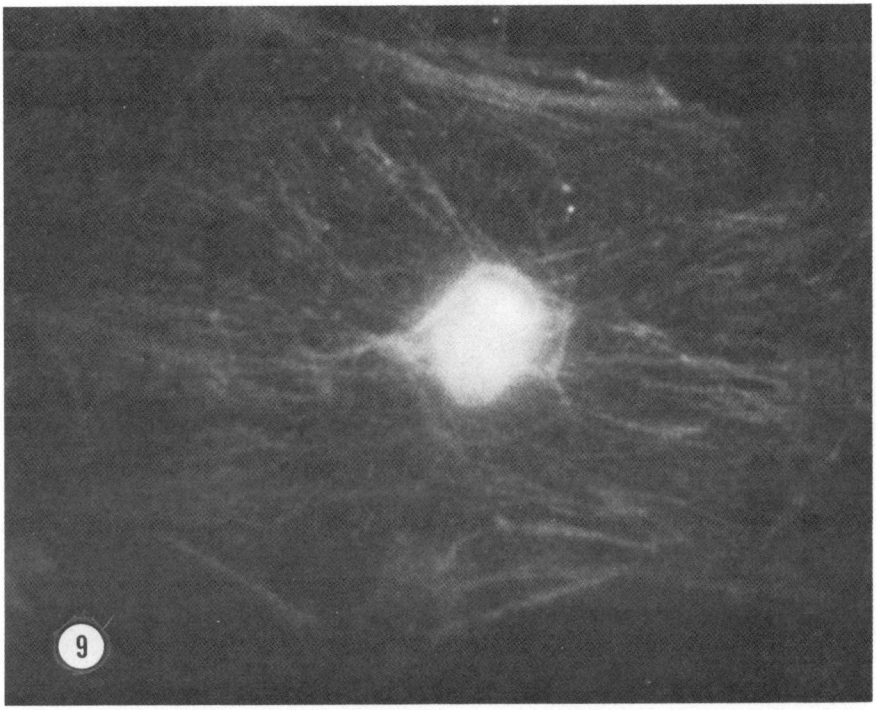

Fig. 9. The distribution of calmodulin, a calcium-mediated regulatory protein found in most cells, is similar to that of the actin cytoskeleton when viewed with immunofluorescence techniques [Means et al., 1982]. Here it appears as a delicate pattern of fluorescence throughout the cytoskeleton. When many identical cells are lysed in detergent to produce the equivalent of what is shown in Figure 5 or 6 and assayed for the distribution of calmodulin via SDS gels, the calmodulin is present in both the detergent-soluble and -insoluble fractions of both morphologies (see Fig. 10), indicating that some of the calmodulin may have a cytosolic distribution and is not bound to the actin cytoskeleton [Edds and Venuti-Henderson, 1982]. Calmodulin may, furthermore, be involved in regulating more than one cellular function, and this may be reflected in its differential distribution throughout the cell. ×2,400.

gists have sought the nature of such a link in nonerythroid cells for several years. In most instances it has not even been possible to visualize substantial linking structures between the cytoskeleton and the membrane with a variety of ultrastructural methods. There was growing circumstantial evidence in many cell types, however, that such linkages had to exist. The physical basis of that link may still require new methods for visualization but the most recent evidence points toward the identification of at least some of the molecular components of that link, i.e., α-spectrin.

Fig. 10. Whole cells were lysed in Laemmli sample buffer [Laemmli, 1970] and the components were separated on 15% SDS gels. Actin is by far the major protein observed in these cells, making up approximately 14% of total cellular protein. The tubulins, alpha and beta subunits, are also seen (tub), as is a single polypeptide representing calmodulin (cal) at approximately 20,000 daltons.

The evidence for a spectrin-link protein in coelomocytes revolves around the use of an antibody raised in rabbits against avian RBC α-spectrin. This antibody has been produced and characterized by others [Repasky et al., 1982] and was a gift from E. Repasky. When applied to transforming coelomocytes and visualized with indirect immunofluorescence techniques we see that in petaloid cells a diffuse fluorescence is present throughout the cytoplasm, indicating a diffuse distribution of a coelomocyte α-spectrin homolog. Concomitant with the appearance of filopodia we see a concentration of the anti-α-spectrin antibody at the point of filopodial emergence (Fig. 11). As the filopodia elongate, so does the region of intense fluorescence

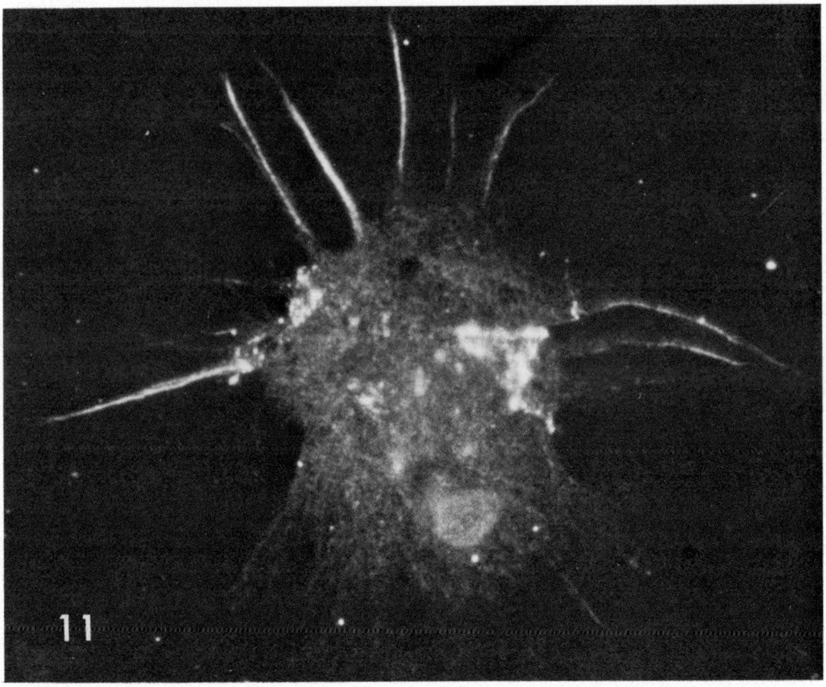

Fig. 11. Not only is calmodulin an actin-binding protein, but α-spectrin also appears to bind to actin in some cells. We have utilized an α-spectrin antibody directed against chicken RBC α-spectrin and standard immunofluorescence techniques to localize spectrin as the filopodia are formed. The antibody was a gift of Dr. E Repasky and has been characterized by her [Repasky et al., 1982]. As the coelomocyte filopodia are forming, there is a concomitant appearance of the α-spectrin homolog in these linear cell protrusions. Sections of the cell that have not yet formed filopodia presumably also contain the α-spectrin-like protein but in a less concentrated distribution, as indicated here by the central diffuse fluorescence in the lower half of the cell. ×1,250.

(Fig. 12), indicating a recruitment and concentration of α-spectrin at those sites. We have probed, with Western blots of SDS gels, the whole coelomocyte homogenate for proteins that cross-react with this antibody directed against chicken RBC α-spectrin and can demonstrate a single polypeptide at ca 240,000 daltons as the sole cross-reacting species [Edds and Venuti-Henderson, 1983]. The implication of these findings is that spectrin is helping to link the plasma membrane to the actin cytoskeleton, possibly in conjunction with other proteins. We hypothesize that the reason it appears most concentrated in the filopodia is that there is need of a strong molecular link that will hold the retracting membrane close to the cytoskeleton and help form the filopodial structure. We are in the process of investigating if the spectrin also helps to bundle the actin filaments in the axial core bundles or elsewhere in the cytoskeleton (Fig. 12).

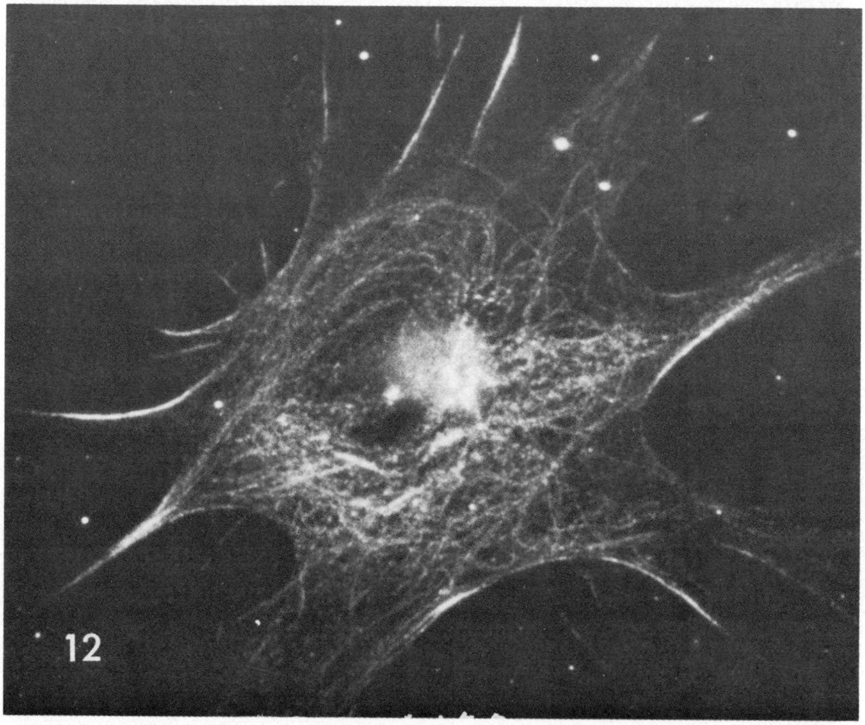

Fig. 12. This anti-α-spectrin immunofluorescence micrograph shows another coelomocyte that has more fully developed filopodia. It is apparent that the α-spectrin is localized most heavily in the filopodia but also to a lesser degree in some other "cytoskeletal elements" seen here encircling the nucleus. There are some reports of spectrin cross-linked to actin in vitro (Mooseker, personal communication) and the pattern observed in the center of this cell may also represent an association of actin bundles and spectrin. Compare with Figures 5 and 6. ×1,100.

There are sure to be other equally exciting and important molecules that are associated with cytoskeletons in nature, and coelomocytes may be a system of choice for some of those studies.

FILOPODIAL FORMATION IN OTHER CELLS

Many cells change shape and in doing so form filopodia or protrusions that are structurally very similar to filopodia, e.g., microvilli. It is of interest to ask whether, being a common structure on many cells, they are formed by the same mechanisms in all cell types or whether different mechanisms have evolved that result in morphologically similar structures. It appears that there are at least three distinct mechansims found in widely divergent cell types that can result in the formation of filopodia-like structures, but most cells will display only two of these mechanisms.

The most unusual method of producing cell extensions is demonstrated by the sperm of the horseshoe crab *Limulus polyphemus*. When activated to undergo the acrosomal reaction, these sperm will generate an acrosomal process out of their anterior end that extends up to 50 μm into the surrounding medium. Tilney and co-workers have investigated this remarkable process and have documented the mechanism for the extension. These sperm have a preformed bundle of actin filaments that, in sperm that are not yet activated, winds around the anterior or head region and is termed the false discharge. When activated, by the presence of egg jelly for example, the relative packing of filaments within the bundle changes abruptly by an unknown mechanism. This causes an extension of most of the bundle out the anterior end of the sperm and, in nature, through an egg's surrounding investments, aiding in the fertilization process [Tilney, 1975; DeRosier et al., 1982; Tilney and Inoue, 1982]. Thus, mechanism 1 involves a change in the packing of actin filaments within pre-formed bundles.

A second, far more common mechanism involves the de novo polymerization of actin monomer into filaments and the simultaneous extension of a cell protrusion. This has been most convincingly documented in the sperm of another invertebrate, the sea cucumber *Thyone*, in which the acrosomal reaction results in the generation of a 90-μm long process in about 2 sec. This same mechanism of explosive polymerization is observed in certain human blood cells. The best-studied of these is, in the case of human blood, the platelet shape transformation that occurs during clot formation or upon rough handling (platelets are very sensitive to most stimuli). Upon settling on a glass surface, for example, the platelets are stimulated to send out several filopodia [Allen et al., 1979]. At the same time there is a dramatic increase in the amount of actin filament formation as assayed by biochemical methods and the appearance of actin filaments in the platelet filopodia [Carlsson et al., 1979; Nachmias, 1980]. Interestingly, platelets are the only other cell type (fragment) so far investigated that appear to utilize an α-spectrin-like molecule in the formation of filopodia [Parysek and Repasky, 1983]. This is especially intriguing, as coelomocytes and human platelets are analogous cell types in their respective organisms, i,e., they help in the formation of cellular clots in response to injury. Other cell types, mainly tissue culture cells, form filopodia as well, but spectrin localization has not yet been observed in those situations. Clearly the near future will be exciting and informative as to the role of actin and spectrin in all cells.

The third type of mechanism of formation of filopodia involves a reorganization of existing filaments into bundles and a concomitant retraction of membrane down over the bundles, as displayed by coelomocytes. As described earlier, the filopodial coelomocytes also actively extend their filopodia and this most likely involves a second mechanism, i.e., the polymerization and incorporation of new actin filaments into the growing bundles. This biphasic filopodial formation involving two discrete mechanisms is quite common and is found in several cell types so far investigated [Small and Celis, 1978; Small et al., 1980].

Recently it has become evident that not all systems conform to one or more of the mechanisms of filopodial formation outlined here. For example, there is now evidence that sea urchin egg microvilli can elongate without actin filament bundle formation [Begg and Hyatt, 1982], although normally they are supported by a stout bundle of actin filaments [Schroeder, 1981; Schroeder and Stricker, 1983]. The list of mechanisms for cellular protrusive activity will continue to grow and be refined, and coelomocytes may be the system of choice for further questions relating to the elucidation of the mechanisms involved.

ACKNOWLEDGMENTS

The author's studies described in this article have been supported by grants from the National Institutes of Health (GM-23351) and the National Science Foundation (PCM 81-19112).

REFERENCES

Allen RD, Zacharski ST, Widirstky ST, Rosenstein R, Zaitlin LM, Burgess DR (1979): Transformation and motility of human platelets. Details of the shape change and release reaction observed in optical and electron microscopy. J Cell Biol 83:126–142.

Begg D, Hyatt H (1982): Changes in actin organization associated with microvillar growth in the sea urchin egg. J Cell Biol 95(2, Pt 2):293a.

Begg D, Rebhun L, Hyatt H (1982): Structural organization of actin in the sea urchin egg cortex: Microvillar elongation in the absence of actin filament bundle formation. J Cell Biol 93:24–32.

Blood Cells of Marine Invertebrates: Experimental Systems in Cell Biology and Comparative Physiology, pages 77–124

Chapter Three
Adhesion and Motility of the Blood Cells of *Limulus*

Peter B. Armstrong

Department of Zoology, University of California–Davis, Davis, California 95616 and the Marine Biological Laboratory, Woods Hole, Massachusetts 02543

INTRODUCTION

Limulus is a large, relatively hardy, and, in the United States, readily obtainable arthropod that probably ranks as the "world champion invertebrate blood donor." I know of no invertebrate from which it is possible to obtain as large a quantity of blood as easily as it is from *Limulus*. A large animal yields 100–150 ml of blood and it is relatively easy to collect one or more liters of blood in an hour or so. Investigators studying blood or blood cells of insects or crustaceans have to view with some envy those of us who have chosen the horseshoe crab as the object of our hematological attentions.

The blood has two phases, the plasma and the blood cells. The plasma contains in solution the respiratory protein hemocyanin, which accounts for 90–95% of the total plasma protein. Based on cell morphology, there appears to be only one blood cell type in the main circulation of the adult intermoult horseshoe crab *Limulus polyphemus*, the granular hemocyte or amebocyte [1–3]. This cell is an oval, plate-shaped structure, 15–20 μm in its longest dimension. The cytoplasm is packed with oval, refractile granules 1–2 μm in length (Fig. 1). As will be discussed below, the amebocyte can be stimulated by a variety of environmental factors to undergo degranulation and become adhesive and acquire the ability to protrude cell processes. These alterations result in a pleiomorphic population (Fig. 2) of cells that are very different in appearance from the parent cells, but nevertheless are derived from them [4–6]. This ability to undergo striking alteration in form led some investigators

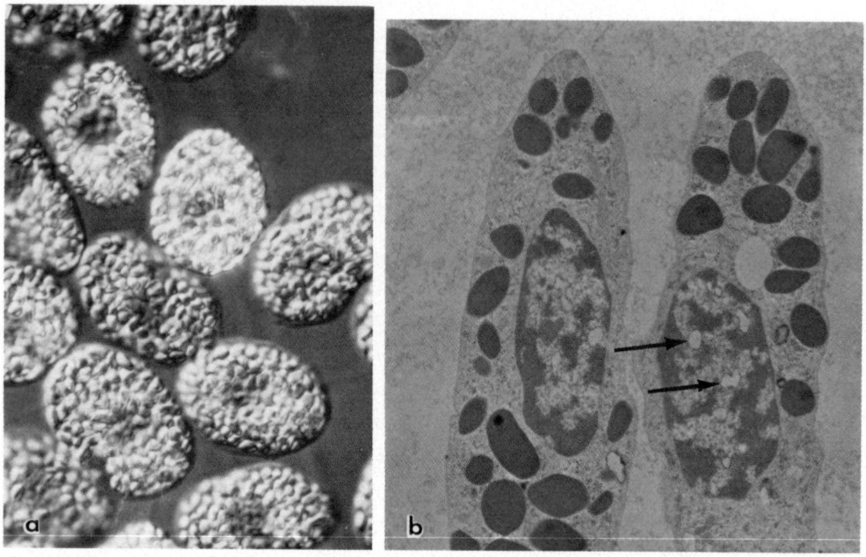

Fig. 1. *Limulus* amebocytes fixed immediately after bleeding to prevent activation. a. Intact cells oriented with the short dimension perpendicular to the optic axis of the microscope. The cytoplasm is packed with oval granules. The fixative was N-ethyl maleimide ×1,243. From Armstrong [4], with permission of Academic Press. b. Transmission electron micrograph of two cells. The plane of section is parallel to the short axis of both cells. The cytoplasmic granules are uniformly electron-dense. The nuclei contain unusual membrane-bound vesicles (arrows). The cells were fixed in OsO_4-glutaraldehyde for 5 min followed by glutaraldehyde, as recommended by Eisenman and Alfert [258]. ×5,300.

to postulate the existence of many cell types in the blood. For example, the small agranular cell reported in freshly prepared films of extravasated blood by Loeb [3], which resembles the prohemocyte of other arthropods, is most likely derived from the granular amebocyte that has undergone degranulation during bleeding (Fig. 2c) [7]. Similarly, the "fragile corpuscle" reported by Gregoire [8–10] to be a distinct cell type is most likely the amebocyte in the process of degranulation following extravasation. The release reaction of amebocytes is a process of exocytosis of cytoplasmic granules rather than one of cell lysis as envisioned by Gregoire [8–10]. This can be observed by electron microscopy [1,11–13], by visual inspection in the optical microscope [14], and by the absence of the cytoplasmic marker lactate dehydrogenase in the external milieu [15] (see also, following sections).

The best way to prevent the morphological changes that follow removal of blood cells from the animal is to collect blood under conditions that inhibit changes in cell form, to bleed directly into fixative, or to examine the blood in situ. In situ examination can conveniently be done in the transparent

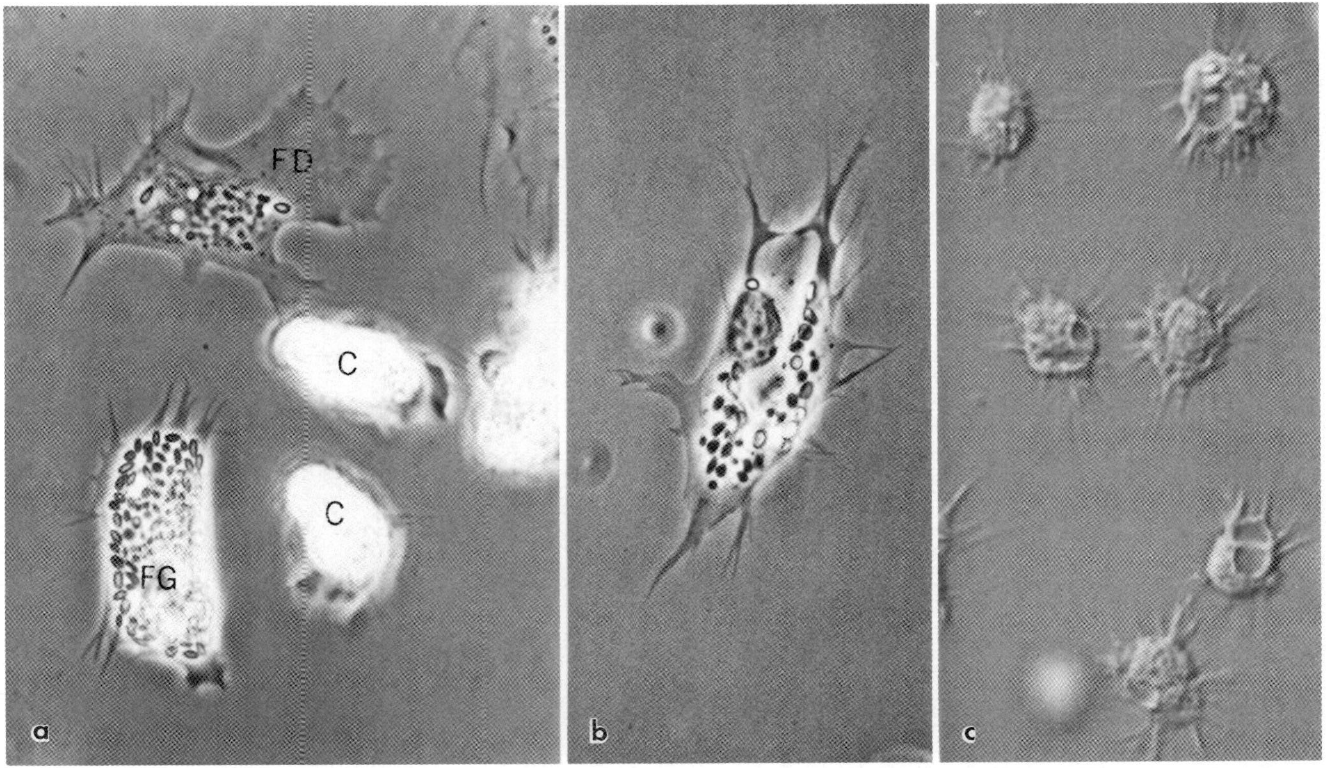

Fig. 2. Following bleeding and subsequent activation, the *Limulus* amebocyte can adopt a variety of forms, depending on the conditions. a. Cells that have migrated onto coverglasses from explants of amebocyte tissue may present the contracted form (C), the flattened granulated form (FG), or the flattened degranulated form (FD). From Armstrong [4], with permission of Academic Press. b. Amebocyte attached to a coverglass that has undergone partial degranulation. c. Cells that have been stimulated to undergo degranulation by bacterial lipopolysaccharide. All figures ×1,046.

abdominal spines of young animals under conditions of transillumination [16]. Young animals can also be injected with formaldehyde and the blood cells can be examined in situ in isolated gill leaves [5,17]. In these cases, a majority of the cells are fully granular and resemble those in Figure 1.

Although, as indicated above, there does appear to be but a single type of cell in the main circulation of the intermoult adult, some variation has been reported within this class of cells. In the Japanese horseshoe crab, *Tachypleus*, two forms of the amebocyte have been distinguished, based on distribution in the cell of the protein coagulogen [18] and on staining properties [19]. According to the immunocytochemical study of Shishikura et al. [18] some cells show coagulogen confined to the granules, others to the cytoplasm. They propose that the cells containing antigen in the cytoplasm are equivalent to the fragile corpuscles of Gregoire [8–10]. Since, as discussed before, the existence of a cell that undergoes release by cytolysis (e.g., the fragile corpuscle) is not supported by our own observations, the study of Shishikura et al. [18] should be repeated. It is possible that the cytoplasmic localization of coagulogen is an artifact of poor fixation. Dumont et al. [1] have reported that just prior to granule release, the morphology of the granule contents undergoes alteration. It is possible that the staining differences in granules [19] is reflective of this change rather than indicative of many classes of cells. According to Shishikura and Sekiguchi [19], only one type of amebocyte is discernible in the blood of *Limulus* by their methods. Some heterogeneity of cells may exist, however. I have observed that in *Limulus* blood, a fraction of the amebocytes contain, in addition to the oval, refractile cytoplasmic granules, smaller inclusions that fluoresce bright red when illuminated with the Zeiss RITC filter set for epillumination (Fig. 3). The inclusions are nonfluorescent in the living cell but become visible after formaldehyde fixation. The number of such inclusions in individual cells varies from zero (a majority of cells), to a few, to many (about 1–2% of the cells) (Fig. 3b).

A second cell, the cyanocyte (Fig. 4), has been described as occurring in restricted areas of the hemocoel, especially the vascular spaces associated with the neural plexus of the compound eyes [20,21]. The cytoplasm of this cell contains crystals of what, based on the distinctive morphology of the subunits, is almost certainly hemocyanin (Fig. 5). Fahrenbach [21] has suggested that these cells synthesize hemocyanin and release it into the blood. The cyanocyte is very rare or absent in the general circulation of intermoult adults, but is present as 1–8% of the hemocytes in the ocular sinusoids and has been reported to occur also in the general circulation of the embryo [22]. A similar cell has been described in spiders [22,23] and crustaceans [24]. Crystal-containing cells have been described in insects [25–27], but these presumably are not cyanocytes because insects lack hemocyanin in the plasma.

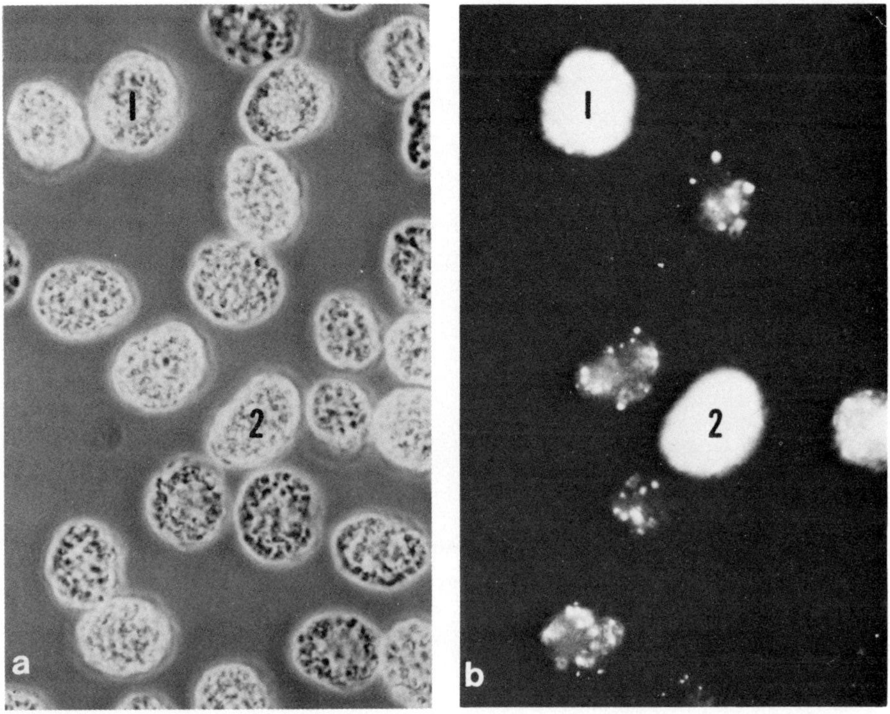

Fig. 3. Unactivated *Limulus* amebocytes fixed in freshly prepared paraformaldehyde and observed by phase-contrast microcscopy (a) and epiillumination (b) with a filter set to reveal red autofluorescence (Zeiss BP5461/12 and LP590). A fraction of the cells contain numbers of particulate cell organelles that show brilliant red autofluorescence after formaldehyde fixation (several are indicated by numbers). The same field is shown in both photomicrographs and the numbers indicate the same cells in panels a and b. The number of autofluorescent cell organelles per cell varies from none (most of the cells do not show fluorescent inclusions), to a few, to many (numbered cells).

The sites of hemocytopoiesis for amebocytes and cyanocytes have not been established in *Limulus*. Specialized hematocytopoietic organs have been described for a variety of other arthropods [24,28–34] and the circulating prohemocyte is also thought to contribute to hemocytopoiesis. This cell is mitotic in the circulation and appears to represent a stem cell population that differentiates into the various other cell types in the circulation [35–43]. As noted above, the prohemocyte is apparently absent from the blood of intermoult adult *Limulus*. The circulating amebocyte in the intermoult adult is apparently nonmitotic [44]. Release of newly produced amebocytes into the circulation of intermoult adults appears to be very low, since isotopically

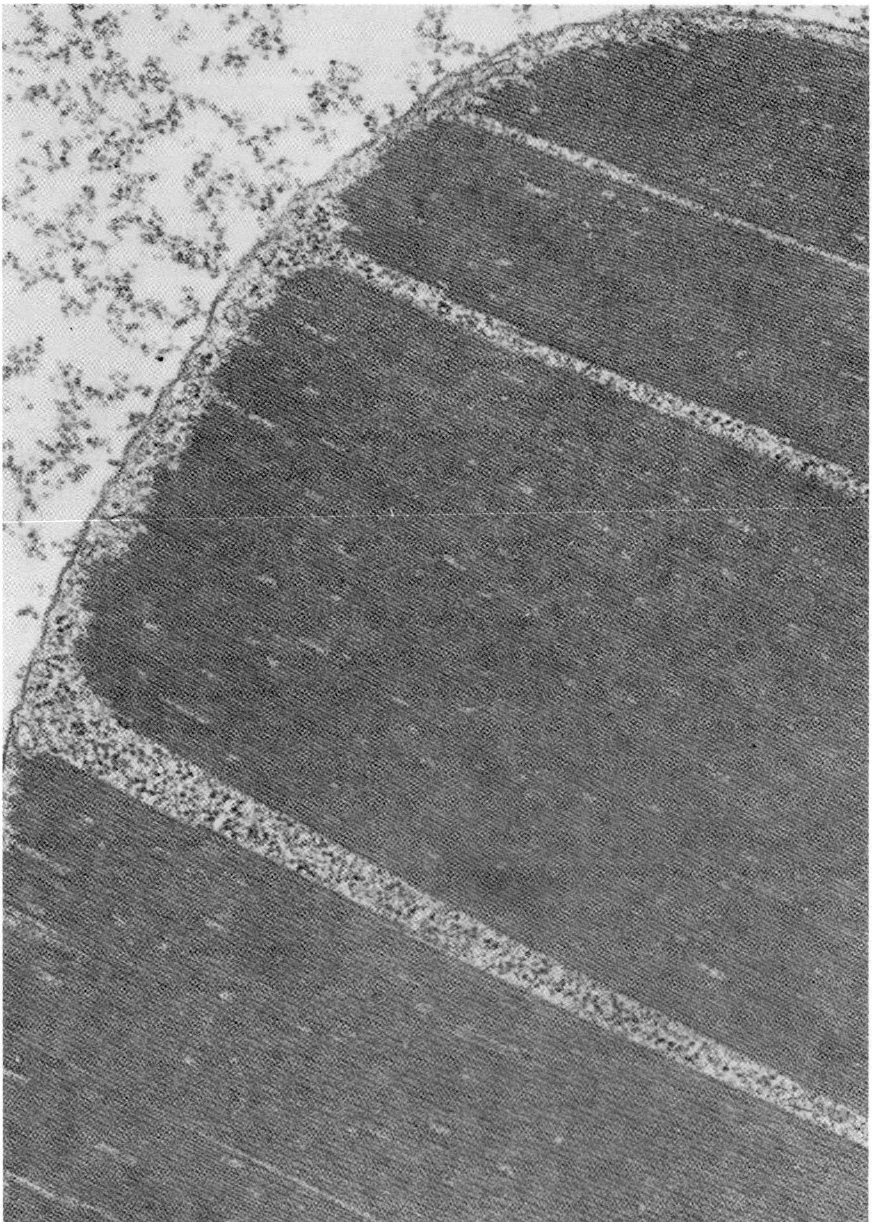

Fig. 4. Electron micrograph of a mature cyanocyte containing several large hemocyanin crystals sectioned parallel to the columns of stacked hemocyanin molecules. ×45,000.

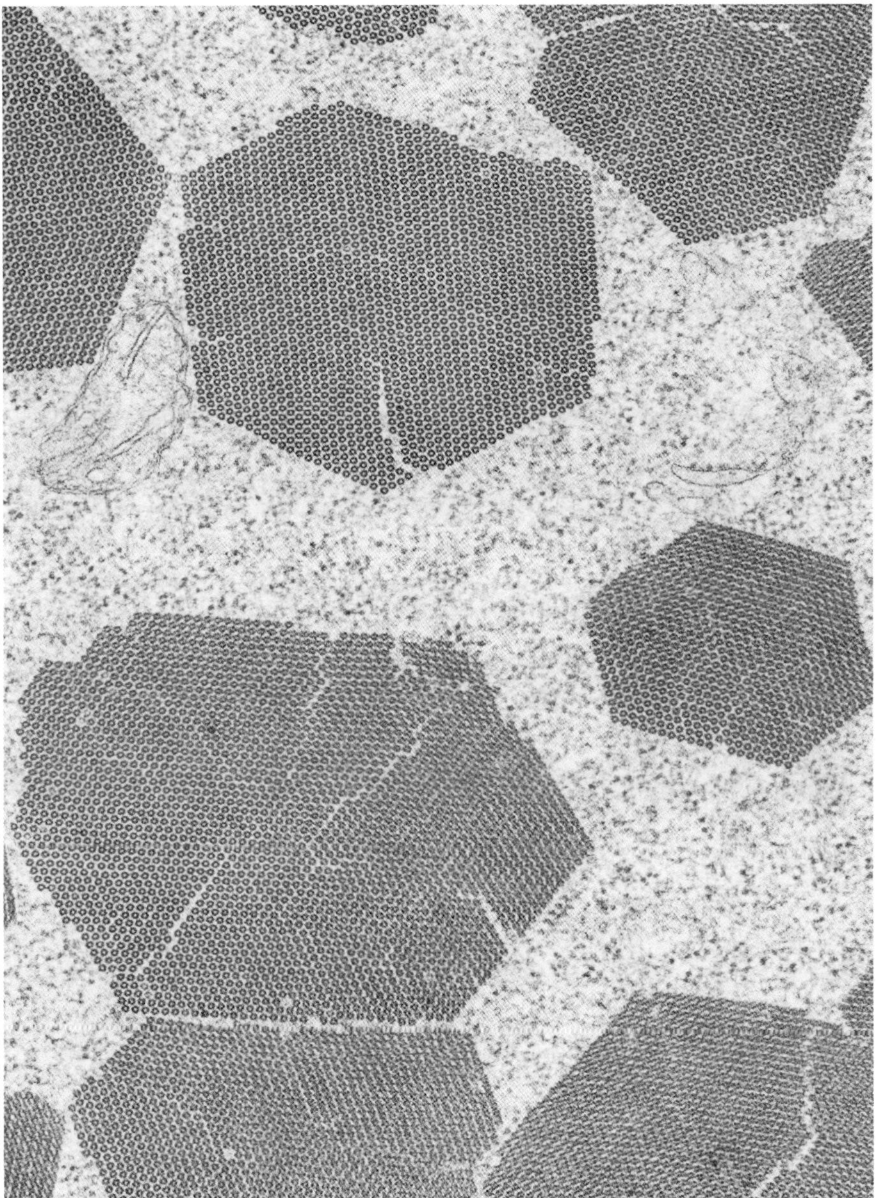

Fig. 5. Electron micrograph of an advanced cyanoblast containing several hemocyanin crystals cut in cross section. ×43,000. The hemocyanin molecule is annular in cross section. Both electron micrographs of the cyanocyte provided by W.H. Fahrenbach. From Fahrenbach [20] with permission of the Rockefeller University Press.

labeled cells were not detected in the blood of adults injected chronically with [^{3}H]-algal protein hydrolysate (Levin, unpublished). It is possible that in the adult, hemocytopoiesis is restricted to the times of moulting.

COMPARATIVE ASPECTS

The amebocyte of *Limulus* resembles morphologically the granular hemocyte of the arthropods most closely related to *Limulus* (e.g., scorpions [45,46] and spiders: the chromophobe of Deevey [47] and the granular hemocyte of Browning [48] and Sherman [22,49]). More distantly related arthropods, including insects [42,50–55] and crustaceans [49,50,54–61] also have a blood cell (the granular hemocyte) morphologically similar to the *Limulus* amebocyte that may be the predominant or even the sole cell in the blood [33,59–61]. As described above, the adult intermoult *Limulus* appears to lack the other cell types that have been described in other arthropods [8–10,24–27,35–58]. The extent of functional similarity of the *Limulus* granular amebocyte and morphologically similar cells in other arthropods has not been thoroughly studied.

ACTIVATION

In the intact circulatory system, the amebocyte is, as indicated previously, an ovoid, plate-shaped cell that has a cytoplasm packed with granules and that is neither adhesive nor motile (Fig. 1). Following extravasation or trauma to the animal, the amebocyte undergoes an activation reaction that leads to the acquisition of adhesiveness, loss of granules by exocytosis, and the protrusion of pseudopods (Fig. 2) [1,3–6,9,11–15,45,62–71]. The activation of a discoid circulating cell upon extravasation to a state capable of adhesion, degranulation, and motility is characteristic of thrombocytic cells in invertebrates [72] and vertebrates [73–85]. Although of profound functional importance (it is essential that thrombocytes be nonadhesive in the undamaged animal, but be able to respond to bleeding by the appropriate functional alterations), the underlying basis of activation is only partially understood, even in a system as well studied as the mammalian blood platelet [74,76,83,85]. In invertebrates in general, and in *Limulus* in particular, our knowledge of the underlying mechanisms of activation is superficial indeed. Of interest are the environmental cues that trigger activation, the cellular pathways by which stimuli impinging on the cell membrane are transduced into the events of activation, and the nature of the changes in the cytoskeleton that lead to pseudopodial protrusion and motility and the changes at the cell surface that lead to cell adhesion.

Little can be said about the kinds of environmental cues that trigger amebocyte activation. Although the amebocyte is responsive to bacterial

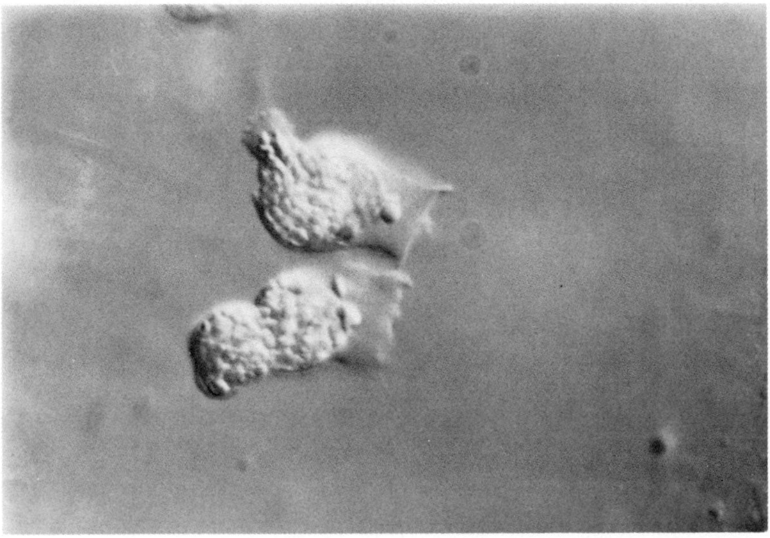

Fig. 6. Activated amebocytes in a gill leaf of a juvenile horseshoe crab viewed in situ. The motile cells are migrating on the lining of the hemocoel. From Armstrong [5], with permission of Company of Biologists, Ltd. ×1,309.

endotoxin (lipopolysaccharide, LPS) [14,16,67,86], the events of activation occur, albeit more slowly, under endotoxin-free conditions [4–6,14]. I have observed that the cells in isolated gill elements sometimes do and sometimes do not undergo activation (as judged by cell clumping and pseudopod-directed migration; Fig. 6) [5]. When bled under sterile, endotoxin-free conditions into shallow dishes, the amebocytes clump over the period of minutes to an hour or more to form a coherent tissue-like mat many cells thick (Fig. 7) [4,17,69–71]. Only the cells of the very bottom layer are in contact with a foreign surface (the dish), but the entire collection of cells eventually does become adhesive [4,5]. Thus, it appears that relatively minor trauma is capable of eliciting the activated state. It is not known whether the activation reaction can be elicited in unactivated cells by contact with cells that have themselves undergone activation, as does occur with the vertebrate platelet [83].

One approach to study of the second messengers involved in the activation response is to determine the effects on activation of appropriately chosen pharmacologic agents. Since exposure of freshly obtained cells to agents that elevate cyclic AMP levels retards activation (Fig. 12d), it can be suggested that a reduction in cAMP levels may play a role in transducing stimuli that impinge on the cell surface into the activation response.

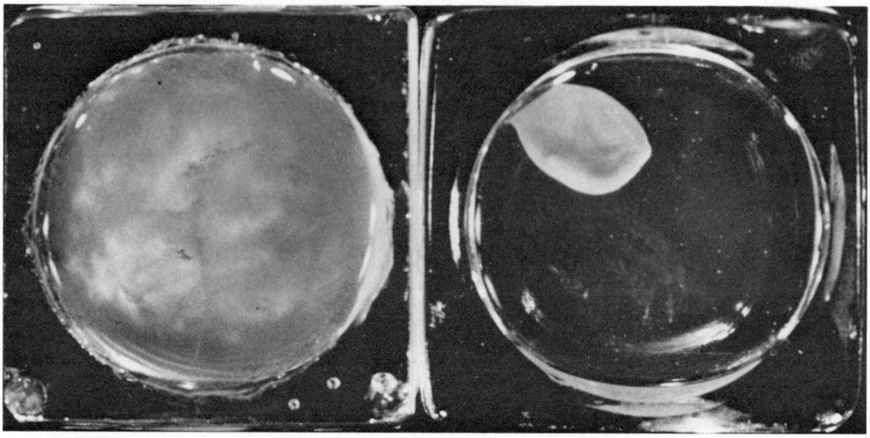

Fig. 7. When blood is collected into sterile, LPS-free embryo watchglasses, the cells settle to the bottom of the dish and cohere to form a tissue-like cellular layer ("amebocyte tissue" [17,69–71]). The blood in the left-hand dish was collected 2 hr previous to photography; that in the right dish, 1 day earlier. The amebocyte tissue in the right dish has undergone contraction. The aggregated blood cells show no signs of the melanization after removal from the animal that is observed in arthropods containing the phenol oxidase activating system. ×1.4.

The activation response results in an alteration in the phenotype of the amebocyte. A formerly nonadhesive, nonmotile cell becomes adhesive and locomotory (Fig. 2). The first alteration presumably involves alterations in the composition and/or organization of the cell surface. The change in shape from the rigid, ovoid disk to that of a polymorphic, readily deformable, ameboid cell presumably involves alterations of the cytoskeleton. The unactivated cell has a circumferential bundle of microtubules (the "marginal band") that breaks down during activation [1,87,88] (see also Chapter One by Cohen and Nemhauser). It has been suggested that, as in nucleated erythrocytes [89], the bundle of microtubules stabilizes the discoid shape of the unactivated cell and that disorganization of the microtubule bundle during activation results in a cell capable of the range of surface deformation necessary for pseudopodal protrusion. Microtubules are apparently reorganized in the activated amebocyte because they are present in modest numbers in locomoting cells. Presumably cytoskeletal actin, myosin, and associated proteins also undergo reorganization during the activation response, but this has not yet been investigated in the amebocyte.

DEGRANULATION

Degranulation of the amebocyte can conveniently be studied by diluting 5–10 drops of freshly drawn blood in 15 ml of a sterile, LPS-free 3% solution

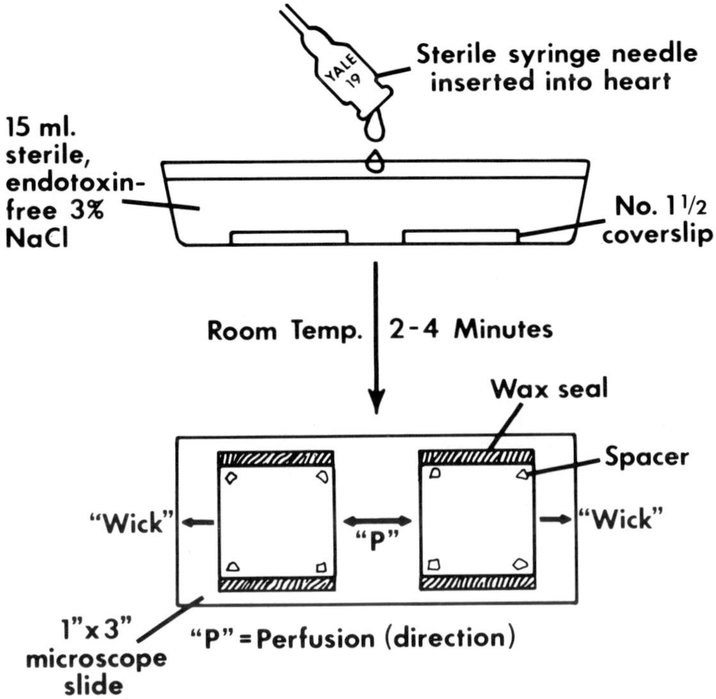

Fig. 8. Preparation of perfusion chamber for the study of exocytosis of the *Limulus* amebocyte. Blood drawn by cardiac puncture is diluted in 15 ml endotoxin-free 3% NaCl in a 90-mm petri dish that contains several 22-mm coverglasses (upper figure). After 2–4 min to allow cell attachment, the coverglasses are inverted on a small pool of 3% NaCl on a sterile 1-in × 3-in microscope slide. The coverglasses are spaced above the slide with fragments of No. 1 1/2 coverglasses at the corners and are sealed along two edges with wax. The chambers can then be perfused by introduction of saline at the inner free edges of the coverglasses and removal with wicks of absorbant tissue at the opposite ends. From Armstrong and Rickles [14], with permission of Academic Press.

of NaCl contained in an LPS-free 90-mm petri dish with four to six 22-mm coverglasses on the bottom. The cells settle and attach to the coverglasses in 1–5 min and can be observed in a simple perfusion chamber constructed by inverting a coverglass over a drop of saline on a sterile, LPS-free microscope slide. The coverglass is supported on fragments of a No. 1 1/2 coverglass. The cells can be presented with various agents dissolved in 3% saline that is perfused beneath the coverglass (Fig. 8). The progress of degranulation is ascertained by microscope examination.

Examination of these preparations reveals that the cells constitute a homogenous population. There is no evidence for different subpopulations of cells, such as cells homologous to the fragile or explosive corpuscles de-

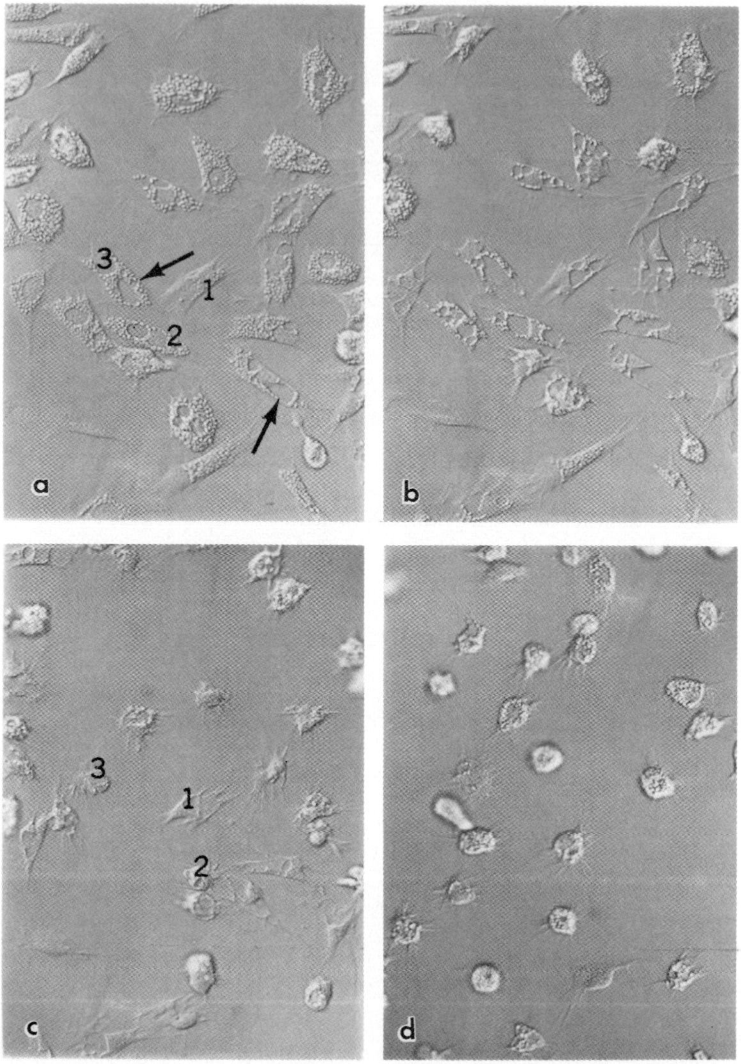

Fig. 9. Exocytosis of the *Limulus* amebocyte induced by bacterial lipopolysaccharide. a–c. Time course of exocytosis at 10 μg/ml LPS. a. t=0. b. t=2 min. c. t=10 min. The cells are spread on a microscope coverglass of an observation chamber constructed as indicated in Figure 8. The oval refractile bodies in panel a are the cytoplasmic granules. Spontaneous degranulation (detected by the domains of exocytotic membrane [arrows]) has occurred to a slight extent. In contrast to the slow time course of spontaneous degranulation, LPS-induced degranulation is evident by 2 min (b) and is complete by 5 min. Nos. 1, 2, and 3 indicate the same individual cells in panels a and c. At low doses of LPS (0.1 μg/ml; panel d), the cells that were spread on the substrate contract but do not degranulate. From Armstrong and Rickles [14], with permission of Academic Press. ×336.

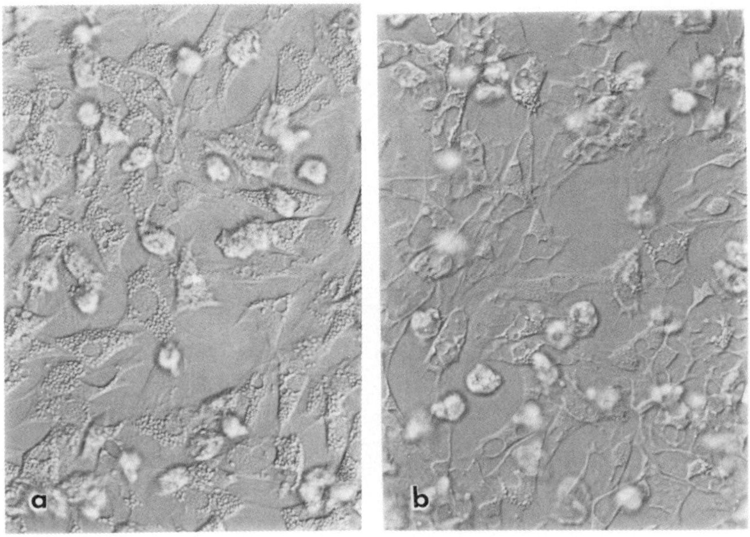

Fig. 10. Exocytosis induced by the ionophore A23187. a. t = 0 min. b.t = 1 min. ×336.

scribed in certain insects and crustaceans [31,54,61,90–97] and in *Limulus* [8–10]. The fragile corpuscle is recognized as a cell that responds to contact with artificial surfaces by cytoplasmic lysis and release of constituents involved in coagulation. Even when the time between bleeding and initial observation was made very short, cells of this type were not seen in *Limulus* (see also Silverberg [98]). The release reaction in *Limulus* involves exocytosis rather than cell lysis [1,11 15,99,100] (see Ornberg, Chapter 4).

Degranulation of the amebocytes can be elicited by specific secretagogs such as bacterial lipopolysaccharide [2,14,101,102] or will occur spontaeously in extravasated cells under LPS-free conditions [14]. Rapid degranulation is seen at 10 μg/ml LPS (Fig. 9a–c). At 1 μg/ml, the response is erratic: Some preparations degranulate; others show cytoplasmic contraction but no appreciable degranulation. At 0.1 μg/ml, cells contract without degranulating (Fig. 9d). LPS is present in the cell wall of all gram-negative bacteria and, as such, serves as the extracellular messenger indicating the presence of gram-negative organisms to effector cells such as the amebocyte. Fungi are also potential pathogens of invertebrates. β-1,3-Glucans are present in the cell wall of most fungi [103] and apparently play an analogous role as a signal molecule in crustaceans [104–106]. In contrast to the responsiveness of amebocytes to LPS, the cells do not degranulate when exposed to β-1,3-glucans or yeast cell walls (Zymosan). As with a variety of cell types, degranulation can be elicited by the ionophore A23187 (Fig. 10), suggesting

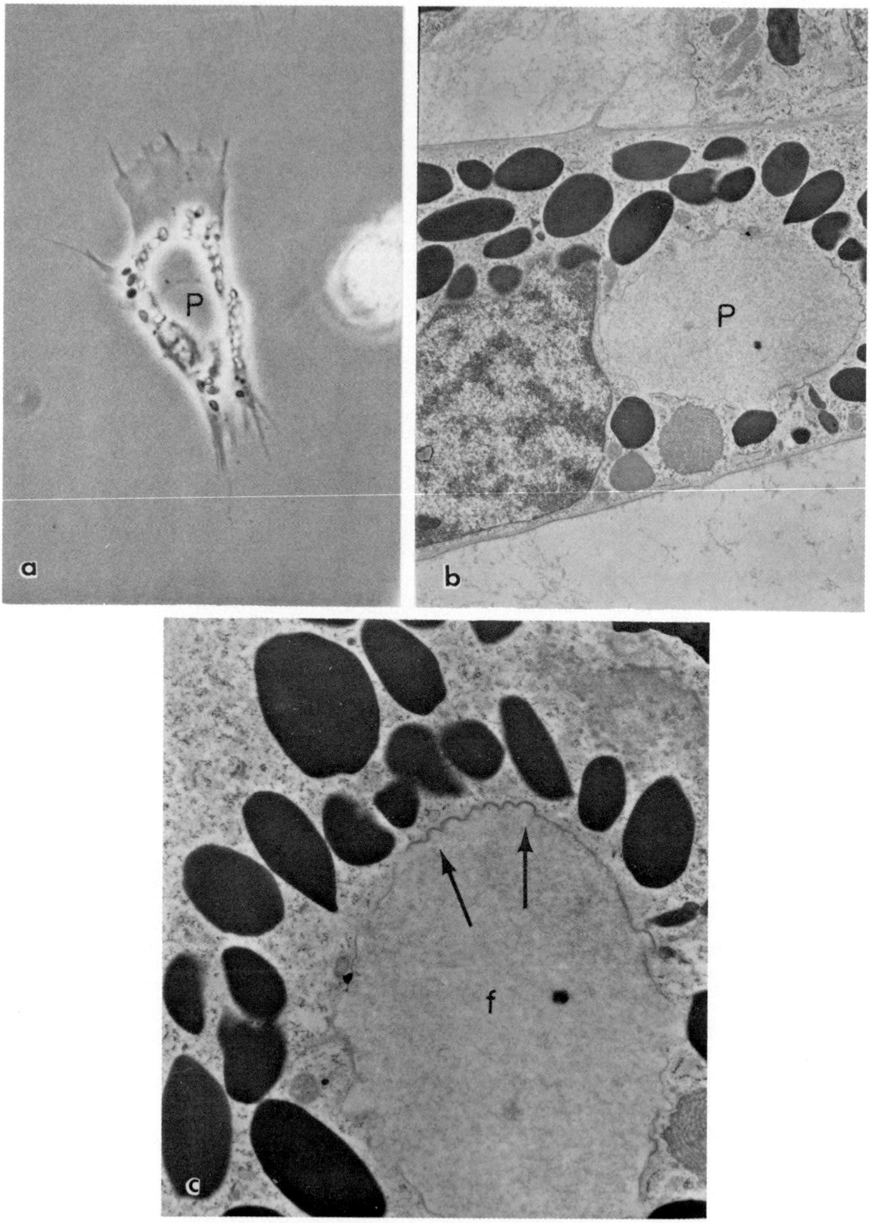

Fig. 11. See legend on facing page.

that the process involves an increase in cytoplasmic Ca^{++} concentration. In the absence of specific secretagogs, isolated amebocytes undergo spontaneous degranulation (Fig. 11). This occurs over a period of hours, rather than over a few minutes, as when triggered by LPS. Exocytosis involves fusion of the granule membranes with either the plasma membrane or the membranes of granules that have already begun the discharge reaction [11–13]. When amebocytes flattened onto microscope coverglasses undergo spontaneous degranulation, large domains of the cell surface of characteristic morphology are established (Fig. 11a). At the fine structural level, these can be seen to be associated with flocculent material at the cell surface (Fig. 11b), presumably material released from the cytoplasmic granules that has subsequently undergone gelation. The cell membrane surrounding such exocytotic plaques has a scalloped appearance with elements that resemble the coated pit (Fig. 11c). Large numbers of endocytotic vesicles are not observed in the cytoplasm.

LPS-induced degranulation is retarded by agents that block anion transport, including sodium isethionate (Fig. 12a), SITS (4-acetoamido-4′-isothiocyano-2,2-disulfonic acid) (Fig. 12b), DNDS (4,4′-dinitro-2,2′-stilbene-disulfonic acid), and suramin (bis(m-amino-m-aminobenzoyl-p-methylbenzyl-1-naphthylamine-4,6,8-trisulfonate) (Fig. 12c) [14]. It has been suggested that anion transport from the bathing medium into the secretory granule generates an osmotic pressure differential that provides the force that expels the granule contents following fusion of granule membrane with the plasma membrane [107] and that inhibition of ion movement suppresses exocytosis. Exocytosis in the dogfish phagocyte [108] and the human blood platelet [109] is similarly sensitive to anion channel blockers. Degranulation of the amebocyte is also suppressed in the presence of agents that elevate cyclic AMP levels (Fig. 12d) [14], suggesting that the degranulation that is elicited by endotoxin requires a fall in cAMP levels. Of possible relevance, Liang et al. [110] have described a Ca^{2+}-activated phosphodiesterase that also binds bacterial lipopolysaccharide [111]. They propose that this protein is associated with the plasma membrane. Unfortunately, the relevant immunocyto-

---

Fig. 11. Spontaneous degranulation during prolonged culture under LPS-free conditions results in the formation of large domains of the cell surface that are associated with the process of exocytosis. a. Phase-contrast light micrograph of flattened, partially degranulated cell. P = exocytotic domain. b. Electron micrograph of a section of a partially degranulated cell showing a region of the cell surface occupied by a plaque of fibrillar material (the exocytotic plaque) (P). The plane of section is parallel to the substratum. The exocytotic plaque is included in the section because the plasma membrane in this region is indented from the dorsal surface. c. Abundant fibrillar or flocculent material comprises the exocytotic plaque (f) and the surface membrane is indented by coated pits (arrows). Magnifications: a, ×850; b, ×5,300; c, ×10,250.

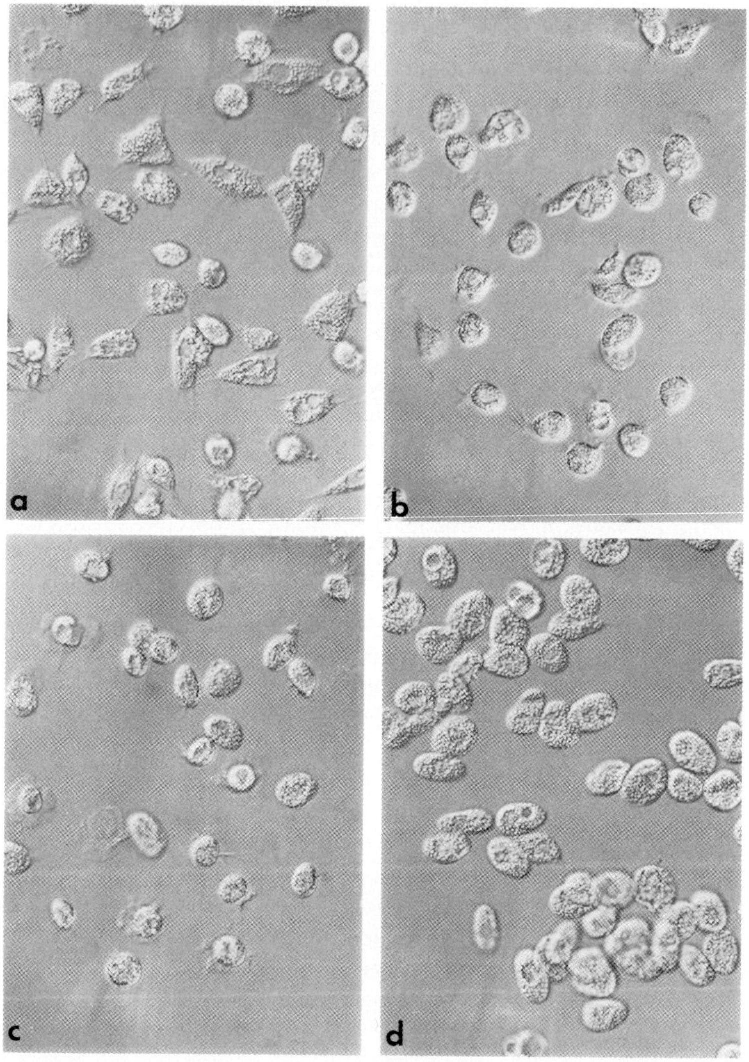

Fig. 12. LPS-elicited exocytosis can be inhibited by the appropriate pharmacologic agents. In this study, the cells were allowed to attach to microscope coverglasses (Fig. 8) and were incubated under LPS-free conditions with the pharmacologic agent for 10–30 min. The cells were then exposed to 10 μg/ml LPS in the presence of the pharmacologic agent and the preparation was examined at successive times with the light microscope (DIC optics) to determine the extent of exocytosis. In all cases, save in panel a, the medium is 3% sterile, LPS-free NaCl. In the absence of the pharmacologic agent, exocytosis was complete within 5 min following the initial exposure to LPS (cf. Fig. 9). a. Cl^- is replaced by isethionate (500 mM), 60 min after addition of LPS. b. SITS is present at 100 μM, 40 min after addition of

chemical localization studies were performed on acetone-permeabilized cells [110], thereby rendering the cytoplasm accessible to antiserum and making it impossible to conclude that the protein resides at the cell surface. It is possible that the phosphodiesterase activity of this protein plays a role in exocytosis, although it is equally plausible that the protein is the lipopolysaccharide-binding component in the cascade that leads to the activation of the protease involved in endotoxin-dependent gelation of amebocyte lysate [112–115] (see Levin, Chapter 5).

The best-studied consequence of degranulation is release of the protein coagulogen [117–123] and a system of proteinases [112–114,124–128] that, as a consequence of a specific proteolytic cleavage of coagulogen, convert it from a soluble protein to one that self-polymerizes to form an insoluble coagulum [119–123,128–130]. In addition to the clottable protein (coagulogen) and the proteinases that activate its polymerization, the cells release a family of proteinase inhibitors, some of which are active against clotting enzyme [15]. The system of proteinases can be activated by bacterial lipopolysaccharide [112,113,125,127,128,131,132] and carboxymethylated (but not native) (1→3)-β-D-glucan [133,134]. The activation of the coagulation system by LPS is the basis for the *Limulus* Amebocyte Lysate (LAL) test for gram-negative bacteria [135]. This test has replaced previous methods of detection and is of considerable commercial importance (Fig. 13). Conversion of coagulogen to a form that can self-polymerize can be achieved by a variety of proteinases [122,125,130,136–139]. The clotting enzyme is a serine proteinase, based on its sensitivity to serine proteinase inhibitors including diisopropyl fluorophosphate, parachloromercuribenzoate and parachloromercuriphenyl sulfonate [127,128]. In the presence of living amebocytes, coagulum formation can occur also in the absence of endotoxin [6,14], presumably under the action of an endotoxin-independent system of proteinases (Fig. 14).

MOTILITY

The active motility of the *Limulus* amebocyte can conveniently be observed in vitro by explanting fragments of amebocyte tissue into chambers in which the tissue fragments are slightly compressed between two coverglasses (Fig. 15) [4,5]. Plasma or endotoxin-free 3% NaCl solution can be used as

---

LPS. c. Suramin is present at 50 μM, 85 min after addition of LPS. d. A cocktail of agents designed to elevate cAMP levels in the cytoplasm (100 μM dibutyryl cAMP + 100 μM prostaglandin Iz + 50 μM theophylline) is present, 70 min after addition of LPS. Elevation of cAMP levels suppresses both initial activation (initiation of cellular locomotion and spreading on the coverglasses) and subsequent exocytosis. From Armstrong and Rickles [14], with permission of Academic Press. ×336.

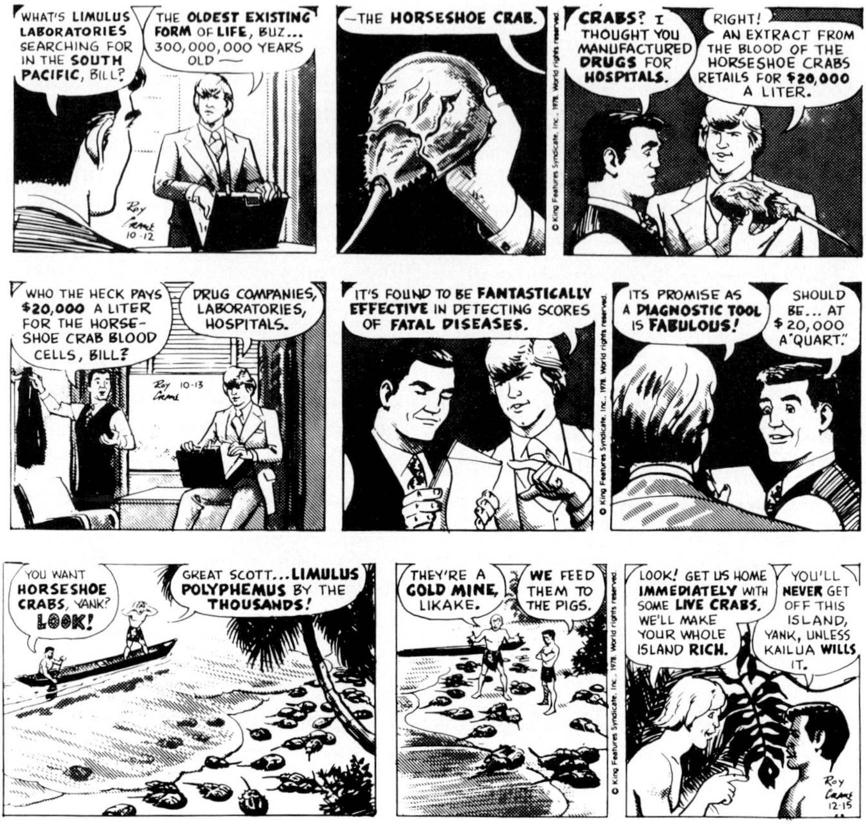
WHAT'S LIMULUS LABORATORIES SEARCHING FOR IN THE SOUTH PACIFIC, BILL?
THE OLDEST EXISTING FORM OF LIFE, BUZ... 300,000,000 YEARS OLD —
—THE HORSESHOE CRAB.
CRABS? I THOUGHT YOU MANUFACTURED DRUGS FOR HOSPITALS.
RIGHT! AN EXTRACT FROM THE BLOOD OF THE HORSESHOE CRABS RETAILS FOR $20,000 A LITER.
WHO THE HECK PAYS $20,000 A LITER FOR THE HORSE-SHOE CRAB BLOOD CELLS, BILL?
DRUG COMPANIES, LABORATORIES, HOSPITALS.
IT'S FOUND TO BE FANTASTICALLY EFFECTIVE IN DETECTING SCORES OF FATAL DISEASES.
ITS PROMISE AS A DIAGNOSTIC TOOL IS FABULOUS!
SHOULD BE... AT $20,000 A "QUART."
YOU WANT HORSESHOE CRABS, YANK? LOOK!
GREAT SCOTT...LIMULUS POLYPHEMUS BY THE THOUSANDS!
THEY'RE A GOLD MINE, LIKAKE.
WE FEED THEM TO THE PIGS.
LOOK! GET US HOME IMMEDIATELY WITH SOME LIVE CRABS. WE'LL MAKE YOUR WHOLE ISLAND RICH.
YOU'LL NEVER GET OFF THIS ISLAND, YANK, UNLESS KAILUA WILLS IT.

Fig. 13. In an adventure in 1978, the comic strip hero Buz Sawyer is enticed to undertake a trip to the South Pacific to discover additional sources of horseshoe crabs for use in the preparation of reagents for the LAL test. Reprinted with special permission of King Features. King Features Syndicate.

the fluid phase. Amebocytes emigrate from the tissue fragments onto the surfaces of the coverglasses (Fig. 16), where they can be studied with the light microscope with phase contrast or differential interference contrast (DIC) optics.

The cells that emerge initially from the tissue explants move rapidly (typically 10–15 μm/min) with hyaline pseudopods (Fig. 17). The cell body is contracted and fully granular. The pseudopods are protruded above the substratum and then are lowered to contact the glass over limited areas (Fig. 18). Forward movement of the cell body involves movement of granular cytoplasm into the pseudopod (Fig. 18c) [4,5,62]. The trailing end is often contracted as a knob-like protrusion that resembles the uropod of the verte-

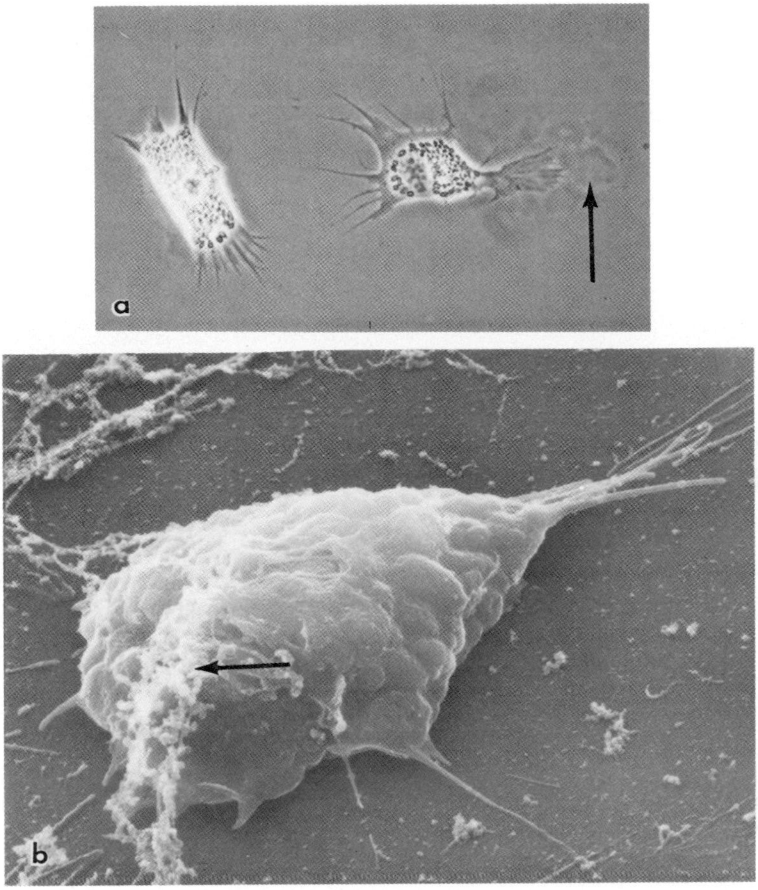

Fig. 14. Formation of coagulum (arrows) in the vicinity of flattened amebocytes maintained in vitro under LPS-free conditions. a. Phase contrast optics, ×600. b. Scanning electron micrograph, ×4,600. From Armstrong [6], with permission of Company of Biologists, Ltd.

brate leukocyte (Fig. 18c). This form of motility—characterized by minimal flattening of the cell on the substratum, forward flow of granular cytoplasm into adherent pseudopods and the presence of a trailing uropod—is strongly reminiscent of that displayed by mammalian granulocytes in vitro [140,141]. In transmission electron micrographs of motile cells, it is apparent that the bulk of the cytoplasm in the pseudopod is unstructured, with free ribosomes as the predominant cell organelle (Fig. 19a). Microfilaments are present in a cortical zone that excludes other cell organelles (Fig. 19b) and as thin linear arrays that originate in filopods and extend back from the leading margin of the main pseudopod into the cell (Fig. 19b).

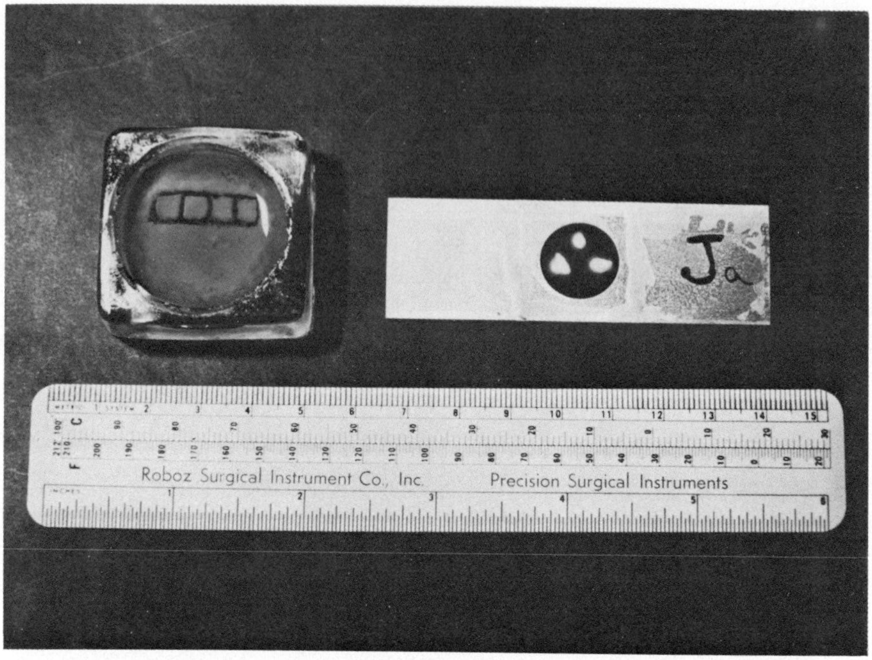

Fig. 15. In order to study the active motility of activated *Limulus* amebocytes, fragments of the coherent mass formed when extravasated amebocytes are allowed to aggregate in vitro ("amebocyte tissue") are explanted into observation chambers constructed by sealing No. 1 1/2 coverglasses above and below a 16-mm hole in a 0.8-mm thick aluminum blank. A chamber with three explants is present in the upper right of the figure. The amebocyte tissue is prepared by collecting 5 ml of blood by cardiac puncture directly into a sterile, endotoxin-free embryo watchglass. The cells settle to the bottom of the dish and aggregate over a period of 1–2 hr at room temperature. A dish containing amebocyte tissue is present in the upper left. Four squares have been trimmed out from the layer of amebocyte tissue covering the bottom of the dish but have not yet been removed to an observation chamber. Under experimental conditions, the watchglass is protected from contamination by being maintained in a sterile 100-mm × 20-mm glass petri dish (not present in the photograph).

After a variable period following the initiation of migration, the cells flatten reversibly on the substrate (Fig. 20). Locomotion continues in the flattened configuration, but the speed of migration decreases markedly. When cell cultures are prepared by allowing freshly collected cells diluted in saline to attach directly to glass surfaces (Fig. 8), many of those cells in direct contact with the glass flatten directly, rather than migrating in the contracted form for a period prior to flattening. If the concentration of cells is high enough to produce multilayering, the cells that do not contact the glass directly migrate for extended periods of time in the contracted form. Even-

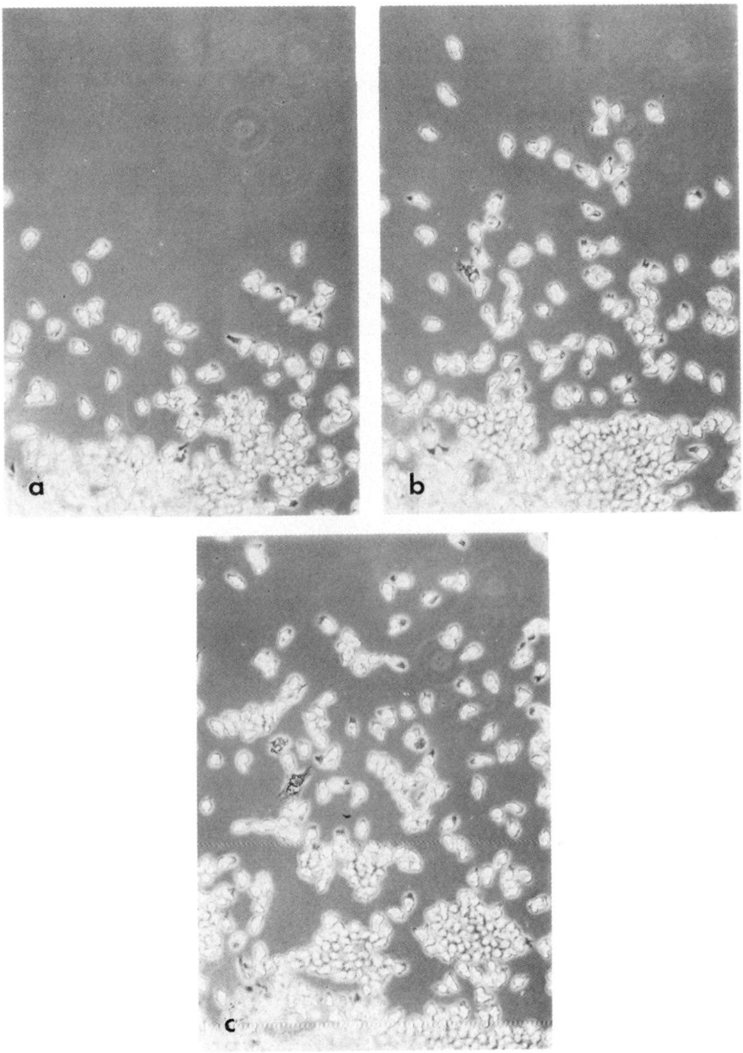

Fig. 16. Sequential photomicrographs showing the migration of *Limulus* amebocytes from an explant of amebocyte tissue on the surface of a microscope coverglass. The explant of amebocyte tissue is at the bottom margin of the photograph. The times after establishment of the culture are 40 min (a), 60 min (b), 100 min (c). Phase contrast optics. From Armstrong [4], with permission of Academic Press.

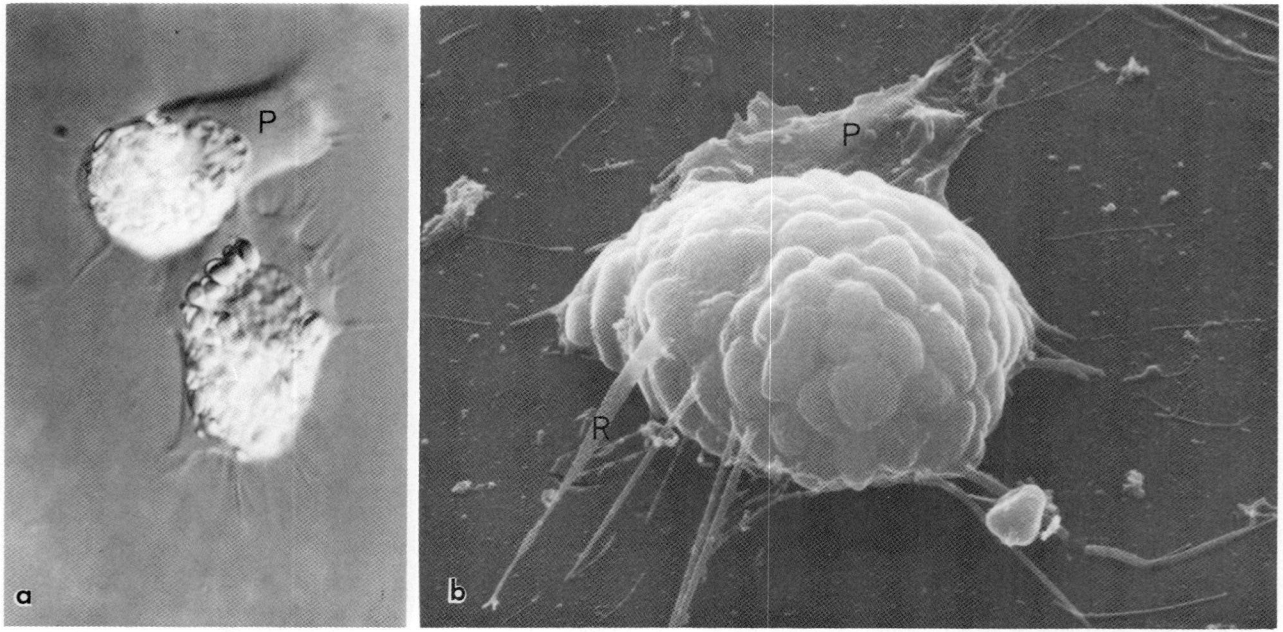

Fig. 17. *Limulus* amebocytes that have emigrated from explants of amebocyte tissue. a. The hyaline pseudopod (P) is prominent. DIC optics. ×1,280. b. Scanning electron micrograph of a migratory cell showing the pseudopod (P) and retraction fibers (R). ×4,600. Locomotion of the amebocyte is accomplished by protrusion of hyaline pseudopods, followed by a forward flow of granular cytoplasm into the basal portion of the pseudopod. From Armstrong [6], with permission of Company of Biologists, Ltd.

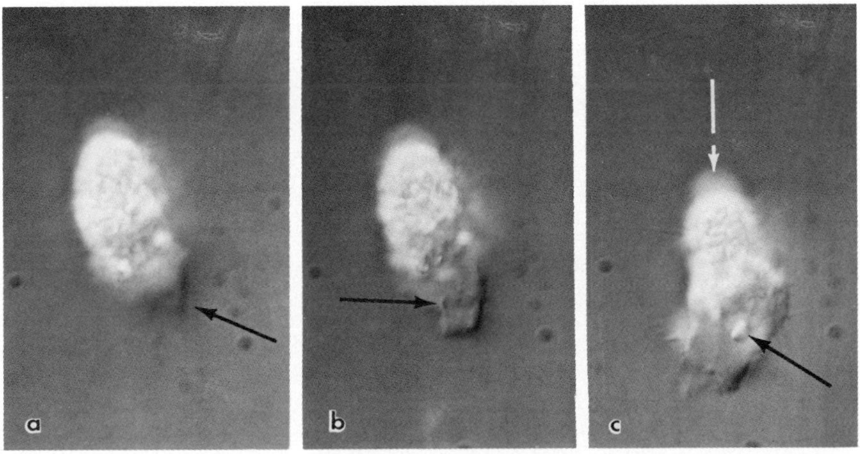

Fig. 18. Sequential DIC photomicrographs of a migrating contracted *Limulus* amebocyte. The plane of focus is at the glass-fluid interface. a. Typically, the pseudopod is protruded initially above the substrate (the pseudopod is out of focus [arrow]). b. It is then lowered to contact the substrate (the initial contact with the substrate occurs along a narrow ridge at the ventral surface of the pseudopod [arrow]). c. The pseudopod then expands over the substrate. A granule can be seen in the process of invading the base of the pseudopod in c (black arrow). The contracted, knob-like uropod at the trailing end is indicated by the white arrow in c. This is held above the substratum, since it remains out of focus during locomotion when the focal plane is at the glass-medium interface. From Armstrong [4], with permission of Academic Press. ×1,326.

tually, the flattened granular cells undergo degranulation (Fig. 21) [4,6]. Migration comes to a halt shortly after this, but the degranulated cells can survive in culture for many days thereafter.

The isolated gill leaves are favorable preparations for the observation of cell migration in vivo [5]. The gill leaves are thin enough that oil immersion objectives and DIC optics can be employed. The trauma of isolation usually induces a fraction of the amebocytes present in the vascular space of the leaf to activate to the motile state. Cell migration occurs over the tissue lining the vascular spaces (Fig. 22). Morphologically, cell motility is identical to that observed in vitro, being accomplished by the protrusion of hyaline pseudopods followed by the flow of granular cytoplasm into those pseudopods (Fig. 6). The amebocytes migrating in the isolated gill leaf can be viewed not only from above but also from the side when an individual cell migrates on the surface of one of the pillars that serve to separate the two faces of the linings of the hemocoel. Observation of cells from the side revealed that hyaline pseudopods often were protruded initially from the anterodorsal surface into the blood-filled space of the gill and only later were lowered to contact the substratum (Fig. 23).

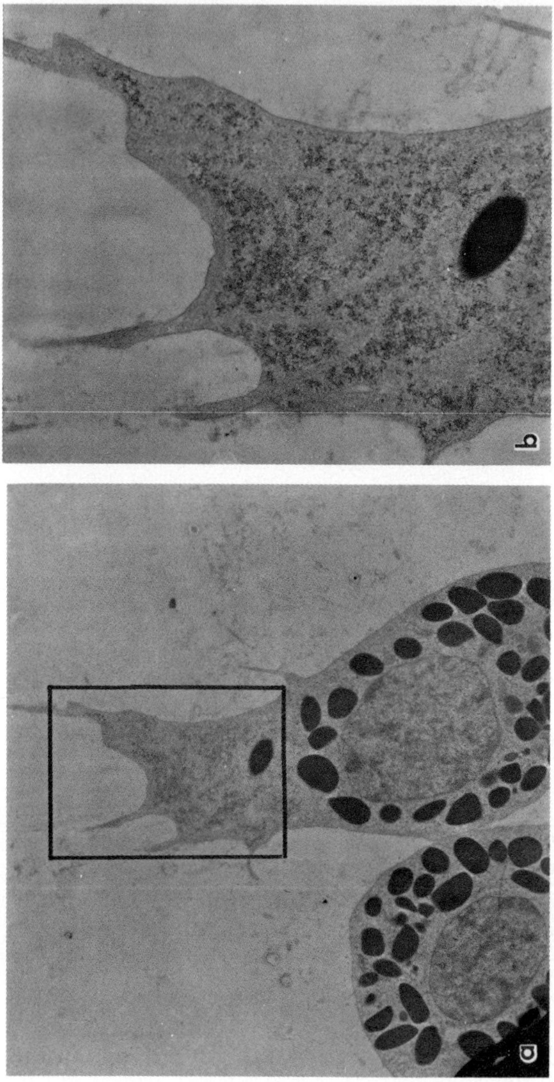

Fig. 19. Transmission electron micrographs of a sectioned locomotory amebocyte from a culture fixed 70 min after preparation. The plane of section is parallel to the substratum. a. Low-magnification view, ×3,000. b. Higher magnification of the area enclosed by the rectangle in panel a, showing the cortical zone of the pseudopod that excludes the cytoplasmic organelles (ribosomes) that occupy the bulk of the pseudopod. ×7,300.

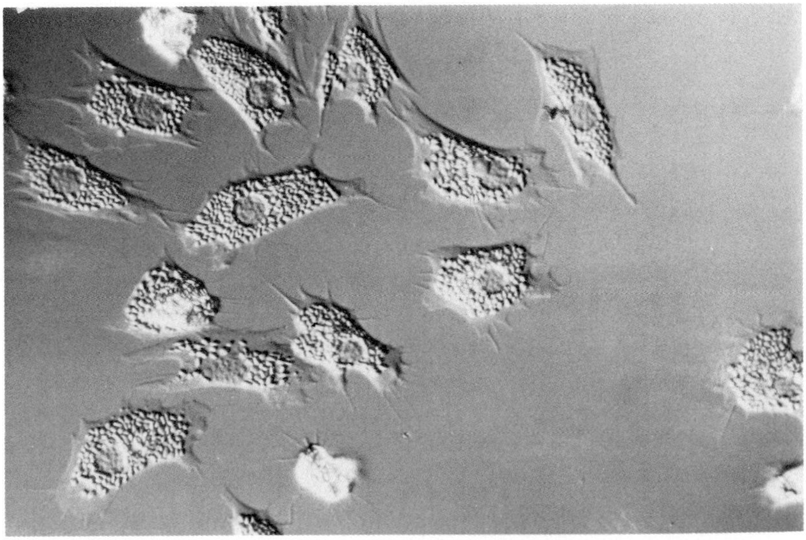

Fig. 20. Granulated amebocytes that have flattened on the substratum. As the cells flatten, the granules become distributed as a single layer and the nucleus becomes visible. Cells in this state are less motile than the contracted cell. In young cultures, cells oscillate between the flattened form and the contracted, rapidly locomoting form, but as the cultures age, progressively more cells are found in the flattened form. DIC optics. From Armstrong [6], with permission of Company of Biologists, Ltd. ×517.

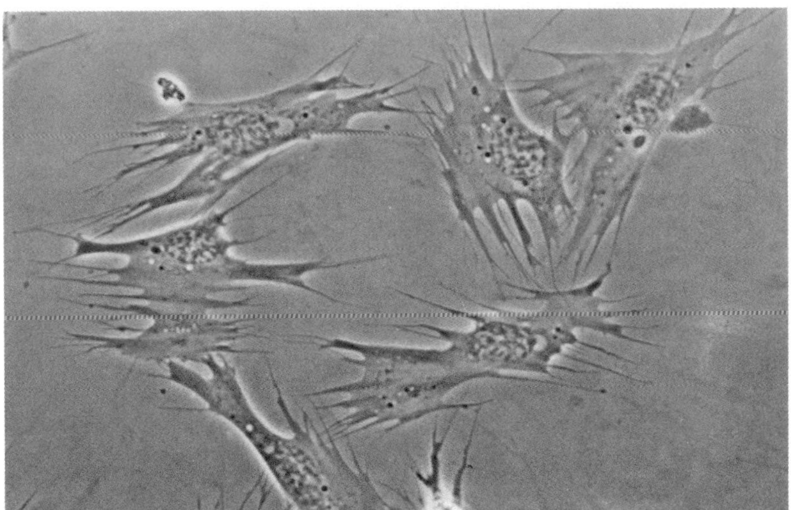

Fig. 21. During degranulation, amebocytes spread on glass surfaces may adopt bizarre shapes, frequently with parallel processes separated by deep clefts. DIC optics. From Armstrong [6], with permission of Company of Biologists, Ltd. ×590.

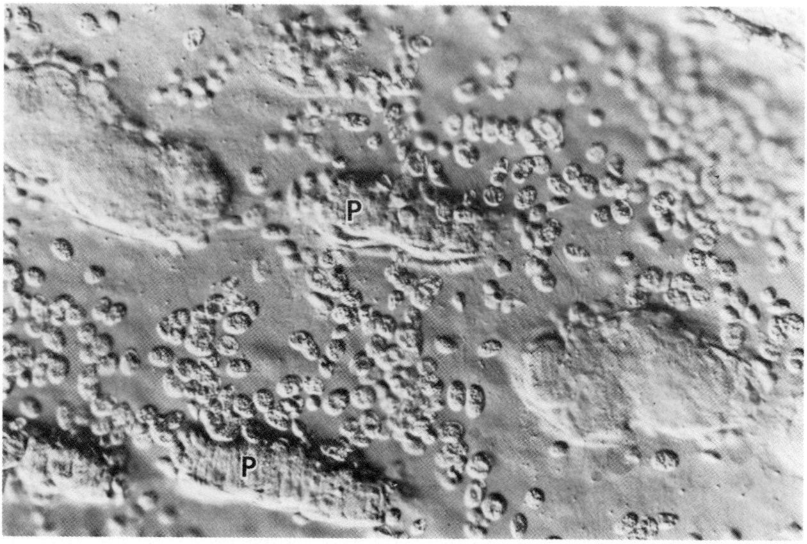

Fig. 22. Low-magnification view of blood cells in the hemocoel of an isolated gill leaf of a juvenile *Limulus*. The gill has been freshly isolated and most of the cells are unactivated. The upper and lower surfaces of the gill leaf enclose the hemocoel and are kept apart by pillars of connective tissue (p). From Armstrong [5], with permission of Company of Biologists, Ltd. ×206.

ADHESION

Activated amebocytes are able to adhere to a wide variety of surfaces including other amebocytes [4], the tissue lining the hemocoel of the gills [5], the gelated clottable protein released from amebocyte granules, and artificial surfaces such as glass, polystyrene, silicone oil, and agarose [6]. Cells can also move and spread on all of these surfaces. The morphology of the attachment sites that cells make with the substrate can be examined by interference reflection microscopy [142,143]. Sites of close approach appear dark grey with this technique. Flattened cells show focal attachment sites (Fig. 24) that resemble those of vertebrate fibroblasts in culture [140,143–145]. In electron micrographs, cell-cell adhesions are characterized by the presence of extended areas of close contact of apposed plasma membrane (Fig. 25). At these sites, adhesion is mediated by direct cell contact, rather than resulting from the action of a voluminous extracellular coagulum that entraps cells in its meshes.

Aggregation of amebocytes can be inhibited by a variety of agents, including drugs that elevate cAMP levels (these inhibit activation [14]), the sulfhydryl reagents dithiothreitol [146] and N-ethylmaleimide [132,146,147] and parachloromercuribenzoate [148], but not iodoacetamide or mercaptoethanol [132,146], high concentrations of the divalent cation chelators ethylenediaminetetraacetate [66,132,148,149] and sodium citrate [68], the protease inhibitors tosyl arginyl methylester and parachloromercuribenzoate [148], the membrane-active agents caffeine and propranolol [150], formaldehyde [68,151], saturated $(NH_4)_2SO_4$ and $MgSO_4$ [64,152], and resorcin, hydroquinone, and pyrrhol [153].

These various inhibitors of aggregation may act on one or more of at least three distinct processes: They may prevent activation of the extravasated blood cells, they may prevent the presumed alterations in the character of the cell surface that allows the activated amebocyte to adhere directly to various surfaces without affecting other aspects of the activation process, or they may suppress the formation of the extracellular coagulum, either by inhibiting exocytosis or by preventing the polymerization of the exocytosed coagulogen. Presumably, inhibition of coagulum formation would not affect aggregation by direct cell-cell adhesion (Fig. 25), but it might minimize the formation of aggregates by the entrapment of amebocytes in a coagulum meshwork.

It seems clear that at least some of the agents listed above prevent activation. Included in this are toxic agents that essentially "fix" the cell such as N-ethylmaleimide [146; Armstrong, unpublished] and formaldehyde. Agents that increase cAMP levels prevent activation in a reversible fashion [14]. A possible role for coagulogen-mediated aggregation is suggested by the observation of Kenney et al., [148] that amebocytes treated with high concentrations of EDTA immediately after bleeding aggregate poorly when the EDTA is removed but aggregate readily if exposed to material released from normally aggregating cells. The factor was purified and had a molecular weight of 17,000, close to that of coagulogen [117,122]. It is essential, in any analysis of the phenomenon of amebocyte aggregation, to determine whether the dominant process being studied is direct cell-cell adhesion or is the entrapment of cells in an extracellular coagulum.

HEMOSTASIS AND WOUND HEALING

One of the principal functions of the amebocyte is to seal leaks in the vascular system. This is achieved in part by the formation of a cellular clot as extravasated blood cells are activated and adhere to the surfaces of the wound and to each other [65,69,70,153,154] (Figs. 7, 25) and in part by the polymerization of a protein (coagulogen) contained within the amebocyte granules and released following bleeding by granule exocytosis [16,63,155]. As noted previously, exocytosis [14] and polymerization of coagulogen are accelerated by the presence of LPS, but both processes occur in its absence

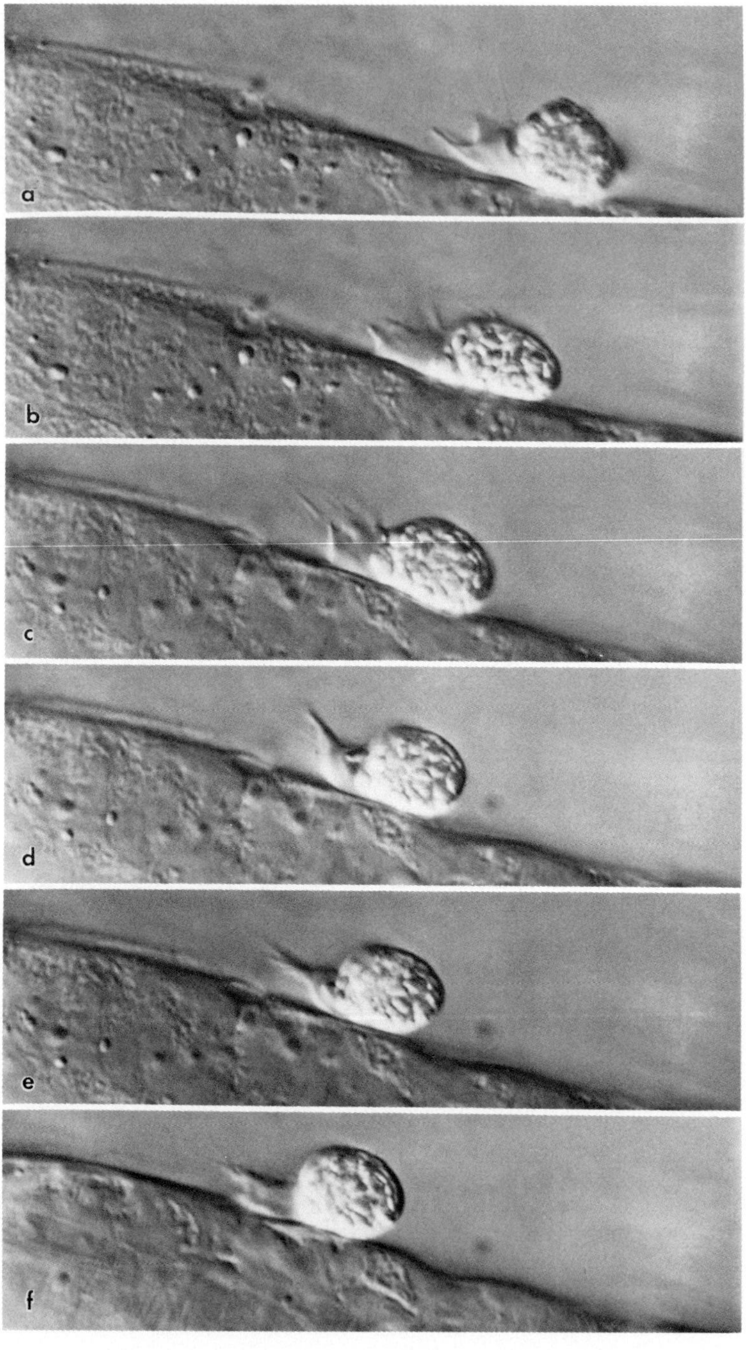
a
b
c
d
e
f

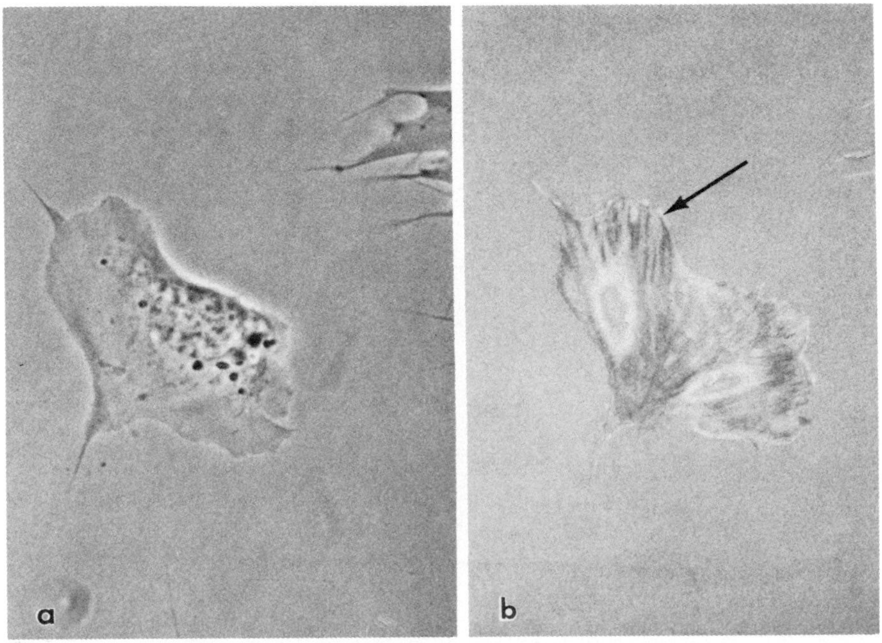

Fig. 24. The contacts established by a flattened, degranulated amebocyte with a microscope coverglass are examined by interference reflection optics. The cell is viewed by phase contrast optics in panel a and by interference reflection optics in panel b. The sites of closest approach appear as dark focal sites (arrow in b). ×1,046.

[6,14]. Cell-free plasma apparently does not contain a system of proteins capable of forming a clot, analogous to the fibrinogens of vertebrates and many arthropods [155–164]. Instead, the entire system is contained within the amebocyte [150]. This includes the protein coagulogen and a protease that transforms the zymogen coagulogen into a form that undergoes self-polymerization to produce the fibrillar elements constituting the clot [165]. The system also includes elements that serve as receptors for LPS and that activate the ultimate protease [112–116]. Gel formation can occur when washed amebocytes are suspended in isotonic saline and then stimulated to degranulate with LPS or are allowed to degranulate spontaneously in the absence of LPS [14], whereas cell-free plasma cannot be induced to form a clot [2,67,139].

Fig. 23. Sequential photomicrographs of an amebocyte migrating in an isolated gill leaf viewed from the side. Hyaline pseudopods are protruded from the anterior margin of the cell initially above the substrate (a,d) and are subsequently lowered to contact the substrate (b,e,f). ×1,432. DIC optics. From Armstrong [5], with permission of Company of Biologists.

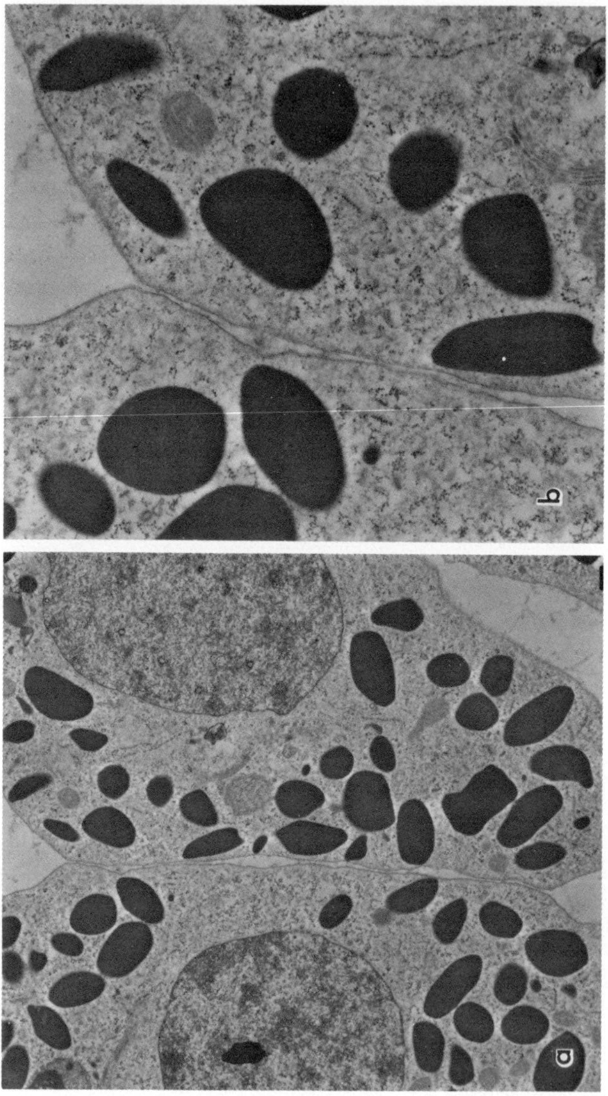

Fig. 25. Electron micrograph of the contact between two amebocytes cultured on a microscope coverglass for 1 hr prior to fixation. The apposed cell membranes are in close contact without a thick layer of intervening extracellular material. (a) × 5,300; (b) × 14,000.

In experimental wounds, a plug of clotted protein forms within 10 min [16,63]. The coagulum is then infiltrated by migratory amebocytes, which replace the clot within 2 days and form a cellular plug with flattened degranulated cells at its surface and granular cells beneath the surface [63]. Epithelial cells later repair the wound by migrating between the degranulated cell layer and the layer of granulated cells. The epithelial cells secrete a cuticle to complete the wound repair process.

DEFENSE AGAINST PATHOGENS

Multicellular organisms are under continual assault by pathogenic organisms, which include prokaryotes (bacteria), single-cell eukaryotes (fungi, protozoa), and multicellular parasites. In order to survive this assault, animals have evolved a diversity of defense mechanisms. The initial barrier to invasion is an epithelial surface that lines the exterior, the gut, the excretory and reproductive systems, and other surfaces that contact the external milieu [166,167]. In arthropods, a tough chitinous cuticle lies above the epithelial lining of the body surface and portions of the gut. This protects the epithelium from mechanical damage and constitutes an additional barrier. Stagner and Redmond [168] have suggested that an additional barrier to bacterial penetration in *Limulus* is provided by a layer of mucus secreted onto the surface of the cuticle by a series of glands that penetrate the epidermis and cuticle (the hypodermal glands). They note that amebocytes migrate into the basal ends of the hypodermal glands and they suggest that these cells may then release the granule contents, thus contributing to the secretions of the hypodermal glands. The aforementioned contribution of the blood cells to wound closure [16,63] certainly functions to restrict the access of pathogens through wounds.

Amebocytes display modest capabilities of phagocytosis of foreign particles (Fig. 26) [169]. Phagocytosis was observed most readily under LPS-free conditions, presumably because degranulated cells (LPS induces degranulation) are nearly or completely immotile and because the extracellular gel that forms in the presence of LPS would be expected to reduce the opportunity for contact between amebocyte and particle. Presumably phagocytosis by amebocytes plays a role in defense against pathogens other than gram-negative bacteria. It has not been established whether any of the fixed tissues in contact with the hemocoel of *Limulus* are phagocytic, in analogy to the reticuloendothelial system of vertebrates and many arthropods [54,55,170–174], but tanned erythrocytes are rapidly cleared from the circulation, even though they apparently are not phagocytosed by the amebocytes [146]. It was not determined whether this removal was a consequence of phagocytosis by a reticuloendothelial organ or simple entrapment in clumps of amebocytes [57,175–179].

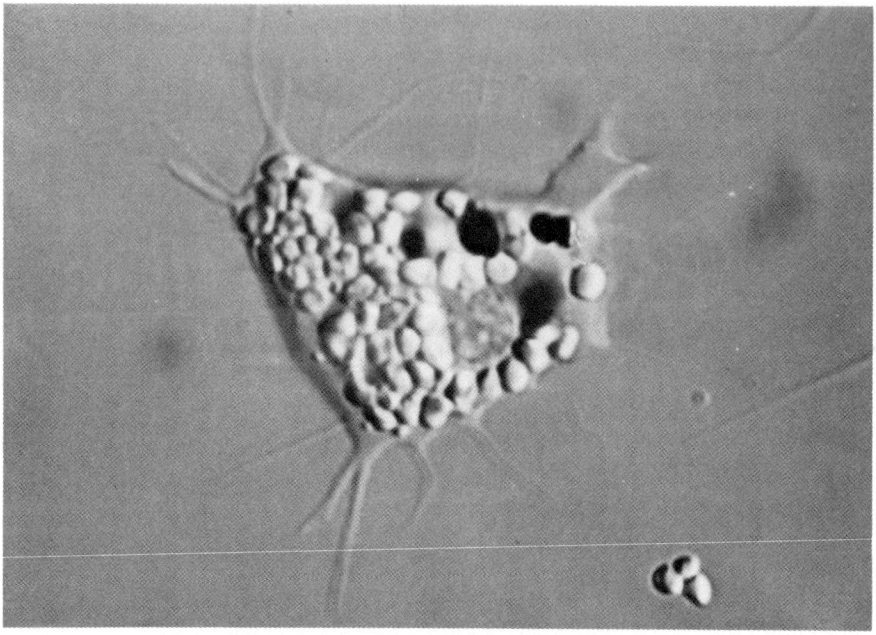

Fig. 26. Amebocyte that has phagocytosed particles of carbonyl iron (black inclusions) in vitro. It has been established that the particles are within the cells, rather than attached to the cell surfaces, by careful focusing with high numerical aperture microscope objectives and because the particles move with the cell as it moves in vitro, flowing with the cytoplasmic granules as the latter invade an extended pseudopod. From Armstrong and Levin [169] with permission of Academic Press. ×2,394.

Gram-negative bacteria constitute an important category of pathogen to marine organisms. The outer cell wall of gram-negative organisms contains LPS, which mediates their pathogenicity [180]. The coagulogen/protease system contained within the granules of the amebocytes [150] is released rapidly from the cells in the presence of microgram quantities of LPS [14] and polymerization of coagulogen and clot formation is triggered by picogram to nanogram quantities of LPS [181]. The gel serves to immobilize bacteria, preventing systemic dissemination in the organism [2,86,101,132,182]. Bacteria enmeshed in the gel are stationary and lack even Brownian movement [86]. Injection of gram-negative bacteria [86,168] or bacterial LPS [16,168] induces cell clumping in vitro and, when bacteria are injected, degranulation and coagulum formation. Fungal pathogens are also potentially important. Crustaceans recognize the presence of fungi by the presence of β-1,3-glucans, a component of the cell walls of most fungi [103]. *Limulus* appears not to respond to β-1,3-glucans in a fashion similar to the response shown by crustaceans. *Limulus* lacks the phenol oxidase defense system of crustaceans; amebocytes are not stimulated to undergo exocytosis when presented with high concentrations of β-1,3-glucans, and native β-1,3 glucans appear unable to activate the coagulum-generating system, although carboxymethylated glucans are active in coagulum generation [133,134].

In addition to the role of polymerized clots of coagulogen in immobilizing bacteria, amebocytes appear capable of killing some types of bacteria. Bactericidal activity has been observed in extracts of amebocytes that had been heated briefly (60°C, 10 min) to inactivate the clotting system. A variety of gram-negative and gram-positive organisms were susceptible if the extracts were dialyzed prior to use to remove a soluble inhibitor of bactericidal activity [183,184]. Amebocytes release a heat-labile bactericidal factor during clotting of the blood [182,185]. The factor exerts its activity only in the presence of plasma [186].

Two potential antibacterial activities are present in the plasma, independent of the amebocytes. The most extensively studied is a bacterial agglutinin activity [187–189]. The second system is a recently discovered proteinase inhibitory activity [190–192].

Limulus plasma can agglutinate a variety of gram-negative and gram-positive bacteria [168,187–189] and contains a LPS-binding activity. Agglutination of gram-negative bacteria appears to be mediated by the lectin limulin [194]. The native form of limulin is a large protein (molecular weight 400,000) composed of 18 identical subunits of a molecular weight of 22,500 [195]. Limulin has been purified by standard biochemical [194–196] and affinity [197–201] methods. Limulin binds sialic acid residues [198,202,203], 2-keto-3-deoxycytonate (KDO) [204], and D-glucuronic acid [205]. It has been postulated that both the LPS-binding activity and agglutination activity directed against gram-negative bacteria found in the plasma are dependent on the KDO-binding activity of limulin [204,206]. KDO links the polysaccharide side chain to the glucosamine backbone of the lipid A residue of LPS [180]. The agglutinin activity against gram-positive organisms may be due to the binding of limulin to sialic acid and D-glucuronic acid residues [198,205] and to a second plasma lectin that recognizes galactosyl residues [207,208]. Following agglutination, bacteria are immobilized, flagellar activity is inhibited, and cells are growth-arrested [168]. It has been suggested that, in addition to direct effects on bacteria, bound plasma lectins operate as opsonins that promote phagocytosis of bacteria either by circulating amebocytes or a system of fixed tissue phagocytes [209].

The blood and tissue fluids are subject to contamination with proteolytic enzymes of endogenous or exogenous origin. Endogenous proteinases include those liberated during blood clotting and released from phagocytic cells. Exogenous proteinases include those released from invading bacteria, fungi, protozoa, and multicellular parasites. Vertebrates are known to possess a variety of proteinase inhibitors free in the plasma that function to regulate those proteinases [210–212]. Recent studies [190–193] have demonstrated that the hemolymph of *Limulus* contains a potent proteinase inhibitory activity that bears a striking resemblance to the α-macroglobulins, an important class of proteinase inhibitors in the blood of vertebrates [213,214]. Features shared by mammalian α_2-macroglobulin and the *Limulus* hemolymph proteinase inhibitor are sensitivity to mild acid treatment and to methylamine, an ability to inhibit the activity of proteinases against macromolecular substrata (e.g., proteins) without affecting activity against low-molecular-weight substrates (e.g., amides and esters), and an ability to inhibit a wide variety of different proteinases of diverse catalytic mechanisms [190–193]. Vertebrates have been separated in evolution from the arthropods by at least 550 million years. It will certainly prove to be an interesting example of evolutionary conservation if further study demonstrates that the α_2-macroglobulin-like inhibitor of *Limulus* is homologous to vertebrate α_2-macroglobulin.

PROBLEMS FOR FURTHER STUDY

The recent interest in the function of blood and blood cells in *Limulus* dates from the characterization of the LPS-responsive coagulation system by Bang [86] and Levin [2,67] and the discovery of plasma lectins by Cohen and others [195,215]. In the period following these reports, our understanding of the function of the various blood components has expanded considerably, settling some outstanding questions, sharpening the nature of others, and revealing unexpected phenomena for study.

One unsolved problem is the site(s) and regulation of hematopoiesis in the adult and the embryologic origin of the hematopoietic tissues. Essentially all of the investigation of the blood has been restricted to the intermoult adult. More attention should be directed to blood cells in embryonic [16] and moulting individuals. Are there categories of blood cells present in the circulation (cyanocytes [22], prohemocytes, etc.) at these stages that are absent from the general circulation of the intermoult adult? Is hematopoiesis in the adult restricted to times of moulting? This is a possibility, since efforts to demonstrate blood cell production in the intermoult adult have not been successful (Levin, unpublished). In other arthropods, blood cells play significant roles in the process of reorganization of the cuticle following ecdysis [47,48,216–218]. To my knowledge, no attempt has been made to look for a similar role for the *Limulus* blood cell. Although adults moult only infrequently, juveniles moult more often and moulting can be induced by injection of the steroid hormone ecdysone [219].

A second category of phenomena of basic interest is that surrounding cell activation following bleeding. The extracellular signals that initiate activation and the character of transmembrane signaling and the second messengers involved are not known (but see Armstrong and Rickles [14]). Also of interest are the character of alterations that occur following activation (viz., acquisition of adhesiveness and the ability to locomote). Presumably the alteration of the amebocyte from the nonadhesive state to the adhesive state is a consequence of alteration in the character of the cell surface (since it is at the cell surface that cells touch when entering into adhesive interactions with adjacent cells). Changes in surface composition during activation could be examined by surface radiolabeling procedures [220,221]. Convincing demonstration of the surface molecules involved in cell-cell adhesion is a demanding exercise. Techniques that have proven useful with other systems include study of surface molecules released by various treatments [222], cell fractionation [223], and use of specific antibodies directed against putative surface adhesive macromolecules for affinity purification and as a probe to interfere with adhesion [224,225].

Active cellular locomotion has been the subject of extensive investigation over the past decade [226,227]. Of interest in the present system is the change in organization of the cytoskeleton and cell membrane during the activation process such that the amebocyte changes from the immotile state, characteristic of the circulating cell, to the motile state, characteristic of the activated cell. The migrating amebocyte resembles at least superficially the migrating vertebrate leukocyte [140,141]. Unanswered questions include the mechanism of pseudopodial protrusion, the organization of the contractile machinery during locomotion, the behavior of the plasma membrane during cycles of pseudopodial protrusion and uropod retraction, and the nature of the adhesive interactions between cell and substratum. Elucidation of a detailed understanding of locomotion in the *Limulus* blood cell should be important to understanding a phenomenon shown by blood cells of other arthropods [33,38,228–234]. The *Limulus* system is attractive for biochemical studies on motility (e.g., isolation of cytoskeleton-associated proteins involved in locomotion [235]) because it is possible to obtain large and homogenous quantities of cells.

The amebocyte is a secretory cell that can be induced to release the cytoplasmic granule contents by the appropriate secretagogs. The cells are responsive to LPS (a soluble signal molecule indicating the presence of gram-negative and potentially pathogenic bacteria) but are not responsive to β-1,3-glucans (soluble molecules released from fungi [103] and treated as extracellular signals by crustacean blood cells [104–106]). There is as yet no full characterization of the factors released during exocytosis. One approach of potential use for such a study is to examine the factors present in the external milieu when a dispersed suspension of freshly collected amebocytes is caused to undergo secretion by the ionophore A23187. Cytolysis is minimal (the supernatant contains a vanishingly small fraction of cellular lactate dehydrogenase [15]). This method has been used to identify a family of proteinase inhibitors, distinct from the plasma α_2-macroglobulin homolog, that regulate the proteinases involved in coagulogen activation [15].

One of the important functions of the blood cell is wound healing. This process has been the subject of but a single histological study [63] and has not been investigated experimentally. Problems of interest include definition of the relative importance of the extracellular coagulum and the cellular plug in wound closure, and a definition of the functional roles of blood cells immobilized at the wound site during the later stages of healing.

In addition to roles in hemostasis and wound closure, the amebocytes function in the defense against pathogens that have gained access to the hemocoel. By far, the best-studied function is the interaction of blood cells with gram-negative organisms [2,14,86,101,181,182]. Less is known of how *Limulus* deals with other classes of bacteria, fungi [236], and protozoa [237–240] of potential pathogenic significance. The reaction of *Limulus* to fungi will be particularly interesting since *Limulus* lacks the prophenoloxidase system that is fungistatic in crustaceans [104–106,241–243]. The role of phagocytosis in defense [169] is not well defined. It has been suggested but not demonstrated that plasma lectins function as opsonins [209]. If not opsonins, then what are the functions of limulin and other plasma lectins? The function of the hypodermal glands in defense [168] is as yet poorly defined.

Finally, a potentially useful approach is the comparison of blood cell structure, behavior, and function between different classes of arthropods. Studies of *Limulus* can serve as a paradigm for study of other arthropods and vice versa. How does the response of the blood cells of other arthropods to LPS (as a signal molecule for gram-negative bacteria) [156,244,245] compare with the already well-studied response in *Limulus* [2,14,101,181,182]? Other arthropods contain secretory blood cells [9,10,42,54,55,246,247]. What are the relevant secretagogs for these cells? What are the functions of the secreted materials in hemostasis and defense? Are claims that the plasma of certain crustaceans and insects contains a fibrin-like molecule [156–164] valid or is clotting in these organisms the province solely of factors released by blood cells following their activation [8–10,61,91–96] as with *Limulus*? Do other classes of arthropods have an α_2-macroglobulin homolog in the plasma? Conversely, does the horseshoe crab show any of the serological defense responses defined in other arthropods [54,237,238,248–250)? The early studies of Noguchi [251] are interesting in this respect. Does *Limulus* possess a system of fixed phagocytic tissues involved in clearance of foreign molecules and/or particles from the blood [170–174]? Does *Limulus* show hemocyte clumping, nodule formation, and encapsulation in response to foreign particles in the hemocoel [51,57,58,167,178,179,252–256]? It has been suggested that the blood cells contribute to the formation of certain internal tissues in insects [38,43,257]. Does an analogous process occur in *Limulus*?

ACKNOWLEDGMENTS

Original research reported in this review was supported by National Science Foundation grant PCM 80-24181.

REFERENCES

1. Dumont JN, Anderson E, Winner G (1966): Some cytologic characteristics of the hemocytyes of *Limulus* during clotting. J Morphol 119:181–208.
2. Levin J, Bang FB (1964): The role of endotoxin in the extracellular coagulation of *Limulus* blood. Bull Johns Hopkins Hosp 115:265–274.
3. Loeb L (1902): On the blood lymph cells and inflammatory processes of *Limulus*. J Med Res 7:145–158.
4. Armstrong PB (1977): Interaction of the motile blood cells of the horseshoe crab, *Limulus*. Studies on contact paralysis of pseudopodial activity and cellular overlapping *in vitro*. Exp Cell Res 107:127–138.
5. Armstrong PB (1979): Motility of the *Limulus* blood cell. J Cell Sci 37:169–180.
6. Armstrong PB (1980): Adhesion and spreading of *Limulus* blood cells on artificial surfaces. J Cell Sci 44:243–262.
7. George WC, Nichols J (1948): A study of the blood of some crustacea. J Morphol 83:425–443.
8. Gregoire C (1952): Sur la coagulation du sang de *Limulus polyphemus*. Arch Int Physiol 60:97–99.
9. Gregoire C (1955): Blood coagulation in arthropods. VI. A study by phase contrast microscopy of blood reactions *in vitro* in Onychophora and in various groups of Arthropods. Arch Biol (Liege) 66:489–508.
10. Gregoire C (1970): Haemolymph coagulation in arthropods. Symp Zool Soc Lond 27:45–74.
11. Ornberg RL, Reese TS (1981): Secretion in *Limulus* amebocytes is by exocytosis. In Cohen (ed): "Biomedical Applications of the Horseshoe Crab (Limulidae)." New York: Alan R. Liss, pp 125–130.
12. Ornberg RL, Reese TS (1981): Beginning of exocytosis captured by rapid-freezing of *Limulus* amebocytes. J Cell Biol 90:40–54.
13. Ornberg RL, Reese TS (1981): Comparison of compound with plasmalemmal exocytosis in *Limulus* amebocytes. Methods Cell Biol 23:301–311.
14. Armstrong PB, Rickles FR (1982): Endotoxin-induced degranulation of the *Limulus* amebocyte. Exp Cell Res 140:15–24.
15. Armstrong PB, Quigley JP (1984): Proteinase inhibitory activity released from the horseshoe crab blood cell during exocytosis. Biochim Biophys Acta (in press).
16. Bang FB (1979): Ontogeny and phylogeny of response to gram-negative endotoxins among the marine invertebrates. In Cohen E (ed): "Biomedical Applications of the Horseshoe Crab (Limulidae)." New York: Alan R. Liss, pp 109–123.
17. Loeb L (1928): Amoebocyte tissue and amoeboid movement. Protoplasma 4:596–625.

18. Shishikura F, Chiba J, Sekiguchi K (1977): Two types of hemocytes in localization of clottable protein in Japanese horseshoe crab, *Tachypleus tridetatus*. J Exp Zool 201:303–308.
19. Shishikura F, Sekiguchi K (1979): Comparative studies on hemocytes and coagulogen of the Asian and the American horseshoe crabs. In Cohen E (ed): "Biomedical Applications of the Horseshoe Crab (Limulidae)." New York: Alan R. Liss, pp 185–201.
20. Fahrenbach WH (1970): The cyanoblast: Hemocyanin formulation in *Limulus polyphemus*. J Cell Biol 44:445–453.
21. Fahrenbach WH (1975): The visual system of the horseshoe crab *Limulus polyphemus*. Int Rev Cytol 41:285–349.
22. Sherman RG (1981): Chilicerates. In Ratacliffe NA, Rowley AF (eds). "Invertebrate Blood Cells." London: Academic, Vol 2, pp 355–384.
23. Midttun B, Jensen H (1978): Ultrastructure of oenocytoids from two spiders, *Pisaura mirabilis* and *Trochosa terricola* (Araneae). Acta Zool (Stockh) 59:157–167.
24. Ghiretti-Magaldi A, Milanesi C, Tognon G (1977): Hemopoiesis in crustacea decapoda: Origin and evolution of hemocytes and cyanocytes of *Carcinus maenus*. Cell Differ 6:167–186.
25. Lai-Fook J (1973): The structure of the haemocytes of *Calpodes ethlius* (Lepidoptera). J Morphol 139:79–104.
26. Neuwirth M (1973): The structure of the hemocytes of *Galleria mellaonella* (Lepidoptera). J Morphol 139:105–124.
27. Raina AK (1976): Ultrastructure of the larval hemocytes of the pink bollworm, *Pectinophora gassypiella* (Saunders) (Lepidoptera: Gelechidae). Int J Insect Morphol Embryol 5:187–195.
28. Akai H, Sato S (1971): An ultrastructural study of the haemopoietic organs of the silkworm, *Bombyx mori*. J Insect Physiol 17:1665–1676.
29. Arvy L (1952): Particularites histologiques des centres leucopoietiques thoraciques chez quelques Lepidopteres. C R Acad Sci Paris 235:1539–1541.
30. Arvy L (1954): Donnes sur la leucopiese chez *Musca domestica*. Proc R Entomol Soc Lond 29A:39–41.
31. Dall W (1964): Studies on the physiology of a shrimp *Metapenaeus masterii* (Haswell) (Crustacen: Decapoda: Penaeidae). Aust J Mar Freshw Res 5:145–161.
32. Hinks CF, Arnold JW (1977): Haemopoiesis in lepidoptera. II. The role of the haemopoietic organs. Can J Zool 55:1740–1755.
33. Lochhead JH, Lochhead MS (1941): Studies on the blood and related tissues in Artemia (Crustacea Anostraca). J Morphol 68:593–632.
34. Stang-Voss C (1974): On the ultrastructure of invertebrate hemocytes: An interpretation of their role in comparative hematology. Contemp Top Immunobiol 4:65–76.
35. Arnold JW (1970): Haemocytes of the Pacific bettle cockroach, *Diploptera punctata*. Can Entomol 102:830–835.
36. Arnold JW (1972): A comparative study of the haemocytes (blood cells) of cockroaches (Insecta: Dictyoptera: Blattaria), with a view of their significance in taxonomy. Can Entomol 104:309–348.
37. Arnold JW (1974): The hemocytes of insects. In Rockstein M (ed): "The Physiology of Insecta." 2nd Ed. New York: Academic, Vol 5, pp 201–254.
38. Clark RM, Harvey WR (1965): Cellular membrane formation by plasmatocytes of diapausing cecropia pupae. J Insect Physiol 11:161–175.
39. Jones JC (1962): Current concepts concerning insect hemocytes. Am Zool 2:209–246.
40. Jones JC (1970): Hemocytopoiesis in insects. In Gordon AS (ed): "Regulation of Hematopoiesis." New York: Appleton-Century Crofts, Vol 1, pp 7–65.

41. Kurtti TJ, Brooks MA (1970): Growth of lepidopteran epithelial cells and hemocytes in primary culture. J Invertebr Pathol 15:341–350.
42. Rowley AF, Ratcliffe NA (1981): Insects. In Ratcliffe NA, Rowley AF (eds): "Invertebrate Blood Cells." London: Academic, Vol 2, pp 421–488.
43. Wigglesworth VB (1956): The haemocytes and connective tissue formation in an insect, *Rhodnius prolixus* (Hemiptera). J Microsc Sci 97:89–98.
44. Yeager JF, Tauber OE (1935): On the hemolymph cell counts of some marine invertebrates. Biol Bull (Woods Hole) 69:66–70.
45. Lankester ER (1884): On the skeleto-trophic tissues and coaxial glands of Limulus, Scorpio, and Mygale. Q J Microsc Sci 24:129.
46. Ravindranath MH (1974): The hemocytes of a scorpion *Palamnaeus swamnerdani*. J Morphol 144:1–10.
47. Deevey GB (1941): Blood cells of the Haitian tarantula and their relation to the moulting cycle. J Morphol 68:457–491.
48. Browning HC (1942): The integument and moult cycles of *Tegenaria atrica* (Araneae). Proc R Soc Lond Ser B 131:65–86.
49. Sherman RG (1973): Ultrastructurally different hemocytes in a spider. Can J Zool 51:1155–1159.
50. Gupta AP (1979): Arthropod hemocytes and phylogeny. In Gupta AP (ed): "Arthropod Phylogeny." New York: Van Nostrand, pp 669–735.
51. Jones JC (1975): Forms and functions of insect hemocytes. In Maramorosch K, Shope RE (ed): "Invertebrate Immunity." New York: Academic, pp 119–128.
52. Moran DT (1971): Fine structure of cockroach blood cells. Tissue Cell 3:413–422.
53. Price CD, Ratcliffe NA (1974): A reappraisal of insect haemocyte classification by the examination of blood from fifteen insect orders. Z Zellforsch 147:537–549.
54. Ratcliffe NA, Rowley AF (1979): A comparative synopsis of the structure and function of the blood cells of insects and other invertebrates. Dev Comp Immunol 3:189–243.
55. Ratcliffe NA, White KN, Rowley AF, Walters JB (1982): Cellular defense systems of the arthropods. In Cohen N, Sigel MM (eds): "The Reticuloendothelial System, A Comprehensive Treatise," Vol 3: "Phylogeny and Ontogeny." New York: Plenum, pp 167–255.
56. Ravindranath MH (1977): A comparative study of the morphology and behavior of granular haemocytes of arthropods. Cytologia 42:743–751.
57. Smith VJ, Ratcliffe NA (1978): Host defense reactions of the shore crab, *Carcinus maenas*. J Mar Biol Assoc UK 58:367–379.
58. Bauchau AG (1981): Crustaceans. In Ratcliffe NA, Rowley AF (eds): "Invertebrate Blood Cells." London: Academic, Vol 2, pp 385–420.
59. Cohen WD, Nemhauser I, Cohen MF (1983): Marginal bands of lobster blood cells: Disappearance associated with changes in cell morphology. Biol Bull (Woods Hole) 164:50–61.
60. Snyder M, Stanley M (1973): Are all hemocytes of the blue crab of one basic type? Virginia J Sci 24:129 (abstract).
61. Hardy WB (1892): The blood corpuscles of the cruastacea, together with a suggestion as to the origin of the crustacean fibrin-ferment. J Physiol 13:165-190.
62. Armstrong PB (1979): Motility of the *Limulus* amebocyte. In Cohen E (ed): "Biomedical Applications of the Horseshoe Crab (Limulidae)." New York: Alan R. Liss, pp 73–92.
63. Bursey CR (1977): Histological response to injury in the horseshoe crab, *Limulus polyphemus*. Can J Zool 55:1158–1165.
64. Copley AL (1974): The clotting of limulus blood. Fed Proc 6:90–91 (abstract).
65. Howell WH (1885): Observations on the chemical composition and coagulation of the

blood of *Limulus polyphemus, Callinectes hastatus*, and *Cucumaria* sp. Johns Hopkins Univ Circulars 5:4–5.

66. Kenney DM, Belamarich FA, Shepro D (1972): Aggregation of horseshoe crab (*Limulus polyphemus*) amebocytes and reversible inhibition of aggregation by EDTA. Biol Bull (Woods Hole) 143:548–567.
67. Levin J, Bang FB (1964): A description of cellular coagulation in the *Limulus*. Bull Johns Hopkins Hosp 115:337–345.
68. Loeb L (1905): Studies on cell granula and amoeboid movements of the blood cells of *Limulus*. Univ Pa Med Bull May 1905:1–34.
69. Loeb L (1920): The movements of the amoebocytes and the experimental production of amoebocyte (cell fibrin tissue). Washington Univ Studies 8:3–79.
70. Loeb L (1921): Amoeboid movement, tissue formation and consistency of protoplasm. Am J Physiol 56:140–167.
71. Loeb L (1928): Amoeboid movement and agglutination in amoebocytes of *Limulus* and the relation of these processes to phagocytosis, tissue formation and thrombosis. In Alexander J (ed): "Colloid Chemistry." New York: Chemical Catalogue Co., Vol 2, pp 487–514.
72. Andrew W (1965): "Comparative Hematology." London: Grune & Stratton.
73. Allen RD, Zacharski LR, Widirstky ST, Rosenstein R, Zaitlin LM, Burgess R (1979): Transformation and motility of human platelets. Details of the shape change and release reactions observed by optical and electron microscopy. J Cell Biol 83:126–142.
74. Belamarich FA, Stiller RA, Shepro D (1973): The release reaction: Is it a common mechanism in all types of hemostatic cells? Ser Haematol 6:418–428.
75. Doolittle RF, Surgenor DM (1962): Blood coagulation in fish. Am J Physiol 203:964–970.
76. Holmsen H, Salganicoff L, Fukami MH (1977): Platelet behavior and biochemistry. In Ogston D, Bennett R (eds): "Haemostasis: Biochemistry, Physiology and Pathology." London: Wiley, pp 239–319.
77. Loewenhaupt RW, Glueck HJ, Miller MA, Kline DL (1977): Factors which influence blood platelet migration. J Lab Clin Med 90:37–45.
78. Loewenhaupt RW, Miller MA, Glueck HI (1973): Platelet migration and chemotaxis demonstrated *in vitro*. Thrombos Res 3:477–487.
79. Pollard TD, Fujiwara K, Handin R, Weiss G (1977): Contractile proteins in platelet activation and contraction. Ann NY Acad Sci 283:218–239.
80. Shepro D, Belamarich FA, Branson R (1966): The fine structure of the thrombocyte in the dogfish (*Mustelus canis*) with special reference to microtubule orientation. Anat Rec 156:203–214.
81. Shepro D, Belamarich FA, Merk FB, Chao FC (1969): Changes in thrombocyte ultrastructure during clot retraction. J Cell Sci 4:763–779.
82. Stalsberg H, Prydz H (1963): Studies on chick embryo thrombocytes. II. Functions in primary hemostasis. Thomb Diath Haemorrh 9:291–299.
83. Weiss HJ: Platelet physiology and abnormalities of platelet function (first of two parts). N Engl J Med 293:531–541.
84. White JG (1971): Platelet morphology. In Johnson SA (ed): "The Circulating Platelet." New York: Academic, pp 45–121.
85. Zucker MB (1980): The functioning of blood platelets. Sci Am 242(6):86–103.
86. Bang FB (1956): A bacterial disease of *Limulus polyphemus*. Bull Johns Hopkins Hosp 98:325–351.
87. Cohen WD, Nemhauser I, Jaeger R (1977): Rapid visualization of the marginal band system in blood cells of marine species. Biol Bull (Woods Hole) 153:420 (abstract).
88. Nemhauser I, Ornberg R, Cohen WD (1980): Marginal bands in blood cells of invertebrates. J Ultrastruct Res 70:308–317.

89. Cohen WD (1978): Observations on the marginal band system of nucleated erythrocytes. J Cell Biol 78:260–273.
90. Ravindranath MH (1974): The hemocytes of an isopod *Ligia exotica* Roux. J Morphol 144:11–22.
91. Ravindranath MH (1980): Haemocytes in haemolymph coagulation in arthropods. Biol Rev Cambr Phil Soc 55:139–170.
92. Rowley AF (1977): The role of haemocytes of *Clitumnus extradentations* in haemolymph coagulation. Cell Tissue Res 182:513–524.
93. Tait J (1910): Crustacean blood coagulation as studied in the arthrostraca. Q J Exp Physiol 3:1–20.
94. Tait J (1911): Types of crustacean blood coagulation. J Mar Biol Assoc UK 9:191–198.
95. Tait J (1918): Capillary phenomena observed in blood cells: Thigmocytes, pagocytosis, amoeboid movement, differential adhesiveness of corpuscles, emigration of leucocytes. J Exp Physiol 12:1–33.
96. Tait J, Gunn JD (1918): The blood of *Astacus fluviatilis*: A study in crustacean blood, with special reference to coagulation and phagocytosis. J Exp Physiol 12:35–80.
97. Yeager JF, Shull WE, Farrar MD: On the coagulation of blood from the cockroach, *Periplaeta orientalis* (Linn.), with special reference to blood smears. Iowa State Coll J Sci 6:325–345.
98. Silberberg M (1938): The causes and mechanisms of thrombosis. Physiol Rev 18:197–228.
99. Belamarich FA (1976): Nature of the contents of large granules of *Limulus* amebocytes. In: "Animal Models of Thrombosis and Hemorrhagic Diseases." DHEW Publ. No. (NIH) 76-892. Washington: U.S. Dept. of Health, Education and Welfare, pp 101–102.
100. White JG (1976): A comment on the ultrastructure of amebocytes from the horseshoe crab (*Limulus polyphemus*). In "Animal Models of the Thrombosis and Hemorrhagic Diseases." DHEW Publ. No. (NIH) 76–982. Washington DC: U.S. Department of Health, Education and Welfare, pp 97–101.
101. Levin J (1967): Blood coagulation and endotoxin in invertebrates. Fed Proc 26:1707–1712.
102. Levin J (1976): Blood coagulation in the horseshoe crab (*Limulus polyphemus*): A model for mammalian coagulation and hemostasis. In "Animal Models of Thrombosis and Hemorrhagic Disease." DHEW Publication No. (NIH) 76–982. Washington, DC: U.S. Department of Health, Education and Welfare pp 87–102.
103. Bartnicki-Garcia S (1972): Cell wall composition and other biochemical markers in fungal phylogeny. In Harborne JB (ed): "Phytochemical Phylogenic Symposium." New York, London: Academic, pp 82–103.
104. Smith VJ, Soderhall K (1983): β-1,3 Glucan activation of crustacean hemocytes *in vitro* and *in vivo*. Biol Bull (Woods Hole) 164:299–314.
105. Unestan T, Soderhall K (1977): Soluble fragments from fungal cell walls elicit defense reactions in crayfish. Nature (Lond)267:45–46.
106. Soderhall K (1981): Fungal cell wall β-1,3 glucans induce clotting and phenoloxidase attachment to foreign surfaces of crayfish hemocyte lysate. Dev Comp Immunol 5:565–573.
107. Pollard HB, Pagoles CJ, Creutz CE, Zinder O (1979): The chromaffin granule and possible mechanisms of exocytosis. Int Rev Cytol 58:159–197.
108. Dunham P, Arvan P, Falkow S, Hoffstein S, Weissman G (1979): Inhibitors of membrane transport reduce lysosomal enzyme secretion from dogfish phagocytes and their killing of sea urchin eggs. Proc Natl Acad Sci USA 76:1873–1877.
109. Pollard HB, Tack-Goldman K, Pazoles CJ, Creutz CE, Shulman NR (1977): Evidence for control of serotonin secretion from human platelets by hydroxyl ion transport and osmotic lysis. Proc Natl Acad Sci USA 74:5295–5299.

110. Liang S-M, Liang C-M, Liu T-Y (1981): Studies on *Limulus* amoebocytes. Isolation and identification of a membrane-bound protein activator of cyclic nucleotide phosphodiesterase from *Limulus* amoebocyte. J Biol Chem 256:4968–4972.
111. Liang S-M, Sakmar TP, Liu T-Y (1980): Studies on *Limulus* amoebocyte lysate. III. Purification of an endotoxin-binding protein from *Limulus* amoebocyte membranes. J Biol Chem 255:5586–5590.
112. Nakamura S, Levin J (1982): Fractionation of *Limulus* amoebocyte lysate. Characterization of activation of the proclotting enzyme by an endotoxin-mediated activator. Biochim Biophys Acta 707:217–225.
113. Nakamura S, Levin J (1982): Endotoxin-mediated *Limulus* proclotting enzyme activator and detection of a previously undescribed protease (protease N). Biochem Biophys Res Commun 108:1619–1623.
114. Nakamura S, Morita T, Harada-Suzuki T, Iwanaga S, Takahashi K, Niwa M (1982): A clotting enzyme associated with the hemolymph coagulation system of a horseshoe crab (*Tachypleus tridentatus*): Its purification and characterization. J Biochem (Tokyo) 92:781–792.
115. Ohki M, Nakamura T, Morita T, Iwanga S (1980): A new endotoxin sensitive factor associated with hemolymph coagulation system of horseshoe crab (Limulidae). FEBS Lett 120:217–220.
116. Tanaka S, Nakamura T, Morita T, Iwanga S (1982): *Limulus* anti-LPS factor: An anticoaguluant which inhibits the endotoxin-mediated activation of *Limulus* coagulation system. Biochem Biophys Res Commun 105:717–723.
117. Mosesson MW, Wolfenstein-Todel C, Levin J, Bertrand O (1979): Characterization of amebocyte coagulogen from the horseshoe crab *Limulus polyphemus*. Thrombosis Res 14:765–779.
118. Nakamura S, Iwanga S, Harada T, Niwa M (1976): A clottable protein (coagulogen) from amebocyte lysate of Japanese horseshoe crab (*Tachypleus tridentatus*). Its isolation and biochemical properties. J Biochem (Tokyo) 80:1011–1021.
119. Nakamura S, Iwanaga S, Niwa M, Harada T (1977): A clottable protein (coagulogen) from hemocyte lysate of Japanese horseshoe crab (*Tachypleus tridentatus*): Isolation, properties and gel formation. Jpn J Med Sci Biol 30:74–77.
120. Nakamura S, Takagi T, Iwanaga S, Niwa M, Takahashi K (1976): A clottable protein (coagulogen) of horseshoe crab hemocytes. Structural change of its polypeptide chain during gel formation. J Biochem (Tokyo) 80:649–652.
121. Nakamura S, Takagi T, Iwanaga S, Niwa M, Takahashi K (1976): Amino acid sequence studies on the fragments produced from horseshoe crab coagulogen during gel formation: Homologies with primate fibrinopeptide B. Biochem Biophys Res Commun 72:902–908.
122. Tai JY, Seid RC, Huhn RD, Liu TY (1977): Studies on *Limulus* amoebocyte lysate. II. Purification of the coagulogen and the mechanism of clotting. J Biol Chem 252:4773–4776.
123. Takagi T, Hokama Y, Morita T, Iwanaga S, Nakamura S, Niwa M (1979): Amino acid sequence studies on horseshoe crab (*Tachypleus tridentatus*) coagulogen and the mechanism of gel formation. In Cohen E (ed): "Biomedical Applications of the Horseshoe Crab (Limulidae)." New York: Alan R. Liss, pp 169–184.
124. Harada T, Morita T, Iwanga S, Nakamura S, Niwa M (1979): A new chromogenic substrate method for assay of bacterial endotoxins using *Limulus* hemocyte lysate. In Cohen E (ed): "Biomedical Applications of the Horseshoe Crab (Limulidae)." New York: Alan R. Liss, pp 209–220.
125. Liu T-Y, Seid RS, Tai JY, Liang S-M, Sakmar TP, Robbins JB (1979): Studies on *Limulus* lysate coagulating system. In Cohen E (ed): "Biomedical Applications of the Horseshoe Crab (Limulidae)." New York: Alan R. Liss, pp 147–158.

126. Sullivan JD, Watson WS (1975): Purification and properties of the clotting enzyme from *Limulus* lysate. Biochem Biophys Res Commun 66:848–855.
127. Tai JY, Liu T-Y (1977): Studies on *Limulus* amoebocyte lysate. Isolation of pro-clotting enzyme. J Biol Chem 252:2178–2181.
128. Young MS, Levin J, Prendergast RA (1972): An invertebrate coagulation system activated by endotoxin: Evidence for enzymatic mediation. J Clin Invest 51:1790–1797.
129. Shishikwa F, Nakamura S, Takahashi K, Sekiguchi K (1982): Horseshoe crab phylogeny based on amino acid sequences of the fibrinopeptide-like peptide C. J Exp Zool 223:89–91.
130. Solum NO (1973): The coagulogen of *Limulus* polyphemus hemocytes. A comparison of the clotted and non-clotted forms of the molecule. Thromb Res 2:55–70.
131. Levin J (1979): The reaction between bacterial endotoxin and amebocyte lysate. In Cohen E (ed): "Biomedical Applications of the Horseshoe Crab (Limulidae)." New York: Alan R. Liss, pp 131–146.
132. Levin J, Bang FB (1968): Clottable protein in *Limulus*: Its localization and kinetics of its coagulation by endotoxin. Thromb Diath Haemorrh (Stuttg) 19:186–197.
133. Kakinuma A, Asano T, Toni H, Sugino Y (1981): Gelation of *Limulus* amoebocyte lysate by an antitumor (1-3)-β-D-glucan. Biochem Biophys Res Commun 101:434–439.
134. Morita T, Tanaka S, Nakamura T, Iwanga S (1981): A new (1-3)-β-D-glucan-mediated coagulation pathway found in *Limulus* amebocytes. FEBS Lett 19:318–321.
135. Watson SW, Levin J, Novitsky TJ (1982): "Endotoxins and Their Detection With the *Limulus* Amebocyte Lysate Test." New York: Alan R. Liss.
136. Elin RJ, Wolff SM (1973): Nonspecificity of the *Limulus* amebocyte lysate test: Positive reactions with polynucleotides and proteins. J Infect Dis 128:349–352.
137. Fumarola D, Pasquetto N, Telesforo P, Donati M (1975): Studies on the clotting mechanism of *Limulus polyphemus*. Thromb Res 7:401–408.
138. Niwa M, Hiramatsu T, Waguri O (1975): Quantitative aspects of the gelation reaction of horseshoe crab amoebocyte and bacterial endotoxin. Jpn J Med Sci Biol 28:98–100.
139. Solum NO (1970): Some characteristics of the clottable protein of *Limulus polyphemus* blood cells. Thromb Diath Haemorrh (Stuttg) 23:170–181.
140. Armstrong PB, Lackie JM (1975): Studies on intercellular invasion *in vitro* using rabbit peritoneal neutrophil granulocytes (PMNS). I. Role of contact inhibition of locomotion. J Cell Biol 65:439–462.
141. Zigmond SH (1978): Chemotaxis by polymorphonuclear leukocytes. J Cell Biol 77:269–287.
142. Curtis ASG (1964): The mechanism of adhesion of cells to glass; a study by interference reflection microscopy. J Cell Biol 20:199–215.
143. Izzard CS, Lochner LR (1976): Cell-to-substrate contacts in living fibroblasts: An interference reflection study with an evaluation of the technique. J Cell Sci 21:129–159.
144. Abercrombie M, Dunn GA (1975): Adhesions of fibroblasts to substratum during contact inhibition observed by interference reflection microscopy. Exp Cell Res 92:57–62.
145. Heath JP, Dunn GA (1978): Cell to substratum contacts of chick fibroblasts and their relation to the microfilament system. A correlated interference-reflexion and high-voltage electron-microscope study. J Cell Sci 29:197–212.
146. Chorney MJ (1978): Abstract of MBL Course on Invertebrate Pathology." Woods Hole, MA: Marine Biological Laboratory.
147. Bryan FT, Robinson CW, Gilbert CF, Langdell RD (1964): N-ethylmaleimide inhibition of horseshoe crab hemocyte agglutination. Science 144:1147–1148.
148. Kenney DM, Belamarich FA, Shepro D (1970): Aggregation and inhibition of aggregation of amebocytes of the horseshoe crab *Limulus polyphemus*. Biol Bull (Woods Hole)139:426–427 (abstract).
149. Nandan R, Brown DR (1977): An improved *in vitro* pyrogen test: To detect programs of

endotoxin contamination in intravenous fluids using *Limulus* amoebocyte lysate. J Lab Clin Med 89:910–918.

150. Murer EH, Levin J, Holme R (1975): Isolation and studies of the granules of the amebocytes of *Limulus polyphemus*, the horseshoe crab. J Cell Physiol 86:533–542.
151. Morrison P, Rothman WH (1957): Agglutination of blood cells in *Limulus polyphemus*. Proc Soc Exp Biol Med 94:21–23.
152. Loeb L (1904): On the spontaneous agglutination of blood cells of arthropods. Univ Pa Med Bull, Feb 1904:1–9.
153. Loeb L (1903): On the coagulation of the blood of some arthropods and on the influence of pressure and traction on the protoplasm of the blood cells of arthropods. Biol Bull (Woods Hole) 4:301–318.
154. Maluf MSR (1939): The blood of arthropods. Rev Biol 14:149–191.
155. Laki K (1972): Our ancient heritage in blood clotting and some of its consequences. Ann NY Acad Sci 202:297–307.
156. Barker WH, Bang FB (1966): The effect of infection by gram-negative bacteria, and their endotoxins, on the blood-clotting mechanisms of the crustacean *Sacculina carcini*, a parasite of the crab *Carcinus maenas*. J Invertebr Pathol 8:88–97.
157. Brehelin M (1979): Hemolymph coagulation in *Locusta migratoria*: Evidence for a functional equivalent of fibronogen. Comp Biochem Physiol 62B:329–334.
158. Durliat M, Vranckx R (1976): Coagulation in the crayfish, *Astacus leptodactylus*: Attempts to identify a fibrinogen-like factor in the hemolymph. Biol Bull (Woods Hole) 151:467–477.
159. Gellissen G (1983): Lipophorin as the plasma coagulogen in *Locusta migratoria*. Naturwissenschaft 70:45–46.
160. Ghidalia W, Vendrely R, Montmory C, Coirault Y, Brouard MO (1981): Coagulation in decapod crustacea. Comparative study of the clotting process in species from groups A, B and C. J Comp Physiol B142:473–478.
161. Lorand L: Fibrinoligase (1972): The fibrin-stabilizing factor system of blood plasma. Ann NY Acad Sci 202:6–30.
162. Morrison PR, Morrison KC (1952): Bleeding and coagulation in some Bermudan crustacea. Biol Bull (Woods Hole) 103:395–406.
163. Numanoi H (1938): On crustacean blood coagulation. Jpn J Zool 7:613–641.
164. Stewart JE, Dingle JR, Odense PH (1966): Constituents of the hemolymph of the lobster *Homarus americanus* Milne Edwards. Can J Biochem 44:1447–1459.
165. Holme R, Solum NO (1973): Electron microscopy of the gel protein formed by clotting of *Limulus polyphemus* hemocyte extracts. J Ultrastruct Res 44:329–338.
166. Harvey WR, Blankemeyer JT (1975): Epithelial structure and function. In Maramarosch K, Shope RE (eds): "Invertebrate Immunity." New York: Academic, pp 3–23.
167. Salt G (1970): "The Cellular Defense Reactions of Insects." London, New York: Cambridge University Press.
168. Stagner JI, Redmond JR (1975): The immunological mechanisms of the horseshoe crab, *Limulus polyphemus*. Marine Fish Rev 37:11–19.
169. Armstrong PB, Levin J (1979): *In vitro* phagocytosis by *Limulus* blood cells. J Invertebr Pathol 34:145–151.
170. Aggarwal SK, King RC (1967): The ultrastructure of the wreath cells of *Drosophila melanogaster* larvae. Protoplasm 63:343–352.
171. Bowers R (1964): Coated vesicles in the pericardial cells of the aphid (*Myzus persicae* Suly). Protoplasm 59:351–367.
172. Mills RP, King RC (1965): The pericardial cells of *Drosophila melanogaster*. Q J Microsc Sci 106:261–268.
173. Nutting WL (1951): A comparative anatomical study of the heart and accessory structures of the arthropteroid insects. J Morphol 89:501–598.

174. Wigglesworth VB (1970): The pericardial cells of insects: Analogue of the reticuloendothelial system. J Reticuloendothel Soc 7:208–216.
175. Gagen SJ, Ratcliffe NA (1976): Studies on the *in vivo* cellular reactions and fate of injected bacteria in *Galleria mellonella* and *Pieris brassicae* larvae. J Invertebr Pathol 28:17–24.
176. Johnson PT (1976): Bacterial infection in the blue crab *Callinectes papidus*: Course of infection and histopathology. J Invertebr Pathol 28:25–36.
177. Neuwirth M, Lai-Fork J (1977): Cytochemistry of the early stages of *in situ* coagulation in *Calpodes ethlius* (Lepidoptera). Can J Zool 55:1767–1772.
178. Smith VJ, Ratcliffe NA (1980): Host defense reactions of the shore crab, *Carcinus maenas* (L): Clearance and distribution of injected test particles. J Mar Biol Assoc UK 60:89–102.
179. Smith VJ, Ratcliffe NA (1980): Cellular defense reactions of the shore crab, *Carcinus maenas*: *In vivo* hemocytic and histopathological reactions to injected bacteria. J Invertebr Pathol 35:63–74.
180. Galanos C, Freudenberg, MA, Luderitz O, Rietschel ET, Westphal O (1979): Chemical, physicochemical and biological properties of bacterial lipopolysaccharides. In Cohen E (ed): "Biomedical Applications of the Horseshoe Crab (Limulidae)." New York: Alan R. Liss, pp 321–332.
181. Levin J, Tomasulo PA, Oper RS (1970): Detection of endotoxin in human blood and demonstration of an inhibitor. J Lab Clin Med 75:903–911.
182. Shirodkar MV, Warwick A, Bang FB (1960): The *in vitro* reaction of *Limulus* amebocytes to bacteria. Biol Bull (Woods Hole) 118:324–337.
183. Nachum R (1979): Antimicrobial defense mechanisms in *Limulus polyphemus*. In Cohen E (ed): "Biomedical Applications of the Horseshoe Crab (Limulidae)." New York: Alan R. Liss, pp 513–524.
184. Nachum R, Watson SW, Siegel SE (1980): Antimicrobial defense mechanisms in the horseshoe crab, *Limulus polyphemus*: Effect of sodium chloride on bactericidal activity. J Invertebr Pathol 36:382–388.
185. Furman RM, Pistole TG (1976): Bactericidal activity of hemolymph from the horseshoe crab, *Limulus polyphemus*. J Invertebr Pathol 28:239–244.
186. Pistole TG, Bitko JL (1978): Bactericidal activity of amebocytes from the horseshoe crab, *Limulus polyphemus*. J Invertebr Pathol 31:376–382.
187. Pistole TG (1976): Naturally occurring bacterial agglutinin in the serum of the horseshoe crab, *Limulus polyphemus*. J Invertebr Pathol 28: 153–154.
188. Pistole TG (1978): Broad-spectrum bacterial agglutinating activity in the serum of the horseshoe crab, *Limulus polyphemus*. Dev Comp Immunol 2:65.
189. Pistole TG (1979): Bacterial agglutinins from *Limulus polyphemus*—An overview. In Cohen E (ed): "Biomedical Applications of the Horseshoe Crab (Limulidae)." New York: Alan R. Liss, pp 547–553.
190. Quigley JP, Armstrong PB (1983): An endopeptidase inhibitor, similar to α-2 macroglobulin, present in the plasma of *Limulus polyphemus*. J Biol Chem 258:7903–7906.
191. Quigley JP, Armstrong PB (1983): An endopeptidase inhibitor found in *Limulus* plasma: an ancient form of α-2 macroglobulin. Ann NY Acad Sci 421:119–124.
192. Quigley JP, Armstrong PB (1983): Characterization and isolation of a homologue of alpha-2-macroglobulin from the plasma of the horseshoe crab, *Limulus*. Biol Bull (Woods Hole) 165:488 (abstract).
193. Quigley JP, Armstrong PB, Gallant P, Rickles FR, Troll W (1982): An endopeptidase inhibitor, similar to α-2 macroglobulin, present in the plasma of *Limulus polyphemus*. Biol Bull (Woods Hole) 163:402 (abstract).
194. Roche A-C, Monsigny M (1974): Purification and properties of limulin: A lectin (agglutinin) from hemolymph of *Limulus polyphemus*. Biochim Biophys Acta 371:242–254.

195. Marchalonis JJ, Edelman G (1968): Isolation and characterization of a natural hemagglutinin from *Limulus polyphemus*. J Mol Biol 32:453–465.
196. Kaplan R, Li SS, Kehoe JM (1977): Molecular characterization of Limulin, a sialic acid binding lectin from the hemolymph of the horseshoe crab, *Limulus polyphemus*. Biochemistry 16:4297–4303.
197. Mureson V, Iwanij V, Smith ZDJ, Jamieson JD (1982): Purification and use of limulin: A sialic acid-specific lectin. J Histochem Cytochem 30:938–946.
198. Nowak TP, Barondes SH (1975): Agglutinin from *Limulus polyphemus*. Purification with formalinized horse erythrocytes as the affinity absorbent. Biochim Biophys Acta 393:115–123.
199. Oppenheim JD, Nachbar MS, Salton MRJ, Auell F (1974): Purification of a hemagglutinin from *Limulus polyphemus* by affinity chromatography. Biochem Biophys Res Commun 58:1127–1134.
200. Roche A-C, Schauer R, Monsigny M (1975): Protein-sugar interactions. Purification by affinity chromatography of limulin on N-acylneuraminyl-binding proteins. FEBS Lett 57:245–249.
201. Shimizu S, Ito M, Niwa M (1977): Lectins in the hemolymph of Japanese horseshoe crab, *Tachypleus tridentatus*. Biochim Biophys Acta 500:71–79.
202. Cohen E, Rozenberg M, Massaro EJ (1974): Agglutinins of *Limulus polyphemus* (horseshoe crab) and *Burgus latro* (coconut crab). Ann NY Acad Sci 234:28–33.
203. Roelcke D, Uhlenbruck G, Metaxas MN (1971): Untersuchungen uber die serologische Spezifitat neuraminsaurehaltiger Rezeptoren auf Humanerythrozyten. Z Immunatsforsch 141:141–151.
204. Rostam-Abadi H, Pistole TG (1982): Lipopolysaccharide-binding lectin from the horseshoe crab, *Limulus polyphemus*, with specificity for 2-keto-3-deoxycytonate (KDO). Dev Comp Immunol 6:209–218.
205. Vaith P, Uhlenbruck G, Muller WEG, Cohen E (1979): Reactivity of *Limulus polyphemus* hemolymph with D-glucuronic acid containing glycosubstances. In Cohen E (ed): "Biomedical Applications of the Horseshoe Crab (Limulidae)." New York: Alan R. Liss, pp 579–587.
206. Rostam-Abadi H, Pistole TG (1979): Sites on the lipopolysaccharide molecule reactive with *Limulus* agglutinins. In Cohen E (ed): "Biomedical Applications of the Horseshoe Crab (Limulidae)." New York: Alan R. Liss, pp 537–545.
207. Cohen E, Baldo BA, Uhlenbruck G (1975): Anti-galactan precipitins in the hemolymph of *Tridacna maxima* and *Limulus polyphemus*. In Hildemann WH, Benedict AA (eds): "Immunologic Phylogeny." New York: Plenum, p 13.
208. Gilbride KJ, Pistole TG (1979): Isolation and characterization of a bacterial agglutinin in the serum of *Limulus polyphemus*. In Cohen E (ed): "Biomedical Applications of the Horseshoe Crab (Limulidae)." New York: Alan R. Liss, pp 525–535.
209. Pistole TG (1982): *Limulus* lectins: Analogues of vertebrate immunoglobins. In Bonaventura J, Bonaventura C, Tesh S (ed): "Physiology and Biology of Horseshoe Crabs: Studies on Normal and Environmentally Stressed Animals." New York: Alan R. Liss, pp 283–288.
210. Heimburger M (1975): Proteinase inhibitors of human plasma—their properties and control functions. In Reich E, Rifkin DB, Shaw E (ed): "Proteases and Biological Control." Cold Spring Harbor, New York: Cold Spring Laboratory, pp 367–386.
211. Lasakowski M, Kato I (1980): Protein inhibitors of proteinases. Annu Rev Biochem 49:593–626.
212. Travis J, Salvesen GS (1983): Human plasma proteinase inhibitors. Annu Rev Biochem 52:655–709.
213. Barrett AJ (1981): α_2-Macroglobulin. Methods Enzymol 80:737–754.
214. Starkey PM, Barrett AJ (1977):α_2-Macroglobulin, a physiological regulator of protein-

ase activity. In Barrett AJ (ed): "Proteinases in Mammalian Cells and Tissues." Amsterdam: Elsevier/North-Holland, pp 663–696.

215. Cohen E, Rowe AW, Wissler FC: Heteroagglutinins of the horseshoe crab, *Limulus polyphemus*. Life Sci 4:2009–2016.
216. Browning HC (1942): The integument and moult cycle of *Tegenaria atrica* (Araneae). Proc R Soc Lond Ser B 131:65–86.
217. Deevey GB (1941): Blood cells of the Haitian tarantula and their relation to the moulting cycle. J Morphol 68:457–491.
218. Sewell MT (1955): Lipo-protein cells in the blood of *Carcinus madnas*, and their cycle correlated with the moult. J Microsc Sci 96:73–83.
219. Krishuakumaran A, Schneiderman HA (1970): Control of molting in mandibulate and chelicerate arthropods by ecdysone. Biol Bull (Woods Hole) 139:520–538.
220. Bolton AE: "Radioiodination Techniques." Arlington Heights, IL: The Amersham Corporation.
221. Franker PJ, Speek JC (1978): Protein and cell membrane iodination with a sparingly soluble chloramine, 1,3,4,6-tetrachloro-3a,6a-diphenylglycolaril. Biochem Biophys Res Commun 80:849–857.
222. Humphreys S, Humphreys T, Sano J (1977): Organization and polysaccharides of sponge aggregation factor. In Robbins PW, Fox CF (eds): "Cell Surface Carbohydrates and Biological Recognition." New York: Alan R. Liss, pp 311–323.
223. Vacquier VD, Moy GW (1977): Isolation of bindin: The protein responsible for adhesion of sperm to sea urchin eggs. Proc Natl Acad Sci USA 74:2456–2460.
224. Edelman GM (1983): Cell adhesion molecules. Science 219:450–457.
225. Gerisch G (1980): Univalent antibody fragments as tools for the analysis of cell interactions in *Dictyostelium*. Curr Top Dev Biol 14:243–270.
226. Bellairs R, Curtis A, Dunn G (1982): "Cell Behaviour." Cambridge: Cambridge University Press.
227. Goldman R, Pollard T, Rosenbaum J (1976): "Cell Motility." Cold Spring Harbor Conference on Cell Proliferation, Vol 3. Cold Spring Harbor, NY: Cold Spring Harbor Laboratory.
228. Arnold JW (1959): Observations on living hemocytes in wing veins of the cockroach *Blaberus giganteus* (L.) (Orthoptera: Blattidae). Ann Entomol Soc Am 52:229–236.
229. Arnold JW (1959): Observations on amoeboid motion of living haemocytes in the wing veins of *Blaberus giganteus* (L.) (Orthoptera: Blattidae). Can J Zool 37:371–375.
230. Arnold JW (1961): Further observations on amoeboid haemocytes in *Blaberus giganteus* (L). (Orthoptera: Blattidae). Can J Zool 39:755–766.
231. Baerwald RJ, Boush GM (1970): Time-lapse photographic studies of cockroach hemocyte migration *in vitro*. Exp Cell Res 63:208–213.
232. Bohn H (1977): Differential adhesion of the haemocytes of *Leucophae maderae* (Blattaria) to a glass surface. J Insect Physiol 23:185–194.
233. Judy KJ, Marks EP (1971): Effects of ecdysone *in vitro* on hindgut and hemocytes of *Manduca sexta* (Lepidoptera). Gen Comp Endocrinol 17:351–359.
234. Walters DR (1970): Hemocytes of saturniid silkworms: Their behavior *in vivo* and *in vitro* in response to diapause, development and injury. J Exp Zool 174:441–450.
235. Korn ED (1982): Actin polymerization and its regulation by proteins from nonmuscle cells. Physiol Rev 62:672–737.
236. Johnson TW (1970): Fungi in marine crustaceans. In Snieszko SF (ed): "A Symposium on Diseases of Fishes and Shellfishes." Washington, DC: American Fisheries Society, pp 405–408.
237. Bang FB (1967): Serological responses among invertebrates other than insects. Fed Proc 26:1680–1684.
238. Bang FB (1970): Disease mechanisms in crustaceans and marine arthropods. In Snieszko

SF (ed): "A Symposium on Diseases of Fishes and Shellfishes." Washington, DC: American Fisheries Society, pp 383–404.
239. Sinderman CJ (1970): "Principal Diseases of Marine Fish and Shellfish." New York: Academic, pp 106–202.
240. Sprague V (1970): Some protozoan parasite and hyperparasites in marine decapod crustaceans. In Snieszko SF (ed): "A Symposium on Diseases of Fishes and Shellfishes." Washington, DC: American Fisheries Society, pp 416–430.
241. Soderhall K (1982): Phenoloxidase activity system and melanization—A recognition mechanism of arthropods? Dev Comp Immunol 6:601–611.
242. Soderhall K, Smith VJ (1983): Separation of the haemocyte populations of *Carcinus maenas* and other marine decapods, and prophenoloxidase distribution. Dev Comp Immunol 7:229–239.
243. Taylor RL (1969): A suggested role for the polyprophenol-phenoloxidase system in invertebrate immunity. J Invertebr Pathol 14:427–428.
244. McKay D, Jenkins CR, Tyson CJ (1973): Effect of endotoxin in resistance of the freshwater crayfish (*Parachaeraps bicarinatus*) to infection. J Infect Dis 128:5165–5169.
245. Paterson WD, Stewart JE (1979): Rate and duration of phagocytic increase in lobsters induced by *Pseudomonas peraleus* endotoxin. Dev Comp Immunol 3:353–357.
246. Gregoire C (1974): Hemolymph coagulation. In Rockstein M (ed): "The physiology of Insecta." 2nd Ed. New York: Academic, pp 309–360.
247. Rowley AF, Ratcliffe NA (1976): The granular cells of *Galleira mellonella* during clotting and phagocytic reactions in vitro. Tissue Cell 8:437–446.
248. Chadwick JS (1967): Serological responses of insects. Fed Proc 26:1675–1679.
249. Lackie AM (1980): Invertebrate immunity. Parasitology 80:393–412.
250. Lackie AM (1983): Immunological recognition of cuticular transplants in insects. Dev Comp Immunol 7:41–50.
251. Noguchi H (1903): A study of immunization-haemolysins, agglutinins, precipitins and coagulins in cold-blooded animals. Zentr Bakterio Parasitenk Infekt Abt 1 Orig 33:353–362.
252. Baerwald RJ (1973): Freeze fracture studies of insect hemocyte gap junctions and associated cell membranes. J Cell Biol 59:14a.
253. Salt G (1967): Cellular defense mechanisms in insects. Fed Proc 26:1671–1674.
254. Schmit AR, Ratcliffe NA (1977): The encapsulation of foreign tissue implants in *Galleria mellonella* larvae. J Insect Physiol 23: 175–184.
255. Williams AJ, Lutz PL (1975): The role of the hemolymph in the carbohydrate metabolism of *Carcinus maenas*. J Mar Biol Assoc UK 55:667–670.
256. Williams AJ, Lutz PL (1975): Blood cell types in *Carcinus maenas* and their physiological role. J Mar Biol Assoc UK 55:671–674.
257. Wigglesworth VB (1959): Insect blood cells. Annu Rev Entomol 4:1–16.
258. Eisenman EA, Alfert M (1982): A new fixation procedure for preserving the ultrastructure of marine invertebrate tissue. J Microsc (Oxford) 125:117–120.

EXOCYTOSIS

Blood Cells of Marine Invertebrates: Experimental Systems in Cell Biology and Comparative Physiology, pages 127–142

Chapter Four
Exocytosis in *Limulus* Amebocytes

Richard L. Ornberg

Laboratory of Cell Biology and Genetics, National Institute of Arthritis, Diabetes, Digestive, and Kidney Diseases, National Institutes of Health, Bethesda, Maryland 20205 and the Marine Biological Laboratory, Woods Hole, Massachusetts 02543

INTRODUCTION

The amebocyte blood cell in the horseshoe crab *Limulus polyphemus* is an exciting secretory cell that may be of practical value in the future study of exocytosis and secretion in general. This chapter is a review of studies on the morphology of secretion in amebocytes done in collaboration with Dr. Thomas S. Reese. It is our hope that this review will foster interest and prove useful to future researchers who wish to use *Limulus* amebocytes.

Exocytosis is one of the major mechanisms by which cells secrete internally stored products and waste material into the extracellular space. The secreted material is packaged in granules and is thus separated from the external space by the granule membrane, a cytoplasmic space, and the plasma membrane. The exocytosis process is a complicated one that involves a series of interactions between the granule membrane and plasma membrane, leading to the formation of a pore or lumen through which the granule contents diffuse out. The granule membrane becomes incorporated into the plasma membrane during the process such that the overall integrity of the plasma membrane is not altered. The stimulus to secrete varies with cell type, but cytosolic calcium ions, either entering the cells from the external space or being released from internal stores, are thought to be the stimulus-secretion coupler in most cells studied so far [Baker, et al., 1980; Douglas, 1978; Rubin, 1982; Hopkins and Dunkin, 1979].

An ultrastructural description of the membrane events of exocytosis was proposed some time ago by Palade [1975] and Palade and Bruns [1968] and has received much support from studies of exocytosis in mast cells [Chi et al., 1976; Lawson et al., 1977], pancreatic A-cells [Carpenter et al., 1977], pancreatic B-cells [Orci et al., 1977], neurohypophysis [Theodosis et al., 1978], *Tetrahymena* [Satir et al., 1973], zoopores [Pinto de Silva and Nogueira, 1977], and exocrine cells [Tanaka et al., 1980]. The essential ultrastructural events include 1) the approach of the secretory granule to the plasma membrane to form a heptalaminar apposition, 2) the coalescence or "fusion" of the apposed membranes to form a patch of pentalaminar junctions, which in freeze-etch views is free of intramembranous particles and therefore proteins, 3) the dissolution or rearrangement of the pentalaminar junction patch to form either a lumen through which granule contents pass or a trilaminar unit membrane diaphragm, which subsequently dissolves to form an exocytotic lumen. Despite overwhelming support for this hypothesis, the data on which it is based are derived, technically, from one experimental approach: chemical fixation. Consequently, the consistency of ultrastructural views from cell to cell may reflect the fixation method more than the generality of the cellular physiological processes involved in exocytosis. A more accurate view, free of the poisonous [Smith and Reese, 1980] and artifactual [Chandler and Heuser, 1980; Chandler, 1979] effects of fixation, and more relevant to known physiological and biochemical events [Heuser et al., 1979] is required. Such a view is provided by physical fixation or quick freezing. With this understanding, we studied the ultrastructure of secretion in the amebocyte blood cell of *Limulus polyphemus* in an attempt to examine, at high resolution, the various stages of membrane interactions accompanying exocytosis.

Ameboycte blood cells are multifunctional cells (see Armstrong, this volume) and have a secretory response that releases clotting proteins [Murer et al., 1975] from granule stores into the coelemic fluid space. The natural stimulus for the secretory response is believed to be gram-negative bacterial endotoxin (ETX) which also activates the clotting enzymes. The remaining functions of the cell—aggregation, motility, and phagocytosis, together with secretion—are involved in the overall homeostatic response of the crab to lesions in the exoskeleton whereby the blood spaces are isolated from incoming septic sea water by a wall of clotted protein and flattened ameboid cells. Early and limited morphological data on the secretory response [Bang, 1955] had suggested that the cells simply fell apart, releasing whole intact granules in the presence of endotoxin. However, it became clear to us at the outset and from previous work [Dumont et al., 1966] that endotoxin-induced secretion of the granule contents in amebocytes was by exocytosis [Ornberg and Reese, 1979a].

There are a number of major advantages to studying amebocytes with quick freezing. First, the amebocyte is the only cell type in the horseshoe crab and is in high titer (2×10^7 cells per 1 ml typically). Consequently, exhaustive and possibly detrimental isolation procedures typical of other cell systems are not necessary. Second, the amebocyte secretory response is very rapid (Fig. 1, 2), such that the time needed to degranulate a cell is anywhere from 1 min to 2 min with no lag period between stimulation and secretion. Because of this, a reasonable number of exocytotic events are occurring and can be captured during the brief time it takes to freeze the cells. Third, the amebocyte plasma facilitates the freezing process with its high protein and salt content [Ornberg and Reese, 1979b]. The hemocyanin surrounding the cells provides an excellent marker for ice crystal size and thus, the overall acceptability of the frozen preparation.

EXPERIMENTAL STUDIES AND DISCUSSION

The methods to obtain fresh amebocytes and freeze them for study have been described previously [Ornberg and Reese, 1981a]. Briefly, amebocytes obtained by either cardiac or leg puncture were frozen by pressing them

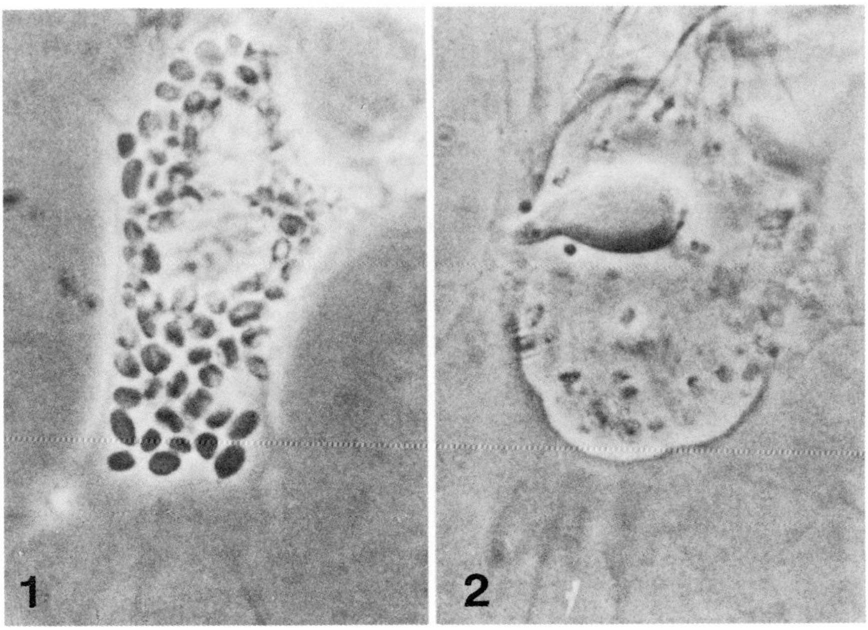

Figs. 1,2. Phase contrast images of a *Limulus* amebocyte attached to glass just prior to (Fig. 1) and 30 sec after (Fig. 2) exposure to endotoxin (1 μg/ml). ×800. From Ornberg and Reese [1981a], The Journal of Cell Biology, with permission of The Rockefeller University Press.

against a liquid helium cooled copper block and were subsequently freeze-substituted for thin sectioning or were freeze-fractured directly. Despite many advantages, the amebocyte preparation did pose subtle problems. Amebocytes are very sensitive to ETX and this necessitates the use of endotoxin-free solutions, glassware, syringes, and needles. In addition, the mechanical agitation accompanying withdrawal of the cells can trigger cell aggregation and clumping in the syringe. These problems can be avoided by minimizing the time between withdrawal and ETX mixing to approximately 10-15 sec. Amebocyte aggregates, once formed, are difficult to disperse even by vigorous shaking, which in fact enhances further aggregation. This aggregating activity makes it impossible to wash the cells for the study of media and drug effects by centrifugation methods. Instead of washing, however, cells can simply be withdrawn and diluted 1:1 into cell-free plasma containing a twofold excess of the drug to be studied. In this way, the effects of calcium-EGTA buffer, cytochalasin D, and propranolol on secretion were studied.

Limulus amebocytes are nucleated cells, approximately 10–20 μm in diameter, with round to oval pleomorphic shapes when suspended in plasma (Figs. 3,4). Amebocytes are filled with numerous secretory granules, mitochondria, and an extensive subsurface smooth endoplasmic reticulum. Golgi apparatus and rough endoplasmic reticulum are rarely seen (Fig. 5). The plasma membrane in the unstimulated cell is smooth, being completely free of microvilli or ruffles, which are common to mast cells and polymorphonuclear leucocytes. Unlike most cells, the plasma membrane, in freeze-etch views, has more intramembrane particles in its external leaflet than in its cytoplasmic leaflet, a feature common only to vertebrate blood platelets. The secretory granules are large, approximately 1 μm in diameter, and pleomorphic with amorphous, osmiophilic contents that completely fill the granule space. The granules are frequently found to be touching one another but are generally separated from the plasma membrane by cytoplasm, which occasionally has a filamentous appearance (Fig. 6).

Upon exposure to endotoxin, amebocytes undergo an immediate transformation and secrete their granule contents. This immediate secretory response is followed in 1-2 min by the appearance of microspikes and the motility

---

Figs. 3,4. Free-floating amebocytes rapid-frozen in whole blood. Amebocytes frozen within seconds of withdrawal in the absence of endotoxin are generally round to oval and are filled with a single type of secretory granule containing clotting proteins (Fig. 3). After 60 sec exposure to endotoxin, massive secretion leading to compound exocytosis is typical (Fig. 4). Differences in the granule density are due to different postsubstitution staining methods used. The amebocyte in Figure 3 was stained with hafnium tetrachloride in acetone to enhance the appearance of granule and plasma membrane and diminish granule matrix staining. In Figure 4, the preparation was stained with uranyl acetate in methanol, which heavily stains the granule matrix. ×25,000.

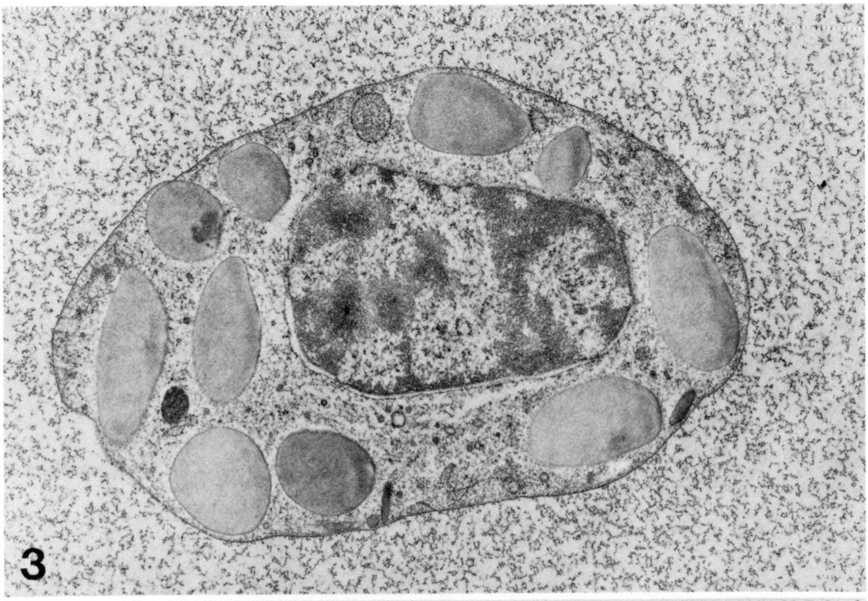

3

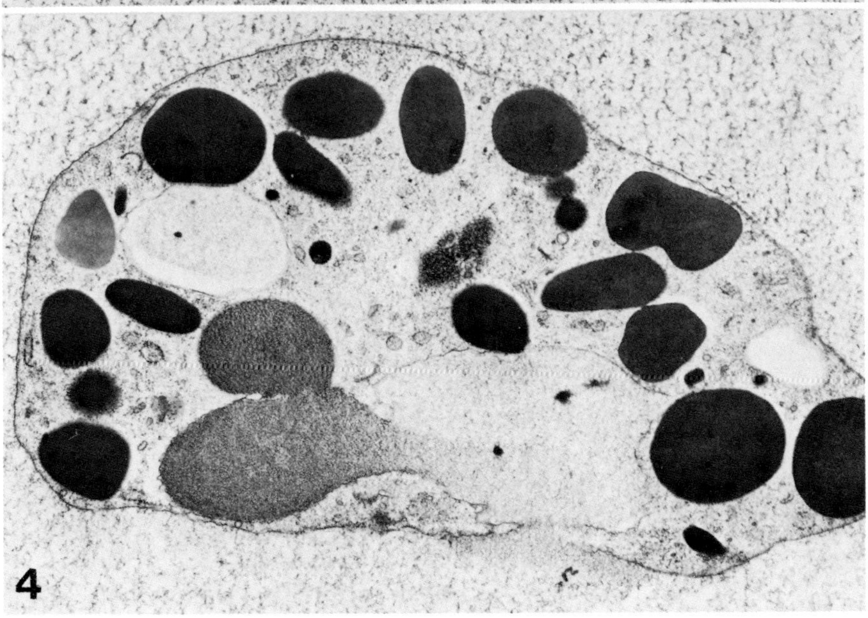

4

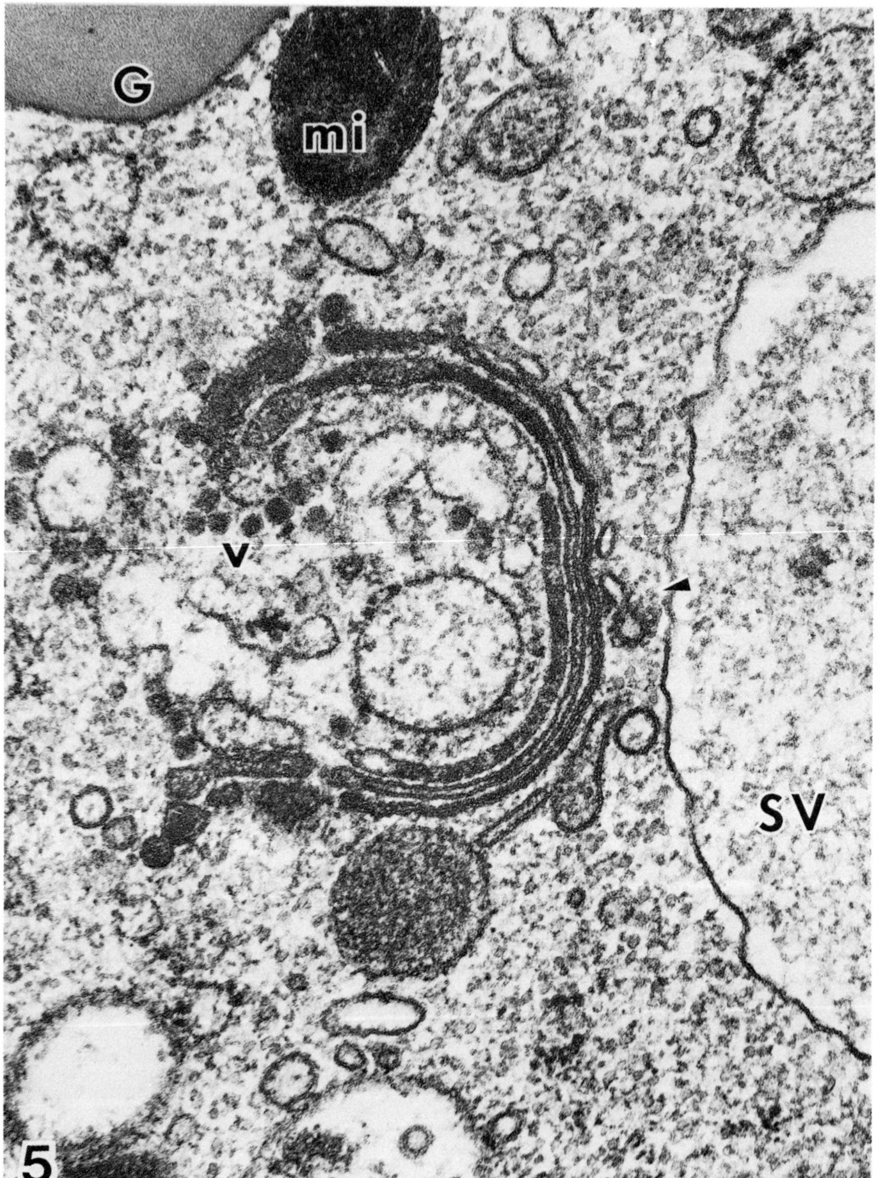

Fig. 5. Rare view of Golgi apparatus near a secretory vacuole (SV) in an amebocyte frozen after 60 sec in endotoxin. A coated vesicle fusing with smooth endoplasmic reticulum on the trans side of the Golgi (arrowhead) presumably supplies membrane from numerous filled vesicles (V), the potential granule precursors, on the cis side of the Golgi. A mature granule (G) is present in the upper left. The origin of the secretory granules is unknown but may be the result of the coalescence of many small vesicles as seen here. ×60,000.

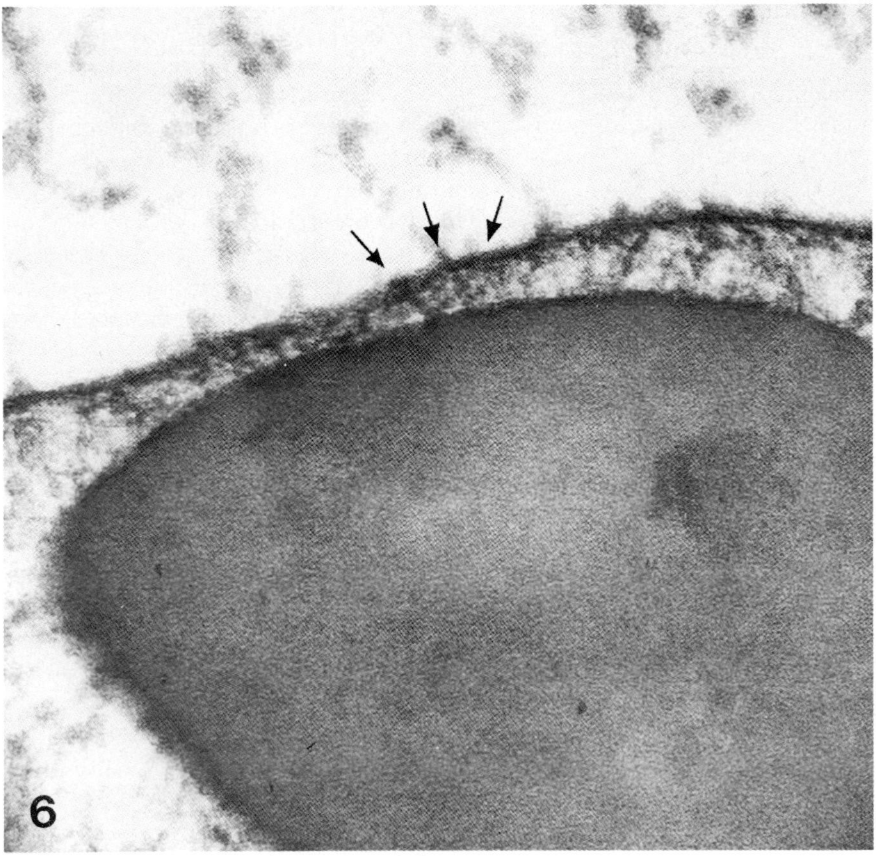

Fig. 6. Relation of a granule membrane to the plasma membrane. Filamentous material bridging the gap of cytoplasm (arrows) is occasionally seen and may be involved in the formation of pedestal appositions. ×175,000.

response. Secretion begins with the discharge of peripheral granules and proceeds radially inward with the discharge of more internal granules into vacuoles created by discharged peripheral granules (Fig. 4). This sequential or compound exocytosis is typical of other secretory cells, having been first described in mast cells [Rohlich et al., 1971]. Once secretion is initiated, the amebocytes release virtually all of their granules and show limited capability to make new granules (Fig. 5). By concentrating on the earliest times after ETX exposure, the critical events of secretory response could be observed without interference by the motility response or the late events of membrane recycling and granule formation, which may follow secretion in this cell as in others [Farquhar, 1981; Holtzman, 1981].

The most important distinction of our work is that previous studies of exocytosis resulted in models constructed from images arranged as they were thought to occur, not necessarily as they naturally occurred. This is due primarily to the slow integrative action of chemical fixatives. Consequently, nothing could be said directly about the timing of the various stages of exocytosis or about which stages were rate-limiting. With the precisely timed fixation of quick freezing and stimulus synchronization of rapid mixing, an accurate sequential process was obvious from views of amebocytes frozen at rest and 1, 5, and 10 sec after mixing with ETX. The membrane events which constitute steps in the granule exocytosis process in amebocytes are best described as follows: 1) the approach step, 2) the contact step, and 3) the pore formation step.

Exocytosis: The Approach Step

The approach step is the process by which the plasma membrane and granule membrane or the granule membrane and neighboring granule membrane come into contact. In amebocytes, this step is evidenced at the earliest times after ETX exposure as a shallow inward depression of the plasma membrane, which forms a flat-bottomed pedestal upon which the granules rest (Fig. 7). Unlike other secretory cells in which secretory granules are thought to move relative to the plasma membrane, the approach step consists of the plasma membrane being pulled into apposition with the granule membrane. A similar phenomenon may occur in mast cells although this has not been explicitly stated [Lawson et al., 1977]. At the level of the more internal granules, an approach step between neighboring granules appears to be circumvented since numerous granule-granule contacts can be seen in resting, unstimulated amebocytes. However, the longevity of such contact may be very short, since the granules are capable of movement relative to one another and thus may undergo several cycles of approach and contact before pore formation occurs.

The mechanism mediating the plasma membrane deformation is not known. A possible structural correlate is the filamentous dense material that connects some peripheral granules with the plasma membrane and neighboring granules. Actin filaments have been observed in mast cells [Rohlich, 1975] and can bind to a variety of secretory granules [Fowler and Pollard, 1982]. These observations supported the hypothesis that an actin-myosin system was involved [Puszkin and Kochwa, 1974], in which granule-bound myosin attached to plasma membrane-bound actin filaments pulled the membranes together in a manner analogous to muscle contraction. However, this hypothesis has fallen into disfavor since numerous attempts have failed to detect myosin on secretory granules or in secretory cells in general [Morgan et al., 1974]. One alternative hypothesis proposes that the filamentous actin

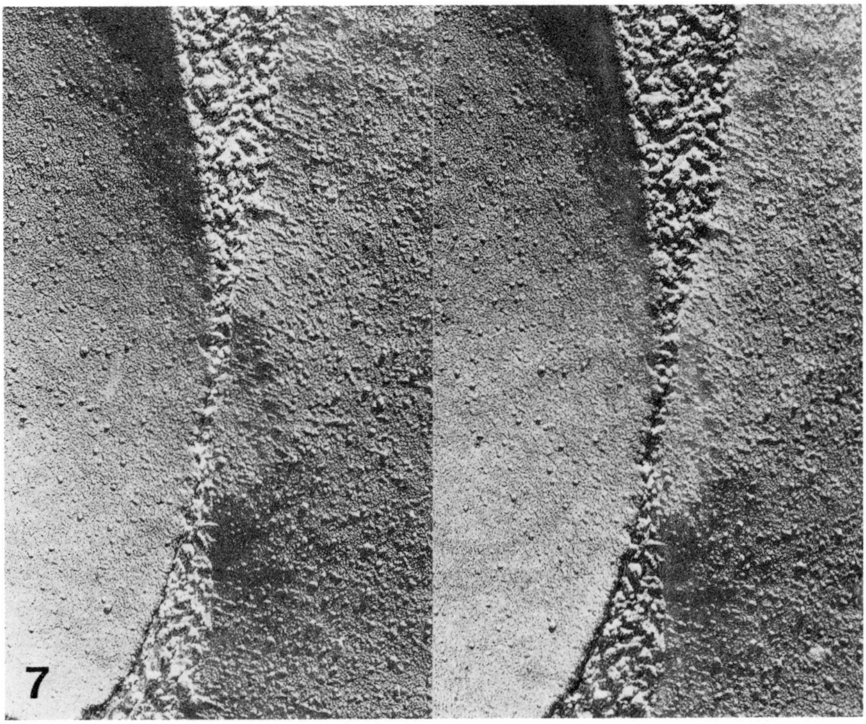

Fig. 7. Stereo view of a pedestal deformation as revealed by freeze-etching, illustrating the relationship of pedestals to secretory granules. The E face of the inward bulge on the right forms the pedestal on which the secretory granule rests for subsequent contact and pore formation. The pedestals generally have flat or, in this case, outwardly curved tops. ×41,000. From Ornberg and Reese [1981a], with permission of The Rockefeller University Press.

network acts as a mechanical barrier to granule movement at rest but transforms from a gel state to a sol state following stimulation to allow granules to approach the plasma membrane by Brownian movement. In an attempt to ascertain whether actin could be involved in exocytosis in amebocytes, we examined the effects of cytochalasin D on secretion. Cytochalasin D is a potent inhibitor of actin polymerization and filament elongation [Schwila, 1982]. While this drug had a dramatic effect on the motile function of the cell, both secretion and plasma membrane deformation were unimpaired [Ornberg and Reese, 1981a]. Thus, the mechanism of the approach step leading to the inward movement of the plasma membrane remains a mystery.

Exocytosis: The Contact Step

The membrane apposition formed within the pedestal depressions of the plasma membrane is the site of intimate contact that leads to pore formation.

The ultrastructure of these contacts differs from that observed previously in other secretory cells in two important ways. First, no expansive pentalaminar junction depicting "fused" membranes was seen. Instead, much of the apposition is in a seven-layered membrane configuration. From both stereo thin section and freeze-etch views, small holes similar in dimension to the punctate contact are seen within some appositions, suggesting that these punctate contacts are indeed precursors of pore formation [Ornberg and Reese, 1981a]. Second, the apposition and contact regions are not cleared of intramembranous particles as described in previous reports of chemically fixed cells [Chi et. al., 1976; Lawson et al., 1977; Orci et al., 1977; Carpenter et al., 1977; Theodosis et al., 1978; Satir et al., 1973; Pinto da Silva and Nogueira, 1977; Tanaka et al., 1980]. In fact, such intramembranous particle clearing has been shown to be an artifact of fixation [Chandler, 1979]. This particular finding is very important since it implies that intramembranous protein does not necessarily have to be moved out of the way for contact to occur and that intramembranous proteins may be involved in the mechanism by which the exocytotic pore is formed.

The membranous appositions between more internal unreleased granules have a pentalaminar appearance similar to that observed in fixed cells. However, appositions between released granules and unreleased granules frequently contained numerous punctate contacts similar to that seen at the plasma membrane [Ornberg and Reese, 1981b]. Consequently, the contact step that serves as the precursor to pore formation involves a very small region of membrane.

Exocytosis: The Pore Formation Step

The final step of pore formation and discharge, referred to as a "fission" in the literature [Palade and Bruns, 1968; Palade, 1975], has only rarely been observed. Consequently, the ultrastructure of the process has been largely hypothesized by biophysical theoreticians rather than observed directly by the electron microscopist. In quick-frozen amebocytes, the pores that form the initial opening for granule content discharge are surprisingly small, having dimensions on the order of a few tens of nanometers. They presumably originate from molecular rearrangements within the punctate contacts in the granule membrane–plasma membrane apposition. Similar small pore openings have been seen in quick frozen mast cells [Chandler and Heuser, 1980]. The lifespan of these pores must be exceedingly short, since they are rarely observed whereas wider openings are more frequent (Fig. 8).

These observations profoundly affect our understanding of membrane interactions accompanying not only exocytosis but also other sites of membrane fusion such as myoblast fusion [Kalderon and Gilula, 1979] and sperm and ovum fusion accompanying the fertilization reaction [Chandler and

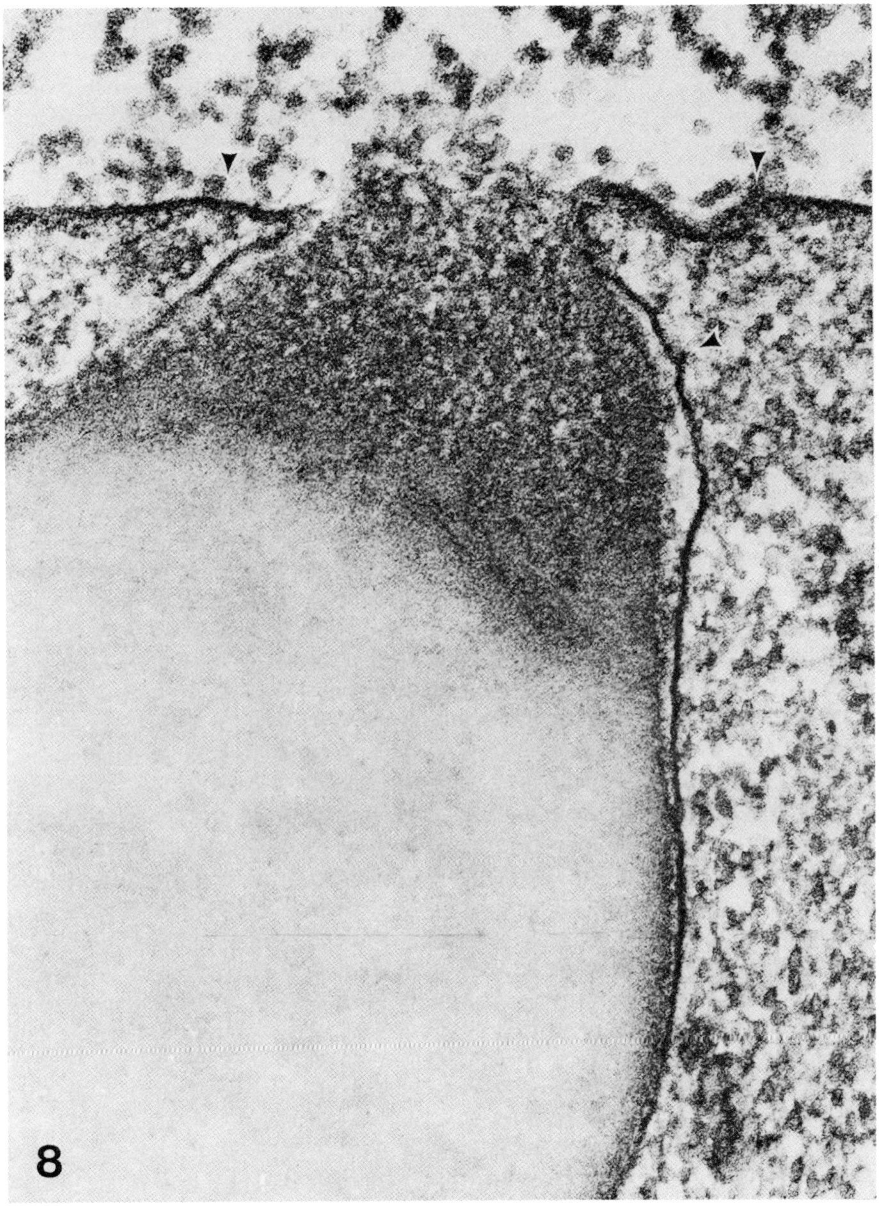

Fig. 8. A large pore in the process of widening to form an exocytotic lumen. This view captured after 5 sec of endotoxin exposure illustrates the rapid dissolution of granule contents into the extracellular space. Shoulders of the original pedestal opposition are still apparent (between arrow heads at top). Based on light microscope measurements of the time for granule dissolution, this particular lumen has been open for only a few tens of milliseconds. ×47,000. From Ornberg and Reese [1981a], with permission of The Rockefeller University Press.

Heuser, 1979]. The small opening suggests that only a few hundred lipid molecules and possibly some protein are involved in the membrane rearrangement of exocytosis. Consequently, previous concepts of expansive pentalaminar junctions, membrane elimination, and the dissolution of membrane diaphragms must be re-examined [Palade, 1975].

In summary (Fig. 9), exocytosis in amebocytes begins immediately after stimulation by ETX with inward movement of plasma membrane to form an apposition with underlying secretory granules. Subsequently, numerous punctate contacts appear within the apposition and indeed may be in a dynamic state of formation and disappearance until a small pore is produced. Once formed, the small pore quickly widens as the granule contents dissolve into the external space.

FUTURE WORK

Physiological processes accompanying these morphological events of exocytosis have been studied to a limited extent in amebocytes. From work in other systems, it is generally accepted that calcium ions act as the stimulus-secretion coupler, not only triggering the initial approach of the secretory granule and plasma membrane but also mediating molecular events within the contact region, leading to pore formation [Heuser and Llinas, 1977]. The source of calcium is generally thought to be the external milieu, although many secretory cells including the amebocyte can secrete in the absence of external calcium [Lowe et al., 1976] and thus possess an internal store of releasable calcium. On the basis of limited studies of calcium distribution in amebocytes, it is qualitatively clear that the secretory granules in resting amebocytes contain calcium [Ornberg and Reese, 1981c]. Furthermore, immediately upon stimulation with ETX, the subsurface endoplasmic reticulum swells dramatically, perhaps as a result of osmotic forces following calcium accumulation. Evidence that endoplasmic reticulum accumulates calcium in other secretory systems [McGraw et al., 1980] analogously to calcium accumulation by the sarcoplasmic reticulum in muscle suggests that internal calcium levels in amebocytes rise with ETX stimulations prior to granule discharge. These ideas obviously need further work.

A second physiological aspect of exocytosis that has only recently received support is the role of osmotic forces. The hypothesis has been put forward that, following the approach and contact steps and just prior to pore formation, a driving force supplied by an intragranular osmolarity increase and a concomitant water influx causes increased intramembranous tension. This then causes pore formation at the contact site [Pollard et al., 1979]. In secretory cells, particularly the adrenal chromaffin cell, the rise in intragranular osmolarity is mediated by a proton influx via an ATPase proton pump

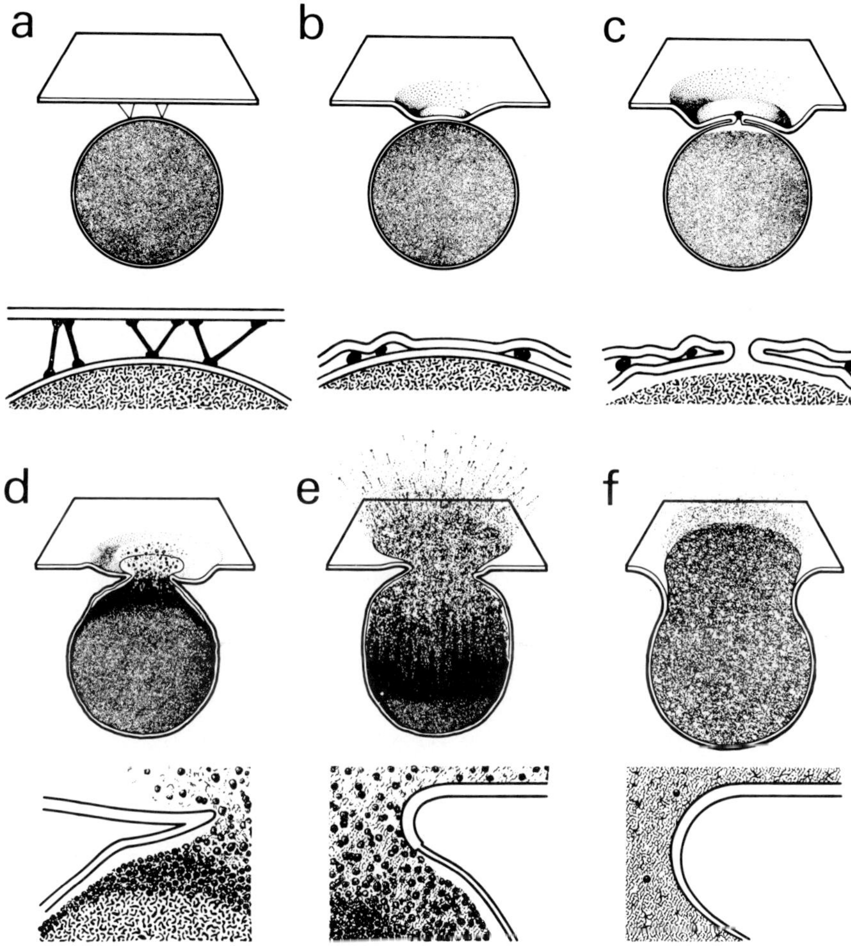

Fig. 9. Hypothetical sequence of the morphological changes that underlie exocytosis of secretory granules at the periphery of *Limulus* amebocytes. Stage a typifies unstimulated cells; b and c, cells stimulated for 1–5 sec; d, cells stimulated for 5–10 sec; e and f, cells stimulated for 10–15 sec. These times, combined with reasonable expectations about the course of exocytosis, are the basis for fitting the morphological changes described here into a sequence. The blood space around the amebocyte is at the top of each drawing. From Ornberg and Reese [1981a], with permission of The Rockefeller University Press.

and a compensatory chloride anion uptake to maintain electroneutrality. Blockers of anion transport in red cells inhibit anion uptake in chromaffin granules and the ATP-dependent lysis of isolated granules, as well as catecholamine release from stimulated chromaffin cells. The anion channel blockers are thought to mediate this effect by preventing the rise in intragranular osmolarity that results from chloride accumulation. In addition, if the extracellular osmolarity is raised by addition of sucrose such that no osmotic pressure gradient exists across the exocytotic junction, catecholamine release is inhibited. Osmotic pressure differences have also been shown to be a requirement for the "exocytosis" of artificial lipid vesicles into artificial black lipid films [Cohen et al., 1980; Zimmerberg et al., 1980]. The role of osmotic forces in amebocyte secretion has been examined with anion channel blockers. Degranulation induced by either endotoxin or the calcium inophore A23187 was inhibited by both anion channel blockers and chloride-free saline, suggesting that anions and presumably osmotic forces are required for amebocyte degranulation [Armstrong and Rickles, 1982].

Further advances in understanding secretion, using amebocytes as an experimental system, will require development of biochemical approaches to studying these cells. An isolation procedure to remove cells from plasma protein would be beneficial in the development of a release assay from which other biological studies can originate. The only release assay presently available is morphological examination, which is not only time-consuming but very nonquantitative. With a suitable assay a broad spectrum of biochemical studies of secretion could examine 1) the role of osmotic forces, 2) energetics, 3) ionic requirements, and 4) macromolecular components of endotoxin stimulation and secretion.

Many morphological issues also remain to be solved. The role of the cytoskeleton in granule movement and exocytosis is particularly important. In addition, the regenerative process of membrane recycling and granule recovery has to be examined. The current idea that amebocytes, once degranulated, never revert to secretory cells is not at all well substantiated. Finally, a careful analytical electron microscope study of the elemental distribution before and after stimulation could provide useful knowledge of the overall physiological processes of secretion. Our present understanding of the *Limulus* amebocyte is almost as primitive as *Limulus polyphemus* itself! Any field of study with respect to secretion in the amebocyte is virtually wide open.

REFERENCES

Armstrong PB, Rickles FR (1982): Endotoxin-induced degranulation of the Limulus amebocytes. Exp Cell Res 140:15–24.

Bang F (1955): A bacterial disease *Limulus polyphemus*. Bull Johns Hopkins Hosp 98:325.

Baker PF, Knight DE, Whittaker MJ (1980): Calcium and the control of exocytosis. In Siegal F (ed): "Calcium Binding Proteins." Amsterdam: Elsevier/North-Holland, pp 47–55.

Carpenter JL, Malaisse-Lagae F, Muller WA, Orci L (1977): Glucagon release from rat pancreatic islets; a combined morphological and functional approach. J Clin Invest 60:1174.

Chandler DE (1979): Quick freezing avoids specimen preparation artifacts in membrane fusion studies. In Rash JE, Hudson CS (eds): "Freeze Fracture: Methods, Artifacts, and Interpretations." New York: Raven, p 81.

Chandler DE, Heuser JE (1979): Membrane fusion during secretion; Cortical granule exocytosis in sea urchin egg as studied by quick freezing fracture. J Cell Biol 83:91–108.

Chandler DE, Heuser JE (1980): Arrest of membrane fusion events in mast cells by quick-freezing. J Cell Biol 86:666.

Chi ET, Langunoff D, Koehler JK (1976): Freeze-fracture study of mast cell secretion. Proc Natl Acad Sci USA 73:2823–2827.

Cohen FS, Zimmerberg J, Finkelstein A (1980): Fusion of phospholipid vesicles with planar phospholipid bilayer membranes. II. Incorporation of a vesicular membrane marker into the planar membrane. J Gen Physiol 75:251–270.

Douglas WW (1978): Stimulus-secretion coupling: Variations on the theme of calcium-activated exocytosis involving cellular and extracellular sources of calcium. In Ciba Foundation Symp 54, "Respiratory Tract Mucus." Amsterdam: Elsevier/Excepta Medica/North-Holland, pp 61–90.

Dumont JN, Anderson E, Winner G (1966): Some cytological characteristics of the hemocytes of *Limulus* during clotting. J Morphol 119:181–208.

Farquhar MG (1981): Membrane recycling in secretory cells: Implications for traffic of products and specialized membranes within the Golgi complex. In Hand AR, Oliver C (eds): "Methods in Cell Biology," Vol. 23, "Basic Mechanisms of Cellular Secretion." New York: Academic, pp 400–427.

Fowler V, Pollard HB: (1982): *In vitro* reconstitution of chromaffin granule-cytoskeleton interactions: Ionic factors influencing the association of F-actin with purified chromaffin granule membranes. J Cell Biochem 18:295.

Heuser JE, Llinas R (1977): "Depolarization-Release Coupling Systems in Neurons." Neurosciences Research Program Bulletin, Vol. 15. Cambridge, MA: MIT press.

Heuser JE, Reese TS, Dennis MJ, Jan Y, Jan L, Evans L (1979): Synaptic vesicle exocytosis captured by quick freezing and correlated with quantal transmitter release. J Cell Biol 81:275–300.

Holtzman E (1981): Membrane circulation: An overview: In Hand AR, Oliver C (eds): "Methods in Cell Biology," Vol 23: "Basic Mechanisms of Cellular Secretion." New York: Academic, pp 379–395.

Hopkins CR, Duncan CJ (eds) (1979): Secretory Mechanism." Symb Soc Exp Biol, Vol 33. Cambridge: Cambridge University Press.

Kalderon N, Gilula NB (1979): Membrane events involved in myoblast fusion. J Cell Biol 81:411–425.

Lawson D, Raff MC, Gomperts B, Fewtrell C, Gilula NB (1977): Molecular events during membrane fusion. A study of exocytosis in rat peritoneal mast cells. J Cell Biol 72:242–259.

Lowe DA, Richardson BP, Taylor P, Donatsch P (1976): Increasing intracellular sodium triggers calcium release from bound pools. Nature 260:337.

McGraw F, Somlyo AV, Blaustein MP (1980): Localization of calcium in presynaptic nerve terminals. An ultrastructural and electron microprobe analysis. J Cell Biol 85:228–241.

Morgan IG, Zanetta JP, Breckenbridge WC, Vincendon G, Gombos G (1974): Adult rat brain synaptic vesicles: Protein and glycoprotein composition. Biochem Soc Trans 2:249.

Murer E, Levin J, Holme R (1975): Isolation and studies of the granules of the amebocytes of *Limulus polyphemus*, the horseshoe crab. J Cell Physiol 86:533–542.

Orci L, Perrelet A, Friend DS (1977): Freeze-fracture of membrane fusions during exocytosis in pancreatic B-cells. J Cell Biol 75:23–30.

Ornberg RL, Reese TS (1979a): Secretion in *Limulus* amebocytes is by exocytosis. In Cohen E (ed): "Progress in Clinical and Biological Research," Vol. 29: "Biomedical Application of the Horseshoe Crab (Limulidae)." New York: Alan R. Liss, Inc., pp 125–130.

Ornberg RL, Reese TS (1979b): Artifacts of freezing in Limulus amebocytes. In Rash JE, Hudson CS (eds): "Freeze Fracture: Methods, Artifacts, and Interpretations." New York: Raven, pp 89–97.

Ornberg RL, Reese TS (1981a): Beginning of exocytosis in *Limulus* amebocytes captured by quick freezing. J Cell Biol 90:49–54.

Ornberg RL, Reese TS (1981b): Comparison of compound with plasmalemmal exocytosis in *Limulus* amebocytes. In Hand AR, Oliver C (eds): "Methods in Cell Biology," Vol 23: "Basic Mechanism in Cellular Secretion." New York: Academic, pp 301–311.

Ornberg RL, Reese TS (1981c): Quick freezing and freeze-substitution for X-ray microanalysis of calcium. In Hutchinson TE, Somlyo AP (eds): "Microprobe Analysis of Biological Systems." New York: Academic, pp 213–223.

Palade GE (1975): Intracellular aspects of protein synthesis. Science 189:347–358.

Palade GE, Bruns RR (1968): Structural modulations of plasmalemmal vesicles. J Cell Biol 37:633–648.

Pinto da Silva P, Nogueira ML (1977): Membrane fusion during secretion. A hypothesis based on electron microscopic observation of *Phytophthora palmivora* zoospores during encystment. J Cell Biol 73:161–181.

Pollard HB, Pazoles CJ, Creutz CE, Ziner O (1979): The chromaffin granule and possible mechanisms of exocytosis. Int Rev Cytol 58:159–197.

Puszkin S, Kochwa S (1974): Regulation of neurotransmitter released by a complex of actin with relaxing protein isolated from rat brain synaptosomes. J Biol Chem 249:7711.

Rohlich P (1975): Membrane-associated actin filaments in the cortical cytoplasm of the rat mast cell. Exp Cell Res 93:293–298.

Rohlich P, Anderson P, Unvas B (1971): Electron microscope observations on compound 48/80-induced degranulation in rat mast cells. J Cell Biol 51:465.

Rubin RP (1982): "Calcium and Cellular Secretory Mechanisms." New York: Plenum.

Satir B, Schooley C, Satir P (1973): Membrane fusion in a model system. Mucocyst secretion in Tetrahymena. J Cell Biol 56:153–176.

Schwila M (1982): Action of cytocholasin D on cytoskeletal networks. J Cell Biol 92:79–91.

Smith JE, Reese TS (1980): Use of aldehyde fixatives to determine the rate of synaptic transmitter release. J Exp Biol 89:19–29.

Tanaka Y, DeCamilli P, Meldolesi J (1980): Membrane interactions between secretion granules and plasmalemma in three exocrine glands. J Cell Biol 84:438–453.

Theodosis DT, Dreiffus JJ, Orci L (1978): A freeze-fracture study of membrane events during neurohypophysial secretion. J Cell Biol 78:542–553.

COAGULATION

Blood Cells of Marine Invertebrates: Experimental Systems in Cell Biology and Comparative Physiology, pages 145–163

Chapter Five
The Role of Amebocytes in the Blood Coagulation Mechanism of the Horseshoe Crab *Limulus polyphemus*

Jack Levin

Departments of Laboratory Medicine and Medicine, University of California School of Medicine, San Francisco, California 94143 and the Marine Biological Laboratory, Woods Hole, Massachusetts 02543

INTRODUCTION

The amebocyte is the only type of circulating cell in the blood of *Limulus polyphemus*, the American horseshoe crab.* It is nucleated and its cytoplasm is packed with granules. When *Limulus* blood is shed or exposed to bacterial endotoxins, there is rapid aggregation of the amebocytes. Aggregation is associated with marked changes in cell shape, which include flattening with an apparent increase in cell diameter, development of long processes that extend from cell to cell, and striking degranulation [Levin and Bang, 1964b; Armstrong and Rickles, 1982]. Morphological descriptions and pictures of amebocytes that demonstrate many of these changes are presented in Chapter Three by Armstrong. As emphasized appropriately by Armstrong, previous investigators incorrectly concluded that there were many types of cells in the blood of *Limulus*, because they observed preparations after the amebocytes had been exposed to foreign surfaces and bacterial endotoxins and accordingly had become altered in content and shape.

*The term *horseshoe crab* is a misnomer in the zoological sense because *Limulus* is not a crustacean, but a member of the class Merostomata (subclass, Xiphosura). The designation *amebocyte* as used in this chapter refers *only* to the circulating cell present in the hemolymph of the horseshoe crab. It should not be inferred that all invertebrate amebocytes are similar cells, since the term *amebocyte* has been utilized generically to identify a wide variety of cells.

However, two types of amebocytes have been described in the Japanese horseshoe crab, *Tachypleus tridentatus*, based on immunocytochemical studies. Shishikura et al. [1977] reported that two different patterns of localization of the clottable protein were detected; one group of cells demonstrated the coagulogen within the cytoplasmic granules, whereas the other type apparently had the coagulogen localized in extragranular cytoplasmic sites. However, these observations may have resulted from alterations in the cells during preparation, and this work should be repeated, particularly since these same workers failed to demonstrate similar findings in *Limulus* [Shishikura and Sekiguchi, 1979].

Another type of cell, designated *cyanoblast*, has been described by Fahrenbach [1970] as rarely occurring in the vascular circulation about the compound eyes. His study demonstrated cells that appeared to contain crystals of hemocyanin in the cytoplasm. However, no quantitative data about the frequency of the cyanoblast in either this localized circulation or in the general circulation were presented, and it is unlikely that the cyanoblast could account for the high concentration of hemocyanin that is present in the blood of *Limulus*.

Although *Limulus* has been used as a source of blood for studies of blood coagulation in invertebrates since the first part of the twentieth century, the exact role of the amebocyte and the source of the clottable protein in *Limulus* remained unknown until approximately 20 years ago. Halliburton [1885], Tait [1911], and Hardy [1892], who studied coagulation in several Crustacea, concluded that the circulating cells provided a "fibrin ferment" (a procoagulant substance that coagulated a fibrinogen-like material in the plasma). However, in contrast, Loeb [1904, 1910], Howell [1885], and Rustum Maluf [1939], all of whom had specifically investigated coagulation in *Limulus*, suggested that the clottable protein was contained in amebocytes and was not present in plasma. The studies of Levin and Bang [1964a, 1968] firmly established for the first time that the amebocytes of *Limulus* contain all of the components of the coagulation system of *Limulus* blood. Not only the clottable protein but all other factors required for coagulation are contained within amebocytes. Cell-free plasma does not clot and is not required for coagulation [Levin and Bang, 1964a; 1968]. These studies provided the basis for an extensive series of investigations in my laboratory and other laboratories that have provided important insights into the blood coagulation mechanism of *Limulus* (and related species of horseshoe crabs), the role of amebocytes in blood coagulation, and the relationships between the blood coagulation mechanism in *Limulus*, which is a primitive invertebrate, and blood coagulation in mammalian systems.

Although the amebocytes of *Limulus* have many physiological functions, including phagocytosis, bacteriostasis, and hemostasis, the multiple functions of this type of cell have been thoroughly reviewed in this volume (see chapter by Armstrong). Accordingly, this chapter will focus on the critical role of the amebocyte in blood coagulation in *Limulus*, and the effects of bacterial endotoxins on this cell and the coagulation mechanism.

EXPERIMENTAL STUDIES

Before considering investigations of blood coagulation in *Limulus*, it is important to discriminate between aggregation with associated release of cellular constituents and true blood coagulation. When blood is removed from *Limulus*, the amebocytes immediately aggregate and subsequently release their contents [Levin and Bang, 1964a,b; 1968]. Although the mechanism(s) by which this occurs in the absence of bacterial endotoxin remains unknown, the speed with which amebocytes aggregate is much greater than is the case for platelets, the comparable cell in mammalian blood. Amebocyte aggregation is not prevented by nonwettable surfaces or by the usual anticoagulants (i.e., sodium citrate, ethylene diamine tetraacetic acid [EDTA], heparin). However, in the absence of bacterial endotoxin, although the components of the coagulation mechanism are released into the medium surrounding the amebocytes, true blood coagulation does not occur. This is an important distinction, not only in regard to an understanding of hemostasis but because it makes possible the study of true blood coagulation as opposed to the preceding step of aggregation and release. Armstrong and Rickles [1982] have claimed that following what they describe as spontaneous degranulation, gelation of materials released by living amebocytes can occur in the absence of detectable concentrations of bacterial endotoxin.

Initial studies of blood coagulation in *Limulus* revealed that the entire coagulation mechanism was released following aggregation of the amebocytes [Levin and Bang, 1964a]. The first series of modern studies indicated that cell-free plasma contained no factors necessary for blood coagulation [Levin and Bang, 1968]. Further progress was aided considerably by the use of N-ethyl maleimide (NEM) to prevent amebocyte aggregation [Levin and Bang, 1968]. This permitted the careful washing of amebocytes without their disruption. Successful utilization of NEM was based on the previous observations of Bryan et al. [1964].

The first description of the fractionation of amebocyte lysate (the term used to describe extracts of amebocytes) clearly indicated the presence of a heat-stable clottable protein and another fraction that contained a relatively heat-labile enzymatic activity [Young et al., 1972]. The rate of the reaction between endotoxin and amebocyte lysate was dependent upon the concentration of the enzymatic fraction [Young et al., 1972] and on the concentration of endotoxin [Levin and Bang, 1968]. Importantly, the enzymatic activity was inhibited by diisopropyl fluorophosphate, para-chloromercuribenzoate, and para-chloro-mercuriphenyl sulfonate, suggesting that the enzymatic activity depended upon serine hydroxyl and sulfhydryl groups. These observations were subsequently confirmed by other investigators [Seid and Liu, 1980]. The reaction between endotoxin and the crude enzymatic fraction was temperature and pH-dependent. Endotoxin apparently did not react directly with the clottable protein. The gel that formed was insoluble in 8 M urea or 2 M 2-mercaptoethanol. The data were correctly interpreted by Young et al. [1972] as suggesting that endotoxin activated an enzyme that then gelled the clottable protein contained in amebocyte lysate.

Enzymatic Mediation of Blood Coagulation in *Limulus*

The initial investigations of blood coagulation in *Limulus* by Young et al. [1972] have been extended and the enzymatic nature of the blood coagulation mechanism in *Limulus* has been confirmed. Amebocyte lysate obtained from *Limulus polyphemus* has been additionally fractionated, by heparin-Sepharose chromatography, into four components. Major coagulation factors (i.e., the proclotting enzyme, coagulogen, and proclotting enzyme-activating factor precursor [proactivator]) were eluted in separate fractions [Nakamura and Levin, 1982a]. The conversion of proactivator to its active form (activator) is an endotoxin-mediated reaction and can be inhibited by polymyxin B. Optimal pH for the activation of the proactivator and the proclotting enzyme are different [Nakamura and Levin, 1982a]. The activator can be inhibited by benzamidine, leupeptin, soybean trypsin inhibitor, and diisopropyl fluorophosphate, suggesting that the activator (like the proclotting enzyme) is a trypsin-type, serine protease. These studies confirmed the preliminary observations of Ohki et al. [1980], based on lysates from *Tachypleus tridentatus*, the Japanese horseshoe crab, that demonstrated the presence of a factor required for the ultimate activation of the proclotting enzyme. Demonstration of an enzyme(s) required for activation of the proclotting enzyme is at variance with the conclusion of Tai and Liu [1977] that endotoxin directly activates the proclotting enzyme.

Other studies have revealed that the proclotting enzyme-activating factor (designated *activator*) has a molecular weight of approximately 50,000, and consists of two identical subunits [Nakamura and Levin, 1982b]. Importantly, the results indicate that the activator molecule does not form a macromolecular complex with bacterial endotoxin (lipopolysaccharide, LPS) but that limited proteolysis occurs during LPS-mediated activation of proactivator. Related investigations have suggested that conversion of the proactivator to an active form is accomplished by another newly described proteolytic enzyme, which appears to be an LPS-dependent protease and is capable of hydrolyzing not only the synthetic substrate S-2222 (as does the clotting

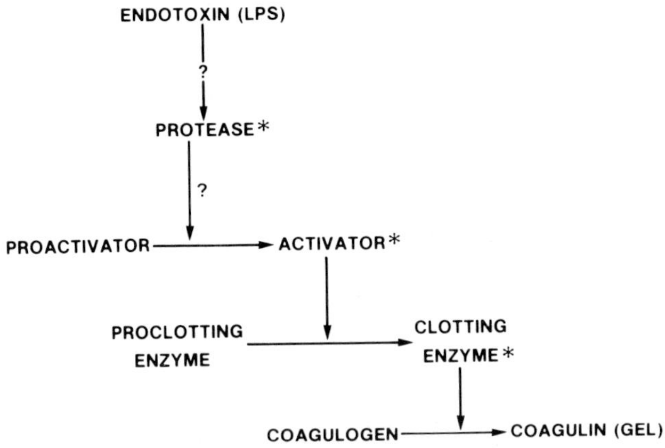

Fig. 1. Activation of blood coagulation in the horseshoe crab by endotoxin. Each of the three enzymes that have been identified is a serine protease (indicated by the asterisks). This enzymatic cascade resembles that which has been described in a variety of mammalian coagulation systems. See Nakamura and Levin [1982a,b] and Torano et al. [1984] for additional data.

enzyme), but also S-2160 and S-2238 [Nakamura and Levin, 1982b]. In contrast, the clotting enzyme hydrolyzes synthetic substrates S-2222, S-2237, S-2422, and S-2423, but not S-2160 and S-2238 [Torano et al., 1984]. All of the synthetic substrates that are susceptible to the clotting enzyme contain arginine and glycine in their P1 and P2 positions, respectively. Therefore, at least three serine proteases have been identified that are required for the activation of *Limulus* blood coagulation by endotoxin [Nakamura and Levin, 1982a,b; Torano et al., 1984]. Current concepts about the biochemistry of coagulation in *Limulus* are shown in Figure 1.

A major technical difficulty in the fractionation of amebocyte lysate is the marked sensitivity of the coagulation mechanism to bacterial endotoxins, which are ubiquitous. Therefore, great care must be taken to establish endotoxin-free conditions for at least some of the purification steps, in order to prepare unactivated fractions that can be experimentally evaluated in a manner that allows the establishment of correct conclusions. Both NaOH in ethanol [Nakamura and Levin, 1982a] and sodium metaperiodate [Tomasulo et al., 1975] have been used successfully to prepare endotoxin-free chromatographic systems.

The time course of generation of clotting enzyme activity in a system consisting of partially purified proclotting enzyme, proactivator, and endotoxin (line A) or a mixture of the proenzyme and activator (line B) is shown in Figure 2. The latter combination produced slightly faster generation of

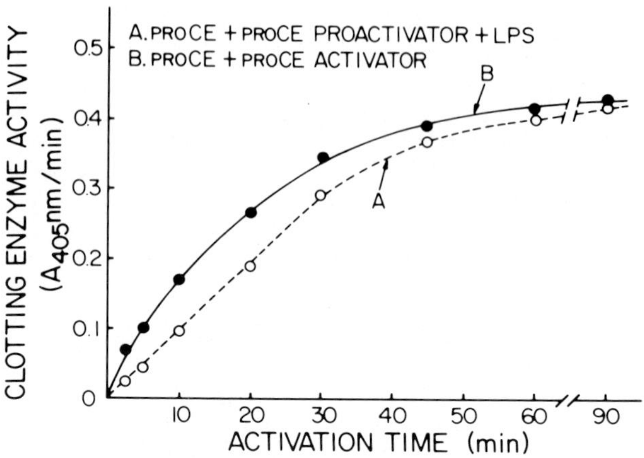

Fig. 2. Time course of clotting enzyme (CE) generation. A (○). Activation mixture: 50 μl of partially purified proclotting enzyme (380 μg protein per 1 ml), 50 μl proactivator (45 μg protein per 1 ml), 50 μl endotoxin (0.1 μg/ml), and 50 μl of 0.1 M Tris-HCl (pH 7.5); B(●). Activation mixture: 50 μl proclotting enzyme and 100 μl of a previously incubated mixture consisting of proactivator and endotoxin (0.1 μg/ml) at a volume ratio of 1:1. Both activation mixtures were incubated for the indicated times, and then generated clotting enzyme activity was assayed with the synthetic chromogenic substrate S-2222. From Nakamura and Levin [1982a] with permission.

clotting enzyme activity than the former, but no initial latent period preceded activation in either reaction. However, a significant initial lag was observed in an activation sample that contained crude proclotting enzyme contaminated by coagulogen [Nakamura and Levin, 1982a]. These results indicated that the latent period observed in a similar reaction mixture by Young et al. [1972] was due to the presence of the coagulogen.

Activation of the proclotting enzyme by other proteases. Different types of proteases were used to examine potential mechanisms of activation of the proclotting enzyme, and the results are summarized in Table I. Activation of proclotting enzyme was observed only at high concentrations of trypsin. Concentrations of trypsin of less than 2 μg/ml, i.e., so-called catalytic amounts with an enzyme:substrate ratio of less than 1:100 (w/w), were ineffective. Interestingly, no significant inactivation of proclotting enzyme was produced by excess concentrations of trypsin, or by high concentrations of α-chymotrypsin, plasmin, or papain [Nakamura and Levin, 1982a], suggesting that the proenzyme has considerable structural stability.

The effect of β-(1,3)-glucans. β-(1,3)-glucans are carbohydrates obtained from fungal cell walls. It has been reported that a carboxymethylated β-(1,3)-D-glucan (CMPS) activates the clotting enzyme in amebocyte lysate via an

TABLE I. Effect of Various Proteases on Proclotting Enzyme Activation

Protease	Concentration	Activation
Thrombin	10–30[a]	No
Urokinase	10–100[a]	No
Trypsin	4–100[b]	Yes
Plasmin	4–400[b]	No
Papain	4–400[b]	No
α-Chymotrypsin	4–100[b]	No

Mixtures consisting of partially purified proclotting enzyme, indicated amounts of protease, and 0.05 M Tris-HCl (pH 7.5) were incubated for 60 min at 37°C. Samples then were assayed with synthetic substrate S-2222 for clotting enzyme activity. Modified from Nakamura and Levin [1982a], with permission.
[a]Units per milliliter.
[b]Micrograms per milliliter.

initial mechanism that is distinct from that which is activated by bacterial endotoxin [Kakinuma et al., 1981; Morita et al., 1981]. The reagent was described as being pyrogen-free and apparently did not produce fever when injected into rabbits. The data were interpreted as indicating that a factor not involved in the endotoxin mediated pathway was required for the reaction between the carboxymethylated glucan and amebocyte lysate [Kakinuma et al., 1981; Morita et al., 1981]. However, unlike endotoxin, CMPS demonstrated an optimal concentration, above which gelation of lysate or activation of the proclotting enzyme did not occur. Furthermore, some of the data indicated that the apparent activation of the proclotting enzyme by CMPS is much less than can be accomplished with endotoxin [Kakinuma et al., 1981]; and other experiments in which CMPS and endotoxin were added sequentially to a preparation of the proclotting enzyme are not consistent with the concept that the gelation observed with CMPS is necessarily the result of the proclotting enzyme [Kakinuma et al., 1981]. More recent experiments have indicated that high concentrations of CMPS cause precipitation of at least some of the proteins contained in amebocyte lysate and importantly that other β-(1,3)-D-glucans do not activate *Limulus* amebocyte lysate (Soderhall, Levin, and Armstrong, unpublished observations). Therefore, the biological significance of the effects of a carboxymethylated β-(1,3)-D-glucan remains unclear, and further study is required to elucidate the mechanism by which preparations of CMPS react with amebocyte lysate.

Studies of the granules of the amebocytes. It has been possible to isolate granules from the cytoplasm of the amebocytes of *Limulus*, following disruption of cells obtained from blood that had been drawn into 2 mM propranolol.

The granules were subsequently purified by centrifugation through sucrose gradients. Transmission and scanning electron microscopy of the granules revealed round or ovoid particles. However, only one type of granule appeared to be present, although this has not been completely documented. Extracts of the granules were prepared by freezing and thawing granule preparations in distilled water [Murer et al., 1975].

Polyacrylamide gel electrophoresis demonstrated patterns similar to those observed with amebocyte lysate. Importantly, extracts of the granules were gelled by bacterial endotoxin, indicating that the granules, which pack the cytoplasm of these cells, contain all of the factors required for the coagulation of blood, including the clottable protein. Shishikura and Sekiguchi [1979] have confirmed that the granules of *Limulus* amebocytes contain the clottable protein. The intracellularly localized coagulation system is released from amebocytes when their granules rupture during cell aggregation [Levin and Bang, 1964b] (see also Chapter Three by Armstrong).

The technique developed for the preparation of intact granules resulted from evaluation of a series of adrenergic blockers. Under strictly defined conditions, propranolol allows disruption of the cell membrane without concomitant disruption of the cytoplasmic granules. However, not all preparative runs are successful, and suspensions of granules often clump during centrifugation in the second sucrose gradient [Murer et al., 1975].

The *Limulus* Amebocyte Lysate Test for Bacterial Endotoxin

Our initial experimental studies of blood coagulation in *Limulus* were undertaken to evaluate the effects of bacterial endotoxin on blood coagulation in this ancient invertebrate and to determine similarities between *Limulus* amebocytes and mammalian blood platelets [Levin and Bang, 1964a,b]. Studies were undertaken because of the previous observations of Bang [1956] that indicated activation of the blood coagulation mechanism in *Limulus* by a pathogenic marine Vibrio species (a gram-negative rod) or heat-stable toxin (an endotoxin) prepared from this bacterium. It is pertinent to this volume that both Frederik Bang [Bang, 1956; Levin and Bang, 1964a,b; 1968] and Leo Loeb [Loeb, 1904, 1910] carried out their studies of blood coagulation in *Limulus* at the Marine Biological Laboratory. After establishing that all of the components of the blood coagulation mechanism in *Limulus* were contained in the amebocytes, the marked sensitivity of this coagulation system to endotoxin and its applicability for the assay of bacterial endotoxins was recognized [Levin and Bang, 1968]. Subsequent investigations from our laboratory [Levin et al., 1970, 1972; Cooper et al., 1971; Tomasulo et al., 1977; Butler et al., 1973; Koster et al., 1978; Levin, 1982] and by others [Elin et al., 1976; Tomasulo, 1979; Rojas-Corona et al., 1969; Young, 1975] established that results of the Limulus Test correlated with other previously established bioassays for endotoxin and that the Limulus Test was useful in a variety of laboratory and clinical settings. The Limulus Test has been successfully utilized for the detection of endotoxin in intravenous solutions, drugs, vaccines, radioisotopes, plasma protein fractions, water supplies, and medical devices; it is also used for the diagnosis of gram-negative bacterial meningitis.

An important application of the Limulus Test is in the detection and quantification of endotoxins in a wide variety of biological reagents that are used in many experimental systems [Rickles et al., 1977, 1979]. Endotoxin is present in many commercially available and extensively used mitogens [Rickles et al., 1977, 1979]. Since endotoxin is itself a mitogen, many studies of mitogens have actually determined the combined effects of the mitogen plus endotoxin. Similarly, erythropoietin is used extensively in studies of hematopoiesis in vitro. We have shown that most batches of erythropoietin are heavily contaminated with endotoxin [Spivak and Levin, 1977; Zuckerman et al., 1979]. Since endotoxins can suppress erythropoiesis, the use of many preparations of erythropoietin results in experiments that simultaneously test the stimulatory effect of erythropoietin and the suppressive effect

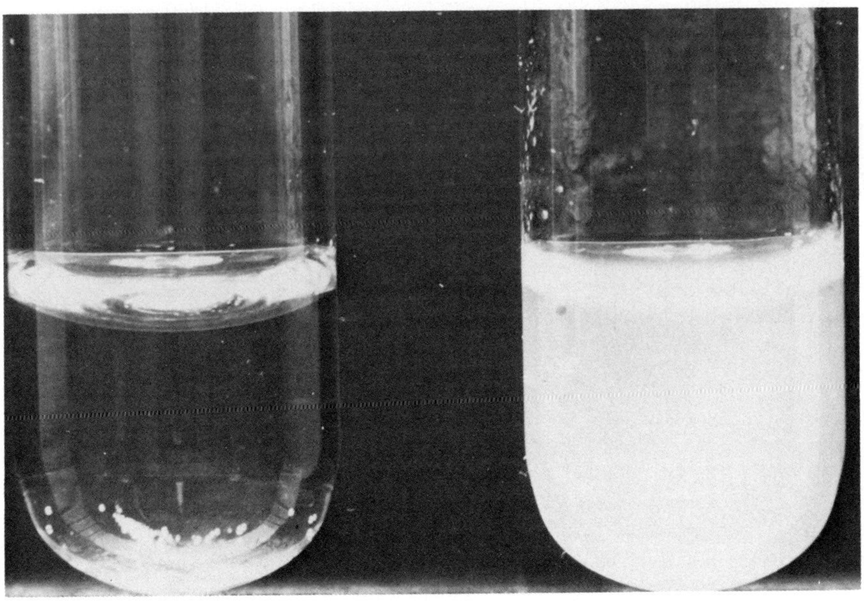

Fig. 3. Amebocyte lysate prepared from *Limulus polyphemus* [Levin and Bang, 1968]. Before addition of bacterial endotoxin, amebocyte lysate is a clear colorless liquid (left). After addition of bacterial endotoxin, a solid gel forms (right).

of endotoxin. Therefore, accurate quantitative relationships between erythropoietin and erythropoiesis cannot be established in the presence of endotoxin. Importantly, it is possible to remove endotoxins from preparations of certain reagents by adsorption with *Limulus* amebocyte lysate [Zuckerman et al., 1979].

Amebocyte lysate, prepared from *Limulus polyphemus* as described previously [Levin and Bang, 1968], is shown in Figure 3. The change from a clear sol to an opaque gel, following the addition of endotoxin, can be utilized to quantitatively measure the reaction between bacterial endotoxin and *Limulus* lysate and to determine the concentration of endotoxin that is present in a solution (Fig. 4) [Levin and Bang, 1968; Levin et al., 1970; Cooper et al., 1971]. Synthetic chromogenic substrates (see above) also are utilized to provide a quantitative endpoint for the Limulus Test [Nakamura et al., 1977; Harada-Suzuki et al., 1982; Homma et al., 1982]. Collected papers that describe various applications of the Limulus Test and methods for its performance are available [Cohen et al., 1979; Watson et al., 1982].

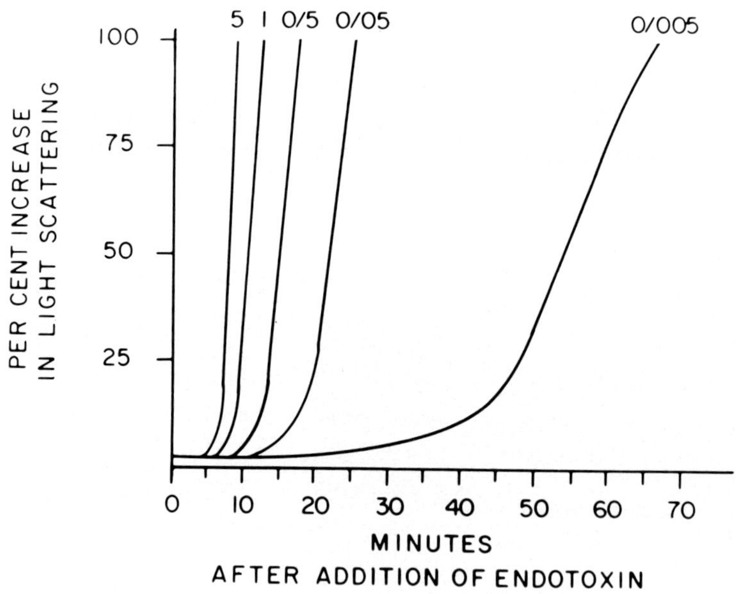

Fig. 4. Increase in light scattering after addition of endotoxin to amebocyte lysate. The record is a direct tracing of continuous recordings of increase in light scattering. Each reaction mixture consisted of 0.9 ml of amebocyte lysate and 0.1 ml of bacterial endotoxin. The final endotoxin concentration in each reaction mixture (μg/ml) is shown along the top. One hundred percent represented the maximum increase in light scattering observed 24 hr after addition of 5 μg/ml of *E. coli* endotoxin to amebocyte lysate. From Levin et al. [1970], with permission.

DISCUSSION

Studies of blood coagulation in *Limulus* have revealed that the coagulation mechanism is present within the granules of the amebocytes, the only type of circulating blood cell. Following aggregation and degranulation of amebocytes, the components of the coagulation mechanism are released into the blood or other suspending medium. This has allowed detailed analysis of this primitive coagulation mechanism. Currently available data indicate that the coagulation system of *Limulus* consists of a clottable protein (designated coagulogen) and a series of enzymes, the sequential activation of which ultimately results in an activated clotting enzyme, which then partially proteolyzes the coagulogen to produce coagulin. Finally, gelation occurs. To date, three enzymes have been identified as playing a role in blood coagulation in *Limulus*, and all are serine proteases [Nakamura and Levin, 1982a,b; Torano et al., 1984; Seid and Liu, 1980]. An essentially identical coagulation mechanism is present in *Tachypleus tridentatus*, the species of horseshoe crab found in Japanese waters.

Since horseshoe crabs live in an environment that contains many gram-negative marine bacteria, the exquisite sensitivity of both amebocytes and the blood coagulation mechanism of these animals to bacterial endotoxins provides the basis for an effective defense mechanism against these organisms and a component of gram-negative bacteria, i.e., bacterial endotoxin or LPS, that produces a variety of pathophysiological effects in many animals. Horseshoe crabs are not unique in the response of their coagulation systems to endotoxin, since a review of the pertinent literature has revealed many other examples of invertebrates with coagulation systems that are activated by endotoxin or bacteria [Levin, 1967] (Table II). Therefore, it is likely that the response of the blood coagulation mechanism, subsequent to activation of the circulating blood cells (when pertinent), to bacteria and their products represents a very ancient defense mechanism (Cyanobacteria, among the most ancient of bacteria, are gram-negative organisms).

Amebocytes and Platelets

Limulus amebocytes not only contain the blood coagulation mechanism, but also contribute to hemostasis by their ability to clump and seal disruptions in the vascular system. In addition, these cells are capable of phagocytosis [Armstrong and Levin, 1979] and possess bactericidal activity [Nachum et al., 1979]. The importance of a factor or factors in plasma contributing to the bactericidal effects of a factor contained in amebocytes requires additional evaluation [Shirodkar et al., 1960; Furman and Pistole, 1976; Pistole and Britko, 1978]. The *Limulus* amebocyte probably represents an example of the precursor of the cell lines that in mammals have diverged to generate white blood cells (primarily involved in antibacterial activities) and throm-

TABLE II. Initiation of Coagulation in Invertebrates by Endotoxin or Bacteria

Animal	Agent
Limulus polyphemus	*Vibrio sp.*
	E. coli
	Shigella
Sacculina carcini	*Vibrio sp.*
	E. coli
	Gaffkya (?)
	Gram-negative bacillus
Homarus americanus	*Shigella*
	Gaffkya
Carcinus maenus	Gram-negative bacillus
Maia squinado	Gram-positive bacillus
Penaeid shrimp	*Vibrio alginolyticus*
	Vibrio anguillarum
	Aeromonas sp.

Modified from Levin [1967], with permission. The original citations from which most of these data were collected are listed in Levin [1967]. See also Stewart [1975] and Lightner and Lewis [1975].

TABLE III. Comparison of *Limulus* Amebocytes and Mammalian Platelets

Characteristics or functions	*Limulus* amebocyte	Mammalian platelet
Hemostasis	Essential	Essential
Blood coagulation	Essential	Ancillary
Clottable protein	Yes	Yes
Nucleus	Yes	No
Viscous metamorphosis	Yes (?)	Yes
Cellular processes	Yes	Yes
Granules	Yes	Yes
Response to endotoxin	Yes	Yes
Phagocytosis	Yes	Yes
Antibacterial function	Yes	Yes
Motility	Yes	Yes

bocytes or platelets (primarily involved in hemostasis and blood coagulation). However, in mammals, the blood coagulation mechanism consists of a series of soluble proteins present in the plasma, although some coagulation factors are associated, at least in part, with platelets and their subcellular organelles [Walsh, 1981; Rao et al., 1982]. It seems likely that hemostatic cells in a variety of species release some of their cytoplasmic contents concomitantly with their physiological actions [Belamarich et al., 1973]. It is noteworthy that platelets are capable of phagocytosis and have a weak bactericidal activity [Levin, 1976; Lewis et al., 1976]. They contain endotoxin-binding substances [Springer and Adye, 1975] and have been shown to interact with bacteria, endotoxin, and viruses [Clawson, 1973; MacIntyre et al., 1977; Levin, 1984]. Under certain conditions, platelets demonstrate a chemotactic response and migrate [Loewenhaupt et al., 1973]. None of these functions would seem to be necessary for the current role of platelets in mammalian hemostasis. Accordingly, it is likely that some of the capabilities of mammalian platelets represent the residua of functions originally present in the more primitive and multicompetent cells from which mammalian blood cells are derived. Table III summarizes and compares some of the functional abilities of *Limulus* amebocytes and human platelets.

Evolution of Blood Coagulation and Relationships Between *Limulus* and Mammalian Coagulation

An important aspect of our increasing knowledge of the basis for the reaction between amebocyte lysate and endotoxin has been recognition of the remarkable similarities between the biochemistry of coagulation in *Limulus* (and *Tachypleus)*, an ancient invertebrate, and mammalian blood coagulation. Our information about coagulation in *Limulus* has been importantly complemented by extensive data obtained from *Tachypleus tridentatus*, a species of horseshoe crab present in the waters adjacent to Japan [Cohen et al., 1979; Shishikura et al., 1983; Nakamura et al., 1982]. It has become apparent that a series of enzymes are responsible for the ultimate clotting of the coagulogen (clottable protein) in the blood of the horseshoe crab and that, like the comparable cascade of enzymes involved in mammalian blood coagulation, the currently identified enzymes are serine proteases [Young et al., 1972; Tai and Liu, 1977; Nakamura and Levin, 1982a,b; Torano et al., 1984; Nakamura et al., 1982]. Synthetic substrates developed for the assay of mammalian coagulation enzymes not only can be utilized for the detection of enzymes required for the coagulation of the blood of the horseshoe crab, but also to distinguish between the various enzymes involved in horseshoe crab coagulation, because of the relative specificities of the latter for different substrates [Nakamura and Levin, 1982b; Torano et al., 1984].

The enzyme responsible for the ultimate step in blood coagulation in *Limulus** and *Tachypleus** not only hydrolyzes the synthetic substrate S-2222, used to detect mammalian Factor X_a, but activates mammalian prothrombin, resulting in the formation of active α-thrombin (just as Factor X_a

*Although complete data are not available for both *Limulus* and *Tachypleus*, the assumption has been made that the coagulation systems of these species are basically similar.

activates prothrombin) [Nakamura et al., 1982]. The *Limulus* clotting enzyme hydrolyzes synthetic substrates that have arginine and glycine in their P1 and P2 positions, respectively [Torano et al., 1984]; and the clotting enzyme of *Tachypleus* cleaves an Arg-Gly bond in the coagulogen [Takagi et al., 1979a]. Recently acquired information about the enzymes required for the coagulation of horseshoe crab blood adds new facts to what we already know about the evolutionary relationships of the serine proteases involved in hemostasis [Hewett-Emmett et al., 1981; de Haen et al., 1975]. Amazingly, although the coagulogens of the four species of horseshoe crabs are single-chain molecules with molecular weights ranging from approximately 15,000 to 24,000, depending on the technique used for measurement and the specific species studied [Shishikura et al., 1983; Nakamura et al., 1980; Tai et al., 1977], and are much smaller than mammalian fibrinogen, the partial proteolysis produced by the reaction between coagulogen and the clotting enzyme results in a proteolytic peptide that has remarkable sequence homology with Rhesus monkey fibrinopeptide B [Takagi et al., 1979a]. Another example of remarkable conservatism is demonstrated by the observation that horseshoe crab coagulogen also contains an amino acid sequence that is homologous with platelet Factor 4 [Takagi et al., 1979b]. However, despite the similarities described, the term *invertebrate fibrinogen* is not appropriate to describe a family of proteins that are so clearly different from mammalian fibrinogen (e.g., the low molecular weight of the coagulogens and the different subunit structures). Collectively, the data suggest that horseshoe crab coagulogen and fibrinogen are derived from a common ancestor or that, alternatively, fibrinogen is derived from horseshoe crab coagulogen. Studies of the evolution of fibrinogen molecules have indicated that the lobster (a true Crustacean) produces a clot by a single enzymatic step that cross-links but does not proteolize the clottable protein of that animal [Doolittle, 1970].

Despite the great development of hemostasis during evolution, there remain striking homologies and similarities between the coagulation mechanism in the horseshoe crab and mammalian blood coagulation. (Collections of references for the comparative physiology of blood coagulation are available [Belamarich, 1976; Macfarlane, 1970; Ratcliffe and Rowley, 1979; Spurling, 1981]). Although coagulation has become extracellular and more complex in higher animals, the activation of blood coagulation in mammals by endotoxin may be derived, in part, from the more primitive mechanism that also serves to control gram-negative infection in the horseshoe crab. A more complete understanding of blood coagulation in the horseshoe crab will provide additional insights into the evolution of blood coagulation mechanisms.

PROBLEMS FOR FUTURE WORK

Although much has been learned about amebocytes and blood coagulation in the horseshoe crab during the last 20 years, as is appropriate, much remains to be understood. Amebocytes aggregate very rapidly, even in the absence of bacterial endotoxin. Nonwettable surfaces do not prevent this phenomenon, which occurs much more rapidly than with mammalian platelets. The membrane of this interesting cell deserves additional study.

Unpublished investigations in our laboratory have indicated that the production of amebocytes is not continuous. Administration of a variety of isotopically labeled amino acids failed to result in detectable isotope in circulating amebocytes. Furthermore, repeated bleeding of *Limuli* during a 4- to 6-week period in July and August results in blood that is essentially devoid of amebocytes. Similarly, hemocyanin disappears and is not replaced. Yet the animals behave normally and do not appear sick or lethargic. When and how are amebocytes replaced (? prior to molting)? How do the animals transport oxygen to tissues (both in and out of water) in the absence of significant levels of circulating hemocyanin, which normally is the dominant plasma protein? Where are amebocytes produced? Although there are many anatomical and physiological atlases that describe *Limulus*, all fail to mention the anatomical location of the site of amebocyte production. There is no evidence that circulating amebocytes are capable of proliferation. What are the bases of the feedback mechanisms that one would expect to be necessary for monitoring the two important physiological functions of oxygen transport and hemostasis?

In regard to the blood coagulation mechanism, the initial reaction between bacterial endotoxin and the coagulation cascade has still not been described. Does endotoxin complex with a factor, which then becomes capable of activating another enzyme? There is no precedent for endotoxin acting enzymatically. Are there other factors in the marine environment that are capable of triggering coagulation in addition to endotoxin? Insight into the mechanism by which endotoxin activates blood coagulation in the horseshoe crab will almost certainly provide important information about the mechanism(s) by which endotoxin activates other physiological cascade systems in mammals, e.g., the blood coagulation, complement, and kallikrein systems.

It will be worthwhile to search for other suitable invertebrates with coagulation systems that respond to bacterial endotoxins in order to gain additional information about this interesting and probably common response to our environment. Such studies also will provide data concerning the evolution of blood coagulation, especially the shift of the clottable protein and other key factors from cellular sites to the plasma. One can be certain that future studies of marine invertebrates will continue to contribute to our understanding of human disease [Bang, 1975].

ACKNOWLEDGMENTS

This study was supported in part by research grant HL 31035 from the National Heart, Lung and Blood Institute, National Institutes of Health, Bethesda, Maryland, and by the Veterans Administration.

REFERENCES

Armstrong PB, Levin J (1979): In vitro phagocytosis by *Limulus* blood cells. J Invertebr Pathol 34:145–151.

Armstrong PB, Rickles FR (1982): Endotoxin-induced degranulation of the *Limulus* amebocyte. Exp Cell Res 140:15–24.

Bang FB (1956): A bacterial disease of *Limulus polyphemus.* Bull Johns Hopkins Hosp 98:325–351.

Bang FB (1975): Comparative pathology of marine invertebrates and the study of human disease. J Pediatr 87:1062–1066.

Belamarich FA (1976): Hemostasis in animals other than mammals: The role of cells. Prog Hemost Thromb 3:191–209.

Belamarich FA, Stiller RA, Shepro D (1973): The release reaction: Is it a common mechanism in all types of hemostatic cells? Ser Haematol 6:418–428.

Bryan FT, Robinson CW Jr, Gilbert CF, Langdell RD (1964): N-ethylmaleimide inhibition of horseshoe crab hemocyte agglutination. Science 144:1147–1148.

Butler T, Levin J, Cu DQ, Walker RI (1973): Bubonic plague: Detection of endotoxemia with the Limulus test. Ann Int Med 79:642–646.

Clawson CC (1973): Platelet interaction with bacteria. III. Ultrastructure. Am J Pathol 70:449–472.

Cohen E, Bang FB, Levin J, Marchalonis JJ, Pistole TG, Prendergast RA, Shuster C Jr, Watson SW, eds (1979): "Biomedical Applications of the Horseshoe Crab (Limulidae)." New York: Alan R. Liss, pp 1–683.

Cooper JF, Levin J, Wagner HN Jr (1971): Quantitative comparison of in vitro and in vivo methods for the detection of endotoxin. J Lab Clin Med 78:138–148.

de Haen C, Neurath H, Teler DC (1975): The phylogeny of trypsin-related serine proteases and their zymogens. New methods for the investigation of distant evolutionary relationships. J Mol Biol 92:225–259.

Doolittle RF (1970): Evolution of fibrinogen molecules. Thromb Diath Haemorrh 39(Suppl):25–42.

Elin RJ, Sandberg AL, Rosenstreich DL (1976): Comparison of the pyrogenicity, Limulus activity, mitogenicity and complement reactivity of several bacterial endotoxins and related compounds. J Immunol 177:1238–1242.

Fahrenbach WH (1970): The cyanoblast: Hemocyanin formation in *Limulus polyphemus.* J Cell Biol 44:445–453.

Furman RM, Pistole TG (1976): Bactericidal activity of hemolymph from the horseshoe crab, *Limulus polyphemus.* J Invertebr Pathol 28:239–244.

Halliburton WD (1885): On the blood of decapod crustacea. J Physiol 6:300–335.

Harada-Suzuki T, Morita T, Iwanaga S, Nakamura S, Niwa M (1982): Further studies on the chromogenic substrate assay method for bacterial endotoxins using horseshoe crab *(Tachypleus tridentatus)* hemocyte lysate. J Biochem 92:793–800.

Hardy WB (1892): The blood-corpuscles of the crustacea, together with a suggestion as to the origin of the crustacean fibrin-ferment. J Physiol 13:165–190.

Hewett-Emmett D, Czelusniak J, Goodman M (1981): The evolutionary relationships of the enzymes involved in blood coagulation and hemostasis. Ann NY Acad Sci 370:511–527.

Homma R, Kuratsuka K, Akama K (1982): Application of the LAL test and the chromogenic substrate test to the detection of endotoxin in human blood products. In Watson SW, Levin J, Novitsky TJ (eds): "Endotoxins and Their Detection With the Limulus Amebocyte Lysate Test." New York: Alan R. Liss, pp 301–317.

Howell WH (1885): Observations upon the chemical composition and coagulation of the blood of Limulus polyphemus, Callinectes hastatus, and Cucumaria sp. Johns Hopkins Univ Circ 5:4–5.

Kakinuma A, Asano T, Torii H, Sugino Y (1981): Gelation of *Limulus* amoebocyte lysate by an antitumor (1→3)-β-D-glucan. Biochem Biophys Res Commun 101:434–439.

Koster F, Levin J, Walker L, Tung KSK, Gilman RH, Rahaman MM, Majid MA, Islam S, Williams RC (1978): Hemolytic-uremic syndrome after shigellosis. Relation to endotoxemia and circulating immune complexes. N Engl J Med 298:927–933.

Levin J (1967): Blood coagulation and endotoxin in invertebrates. Fed Proc 26:1707–1712.

Levin J (1976): Blood coagulation in the horseshoe crab *(Limulus polyphemus):* A model for mammalian coagulation and hemostasis. In "Animal Models of Thrombosis and Hemorrhagic Diseases." (Proceedings of a Symposium of the National Academy of Sciences.) DHEW Publication No. (NIH) 76-982, pp 87–96. Washington, DC: U.S. Department of Health, Education and Welfare.

Levin J (1982): The Limulus Test and bacterial endotoxins: Some perspectives. In Watson SW, Levin J, Novitsky TJ (eds): "Endotoxins and Their Detection with the Limulus Amebocyte Lysate Test." New York: Alan R. Liss, pp 7–24.

Levin J (1984): Bleeding with infectious diseases. In Ratnoff OD, Forbes CD (eds): "Disorders of Hemostasis." Orlando, FL: Grune & Stratton, pp 367–378.

Levin J, Bang FB (1964a): The role of endotoxin in the extracellular coagulation of Limulus blood. Bull Johns Hopkins Hosp 115:265–274.

Levin J, Bang FB (1964b): A description of cellular coagulation in the Limulus. Bull Johns Hopkins Hosp 115:337–345.

Levin J, Bang FB (1968): Clottable protein in Limulus: Its localization and kinetics of its coagulation by endotoxin. Thromb Diath Haemorrh 19:186–197.

Levin J, Tomasulo PA, Oser RS (1970): Detection of endotoxin in human blood and demonstration of an inhibitor. J Lab Clin Med 75:903–911.

Levin J, Poore TE, Young NS, Margolis S, Zauber NP, Townes AS, Bell WR (1972): Gram-negative sepsis: Detection of endotoxin with the Limulus Test. Ann Intern Med 76:1–7.

Lewis JC, Maldonado JE, Mann KG (1976): Phagocytosis in human platelets: Localization of acid phosphatase-positive phagosomes following latex uptake. Blood 47:833–840.

Lightner DV, Lewis DH (1975): A septicemic bacterial disease syndrome of penaeid shrimp. Mar Fish Rev 37:25–28.

Loeb L (1904): On the spontaneous agglutination of blood cells of arthropods. Univ Penn Med Bull 16:441–443.

Loeb L (1910): Uber die blutgerinnung bei wirbellosen. Biochem Z 24:478–495.

Loewenhaupt RW, Miller MA, Glueck HI (1973): Platelet migration and chemotaxis demonstrated *in vitro*. Thromb Res 3:477–487.

Macfarlane RG, ed (1970): "The Haemostatic Mechanism in Man and Other Animals." New York: Academic, pp 1–229.

MacIntyre DE, Allen AP, Thorne KJI, Glauert AM, Gordon JL (1977): Endotoxin-induced platelet aggregation and secretion I. Morphological changes and pharmacological effects. J Cell Sci 28:211–223.

Morita T, Tanaka S, Nakamura T, Iwanaga S (1981): A new (1→3)-β-D-glucan-mediated coagulation pathway found in *Limulus* amebocytes. FEBS Lett 19:318–321.

Murer EH, Levin J, Holme R (1975): Isolation and studies of the granules of the amebocytes of *Limulus polyphemus,* the horseshoe crab. J Cell Physiol 86:533–542.

Nachum R, Watson SW, Sullivan JD Jr, Siegel SE (1979): Antimicrobial defense mechanisms in the horseshoe crab, *Limulus polyphemus:* Preliminary observations with heat-derived extracts of *Limulus* amoebocyte lysate. J Invertebr Pathol 33:290–299.

Nakamura S, Levin J (1982a): Fractionation of *Limulus* amebocyte lysate. Characterization of activation of the proclotting enzyme by an endotoxin-mediated activator. Biochim Biophys Acta 707:217–225.

Nakamura S, Levin J (1982b): Endotoxin-mediated *Limulus* proclotting enzyme activator and detection of a previously undescribed protease (protease N). Biochem Biophys Res Commun 108:1619–1623.

Nakamura S, Morita T, Iwanaga S, Niwa M, Takahashi K (1977): A sensitive substrate for the clotting enzyme in horseshoe crab hemocytes. J Biochem 81:1567–1569.

Nakamura S, Morita T, Harada-Suzuki T, Iwanaga S, Takahashi K, Niwa M (1982): A clotting enzyme associated with the hemolymph coagulation system of horseshoe crab *(Tachypleus tridentatus):* Its purification and characterization. J Biochem 92:781–792.

Nakamura S, Shishikura F, Iwanaga S, Takagi T, Takahashi K, Niwa M, Sekiguchi K (1980): Horseshoe crab coagulogens: Their structures and gelation mechanism. In Liu T-Y, Mamiya G, Yasunobu KT (eds): "Frontiers in Protein Chemistry. Developments in Biochemistry, Vol 10." New York: Elsevier/North Holland, pp 495–514.

Ohki M, Nakamura T, Morita T, Iwanaga S (1980): A new endotoxin sensitive factor associated with hemolymph coagulation system of horseshoe crab (Limulidae). FEBS Lett 120:217–220.

Pistole TG, Britko JL (1978) Bactericidal activity of amebocytes from the horseshoe crab, *Limulus polyphemus.* J Invertebr Pathol 31:376–382.

Rao AK, Schmaier AH, Colman RW (1982): Plasma coagulation proteases, proteolytic inhibitors, and their interaction with platelets. Pathobiol Annu 12:35–64.

Ratcliffe NA, Rowley AF (1979): A comparative synopsis of the structure and function of the blood cells of insects and other invertebrates. Dev Comp Immunol 3:189–243.

Rickles FR, Levin J, Hardin JA, Barr CF, Conrad ME Jr (1977): Tissue factor generation by human mononuclear cells: Effects of endotoxin and dissociation of tissue factor generation from mitogenic response. J Lab Clin Med 89:792–803.

Rickles FR, Levin J, Rosenthal DI, Atkins E (1979): Functional interaction of concanavalin A and bacterial endotoxin (lipopolysaccharide): Effects on the measurement of endogenous pyrogen release, human mononuclear cell tissue factor activation, lymphocyte DNA synthesis, and gelation of Limulus amebocyte lysate. J Lab Clin Med 93:128–145.

Rojas-Corona RR, Skarnes R, Tamakuma S, Fine J (1969): The *Limulus* coagulation test for endotoxin. A comparison with other assay methods. Proc Soc Exp Biol Med 132:599–601.

Rustum Maluf NS (1939): The blood of arthropods. Q Rev Biol 14:149–191.

Seid RC Jr, Liu T-Y (1980): Purification and properties of the *Limulus* clotting enzyme. In Liu T-Y, Mamiya G, Yasunobu KT (eds): "Frontiers in Protein Chemistry. Developments in Biochemistry, Vol 10." New York: Elsevier/North-Holland, pp 481–493.

Shirodkar MV, Warwick A, Bang FB (1960): The in vitro reaction of Limulus amebocytes to bacteria. Biol Bull 118:324–337.

Shishikura F, Sekiguchi K (1979): Comparative studies on hemocytes and coagulogens of the Asian and the American horseshoe crabs. In Cohen E, Bang FB, Levin J, et al (eds): "Biomedical Applications of the Horseshoe Crab (Limulidae)." New York: Alan R. Liss, pp 185–201.

Shishikura F, Chiba J, Sekiguchi K (1977): Two types of hemocytes in localization of clottable protein in Japanese horseshoe crab, Tachypleus tridentatus. J Exp Zool 201:303–308.

Shishikura F, Nakamura S, Takahashi K, Sekiguchi K (1983): Coagulogens from four living species of horseshoe crabs (Limulidae): Comparison of their biochemical and immunochemical properties. J Biochem 94:1279–1287.

Spivak JL, Levin J (1977): Endotoxin contamination of some erythropoietin preparations: Reply No. 2 (letter). Blood 50:549–550.

Springer GF, Adye JC (1975): Endotoxin-binding substances from human leukocytes and platelets. Infect Immun 12:978–986.

Spurling NW (1981): Comparative physiology of blood clotting. Comp Biochem Physiol 68A:541–548.

Stewart JE (1975): Gaffkemia, the fatal infection of lobsters (Genus *Homarus*) caused by *Aerococcus viridans* (var.) *homari:* A review. Mar Fish Rev 37:20–24.

Tai JY, Liu T-Y (1977): Studies on *Limulus* amoebocyte lysate. Isolation of proclotting enzyme. J Biol Chem 252:2178–2181.

Tai JY, Seid RC Jr, Huhn RD, Liu T-Y (1977): Studies on *Limulus* amoebocyte lysate. II. Purification of the coagulogen and the mechanism of clotting. J Biol Chem 252:4773–4776.

Tait J (1911): Types of crustacean blood coagulation. J Mar Biol Assoc 9:191–198.

Takagi T, Hokama Y, Morita T, Iwanaga S, Nakamura S, Niwa M (1979a): Amino acid sequence studies on horseshoe crab *(Tachypleus tridentatus)* coagulogen and the mechanism of gel formation. In Cohen E, Bang FB, Levin J, et al (eds): "Biomedical Applications of the Horseshoe Crab (Limulidae)." New York: Alan R. Liss, pp 169–184.

Takagi T, Nakamura S, Hokama Y, Miyata T, Niwa M, Iwanaga S (1979b): The primary structure of horseshoe crab *(Tachypleus tridentatus)* coagulogen and its homologies with platelet factor 4. Thromb Haemost 42:272 (Abstract).

Tomasulo PA (1979): Correlation of Limulus amebocyte lysate assay with accepted endotoxin assays. In Cohen E, Bang FB, Levin J, et al (eds): "Biomedical Applications of the Horseshoe Crab (Limulidae)." New York: Alan R. Liss, pp 293–302.

Tomasulo PA, March SC, Levin J (1975): Tritiation of endotoxin. Biochim Biophys Acta 400:399–406.

Tomasulo PA, Levin J, Murphy PA, Winkelstein JA (1977): Biological activities of tritiated endotoxins: Correlation of the Limulus lysate assay with rabbit pyrogen and complement activation assays for endotoxin. J Lab Clin Med 89:308–315.

Torano AE, Nakamura S, Levin J (1984): Properties of the clotting enzyme responsible for endotoxin-mediated *Limulus* coagulation. Thromb Res 34:407–417.

Walsh PN (1981): Platelets and coagulation proteins. Fed Proc 40:2086–2091.

Watson SW, Levin J, Novitsky TJ, eds (1982): "Endotoxins and Their Detection With the Limulus Amebocyte Lysate Test." New York: Alan R. Liss, pp 1–409.

Young LS (1975): Opsonizing antibodies, host factors, and the Limulus assay for endotoxin. Infect Immun 12:88–92.

Young NS, Levin J, Prendergast RA (1972): An invertebrate coagulation system activated by endotoxin: Evidence for enzymatic mediation. J Clin Invest 51:1790–1797.

Zuckerman KS, Quesenberry PJ, Levin J, Sullivan R (1979): Contamination of erythropoietin by endotoxin: In vivo and in vitro effects on murine erythropoiesis. Blood 54:146–158.

OSMOTIC REGULATION

Blood Cells of Marine Invertebrates: Experimental Systems in Cell Biology and Comparative Physiology, pages 167–189

Chapter Six
A Comparison of the Water-Regulating Responses of Bivalve and Polychaete Red Cells to Osmotic Stresses

Sidney K. Pierce and Timothy K. Maugel

Department of Zoology, University of Maryland, College Park, Maryland 20742 and the Marine Biological Laboratory, Woods Hole, Massachusetts 02543

INTRODUCTION

The amount of water inside a cell is critical to cellular function. The water dictates intracellular concentrations of all components soluble in it, and in addition the volume of intracellular water controls cell geometry. Over the years the physiological and biochemical bases of cellular water balance have been studied in a wide array of cell types from almost as wide an array of species. There are two main difficulties usually encountered in these sorts of investigations. First, many of these studies utilized solid tissues, or at least pieces or slices of solid tissues, as experimental subjects. While this type of experimental system has contributed a good deal of important information to the understanding of cellular water balance, almost all of the solid tissue preparations suffer a major shortcoming—namely, cell volume cannot be measured directly. The only important exception to that generality is the utilization of some sophisticated, computer-aided optics that seem to give a very reliable measurement of cell volume in some very thin transporting epithelia (for a review see Spring and Ericson [1982]). Second, choosing the most appropriate units to express the presence of intracellular substances is often problematical. Wet weight, dry weight, cell water, and the amounts of most cellular constituents are altered during the response of a cell to an osmotic change. Furthermore, the change in concentration of an intracellular component is often immaterial in such studies; rather the change in absolute amount of the component is the value of importance. These values are usually difficult to obtain with precision in solid tissue preparations. Such problems are minimized by the use of cell suspensions, either various types of blood cells (basically erythrocytes and lymphocytes) or tissue cultured cells that grow in suspension (for example, Erlich ascites cells and mouse lymphoblasts). Since these types of cells are not attached to one another, cell size is easily, rapidly, and accurately measured microscopically, by hematocrit, or electronically by Coulter counter type instruments. In addition, cell numbers are easily determined, thereby permitting accurate measurement of the amount of substances per cell, a sometimes useful means of expressing absolute amounts. Finally, cells in suspension are often easier to handle experimentally, thus facilitating the research.

It is not surprising that many investigators have used cell suspensions for studies of various aspects of cellular water balance. Initially, many of these studies centered on the mammalian erythrocyte. While this cell has been undeniably useful in a variety of studies, including water and ion balance, it is at best an aberrant type of cell and at least potentially atypical in its physiological and biochemical responses. More recent cell water balance studies have turned to other, more morphologically complete vertebrate cell types, such as lymphocytes [Hempling et al., 1977; Ben-Sasson et al., 1975; Hempling et al., 1981; Bui and Wiley, 1982; reviewed by Negendank, 1982], Erlich ascites cells [Hendil and Hoffmann, 1974; Hoffmann and Hendil, 1976; Hoffmann, 1980; Lambert and Hoffmann, 1982], lymphoblasts [Buckhold et al., 1965], dog erythrocytes [Parker et al., 1975, 1977], and nucleated vertebrate erythrocytes such as duck [Kregenow, 1971] and flounder [Fugelli, 1967; Cala, 1977a,b].

While studies on these cell suspensions, in company with those of the solid tissues, have contributed a great deal of information concerning mechanisms of cell water balance, most of the cell types mentioned above are not particularly tolerant of external osmotic variation, a 150–200 mosmolal range on average. In contrast, there are many animal species whose cells are much more tolerant of osmotic concentration variation: the euryhaline osmoconforming invertebrates. In addition, most of these latter species contain blood or coelomic fluid cells of some type and a few have flattened, discoid, hemoglobin-containing cells. Since the cells of these animals can tolerate relatively wide osmotic concentration changes, the responses of the water balance mechanisms should be magnified relative to the vertebrate cell types and, as a result, perhaps more informative to study. The water balance mechanisms of two invertebrate cell suspensions have been examined: the red blood cells of the blood clam *Noetia ponderosa* and the red coelomocyte of the blood worm *Glycera dibranchiata*.

A COMPARISON OF VERTEBRATE AND INVERTEBRATE CELL VOLUME CONTROL MECHANISMS

This subject has been recently reviewed [Pierce, 1982] and thus there is no need to do so in exhaustive detail here. A brief recapitulation seems in order.

That all cells have some capacity to regulate cell volume in response to osmotic stress is well established. Cells swell in response to a hypoosmotic stress and, if the stress does not cause lysis, the cells will recover toward their original volume. The mechanism of volume recovery in response to hypoosmotic conditions utilizes an efflux of one or more intracellular solutes that has the final effect of lowering intracellular osmotic concentrations and causing water to leave the cell. The control of the efflux resides with certain permeability control mechanisms in the surface membrane [Pierce, 1982].

The exact solute utilized for this volume regulating process varies from cell type to cell type, but falls into two main categories: inorganic (usually Na^+, K^+ or Cl^-) and organic (usually low molecular weight, nitrogen-containing compounds: free amino acids or quaternary ammonium compounds). Furthermore, a great deal of the literature suggests that vertebrate cell types use the inorganic solutes for volume control whereas invertebrate cells regulate volume with organic molecules. However, this apparent dichotomy of solute types between phylogenetic groups is probably not real. Recent studies have found vertebrate cells utilizing an organic solute component for volume control and invertebrate cell types regulating volume in part with inorganic ions [Pierce, 1982]. Although perhaps generalities are a bit premature at this point, it seems possible that the volume regulating mechanisms in most cells may turn out to be quite similar, differences in solute being in magnitude rather than type. In any event, the *Noetia* red blood cell and the *Glycera* red coelomocyte stand as interesting models of cell volume regulation in response to osmotic stress. Since these cells are not as well known as some of the others mentioned in this book, they are described briefly below before discussion of the features of their volume regulating systems.

GLYCERA RED COELOMOCYTE

Glycera, unlike most polychaetes, has no circulatory system. Instead, the coelomic fluid serves the circulatory function. There seem to be a variety of cell types suspended in the coelomic fluid of glycerids depending upon the species. For example, the coelomic fluid of *G. convoluta* from the Mediterranean contains hemoglobin-carrying coelomocytes, amoeboid "leukocytes," and large, oval cells with colorless granules [Goodrich, 1899; Romieu, 1923]. The last named cells may be female gametes, but it is impossible to

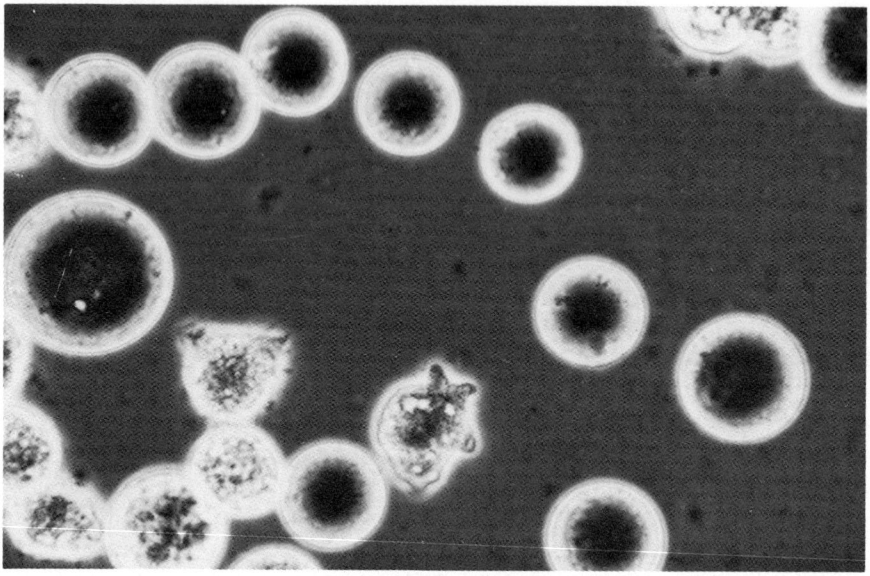

Fig. 1. Phase contrast micrograph of *Glycera dibranchiata* coelomic fluid cells. Amoeboid cells as well as several sizes of the nucleated red coelomocyte are obvious. Cell diameters are in the range of 17–27 μm. Photo by C.J. Costa.

tell from either the descriptions or drawings. The amoeboid cells rapidly take up carmine and india ink, neither of which enter the other two cell types [Goodrich, 1899].

In contrast, most of the coelomic cells in *G. siphonostoma* carry hemoglobin, but in addition are amoeboid. The colorless, amoeboid cells seem to be absent from this species, and the red cells readily phagocytize carmine and india ink [Goodrich, 1899]. At least two types of cells are always found in the coelomic fluid of *G. dibranchiata*: spherical, red hemoglobin-containing erythrocytes and colorless amoebocytes (Fig. 1). Egg cells are also present at various times in the year [Dawson, 1933; Seamonds and Schumacher, 1972; Costa et al., 1980]. The red coelomocytes of *G. dibranchiata* are nucleated and vary considerably in diameter (17–27 μm). The cytoplasm contains some mitochondria, Golgi apparatus, a variety of osmiophilic deposits, and a wide array of vacuoles (Figs. 2,3). No marginal band of microtubules is present. The vacuoles can often be seen fusing with or forming from the surface membrane (Figs. 2,3). When prepared by freeze fracture techniques, the vacuole membrane seems to be composed entirely of particles. Furthermore, at the location on the surface membrane where the vacuole is forming or fusing, the surface membrane particles become a highly ordered

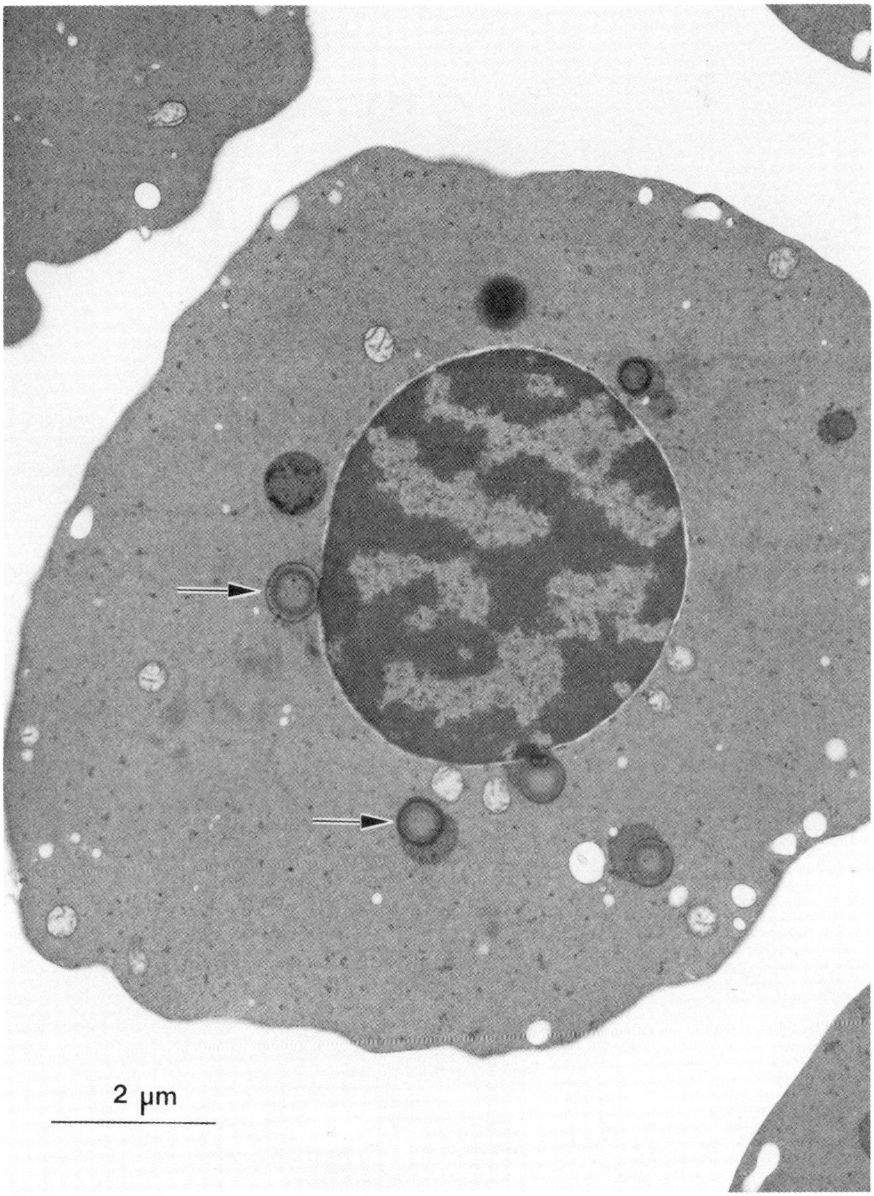

Fig. 2. Electron micrograph of *Glycera dibranchiata* red coelomocytes taken from animals acclimated to full-strength sea water. The nucleus, mitochondria, empty-appearing vacuoles, and diffuse core inclusions (arrows) are obvious.

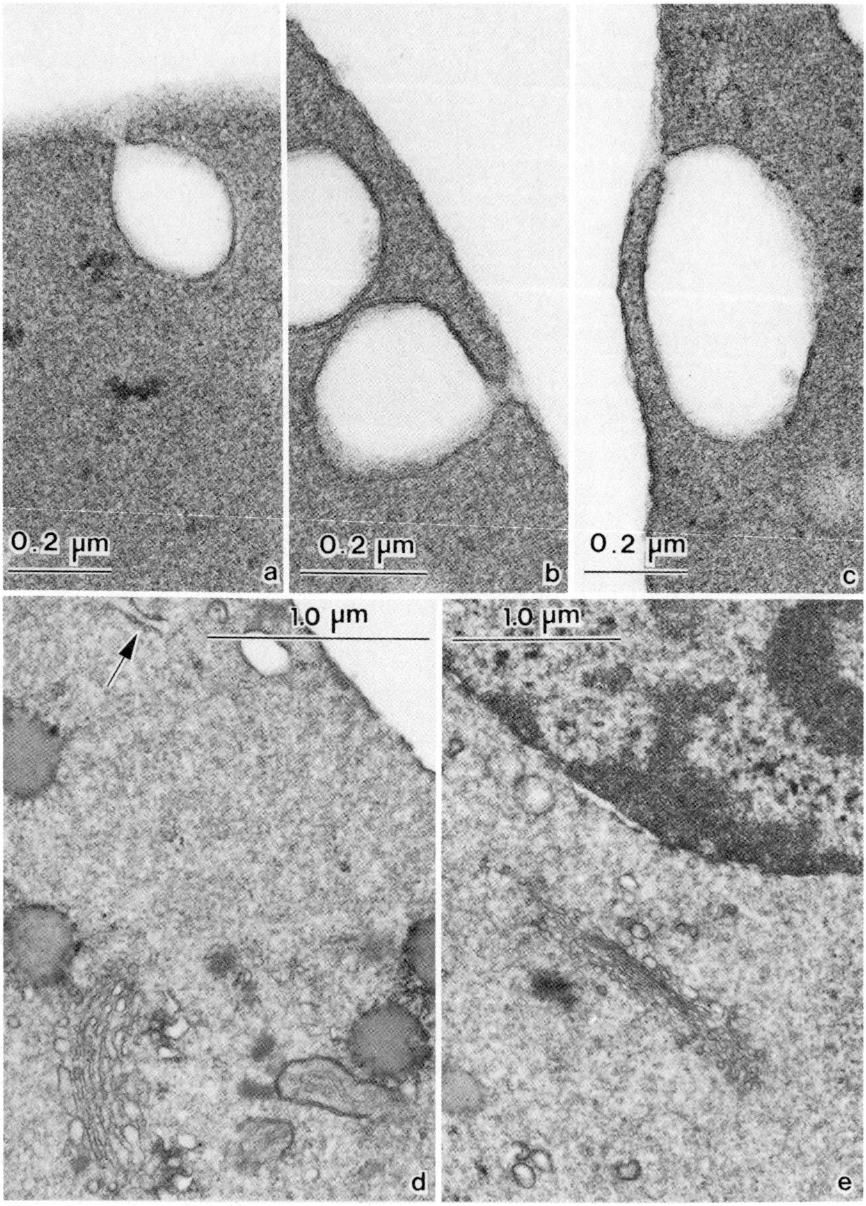

Fig. 3. Higher magnification of *G. dibranchiata* red coelomocytes. Vacuoles are routinely found fused with the surface membrane and open to the outside (a–c). Golgi complexes (d,e) are occasionally observed. On rare occasions, short profiles of rough endoplasmic reticulum (arrow in d) can be found.

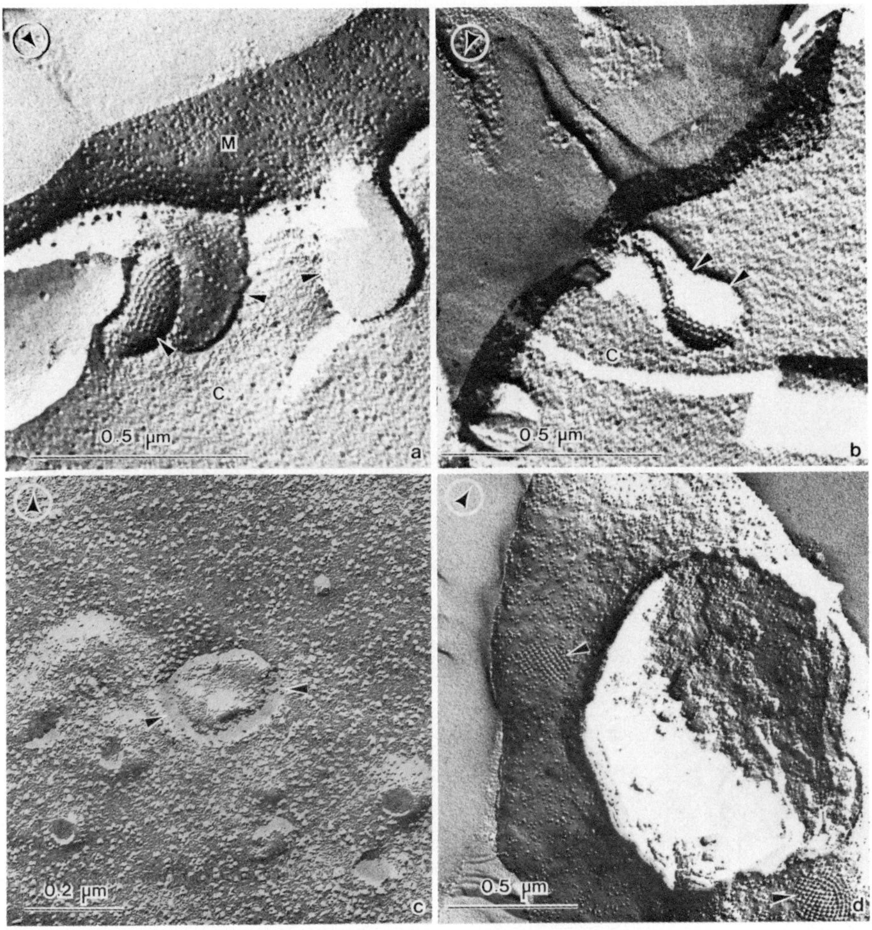

Fig. 4. Freeze-fracture replicas of *Glycera dibranchiata* red coelomocytes. a,b. Particle-lined vacuoles (arrowheads) in the process of forming at the cell membrane (C, cytoplasm; M, membrane). c. P face of the surface membrane showing a forming vacuole (arrowheads) and the vacuolar particles in an array within the surface membrane. d. Lower magnification of a surface membrane fracture showing at least two particle arrays (arrowheads) at presumptive sites of vacuolar formation. Circled arrows indicate the direction of shadow.

array (Fig. 4). The presence of such a large number of vacuoles suggests that the *G. dibranchiata* red coelomocytes might, in addition to their oxygen-carrying role [Hoffmann and Mangum, 1970], be phagocytic or pinocytotic, although an earlier report suggested that they were not [Seamonds and

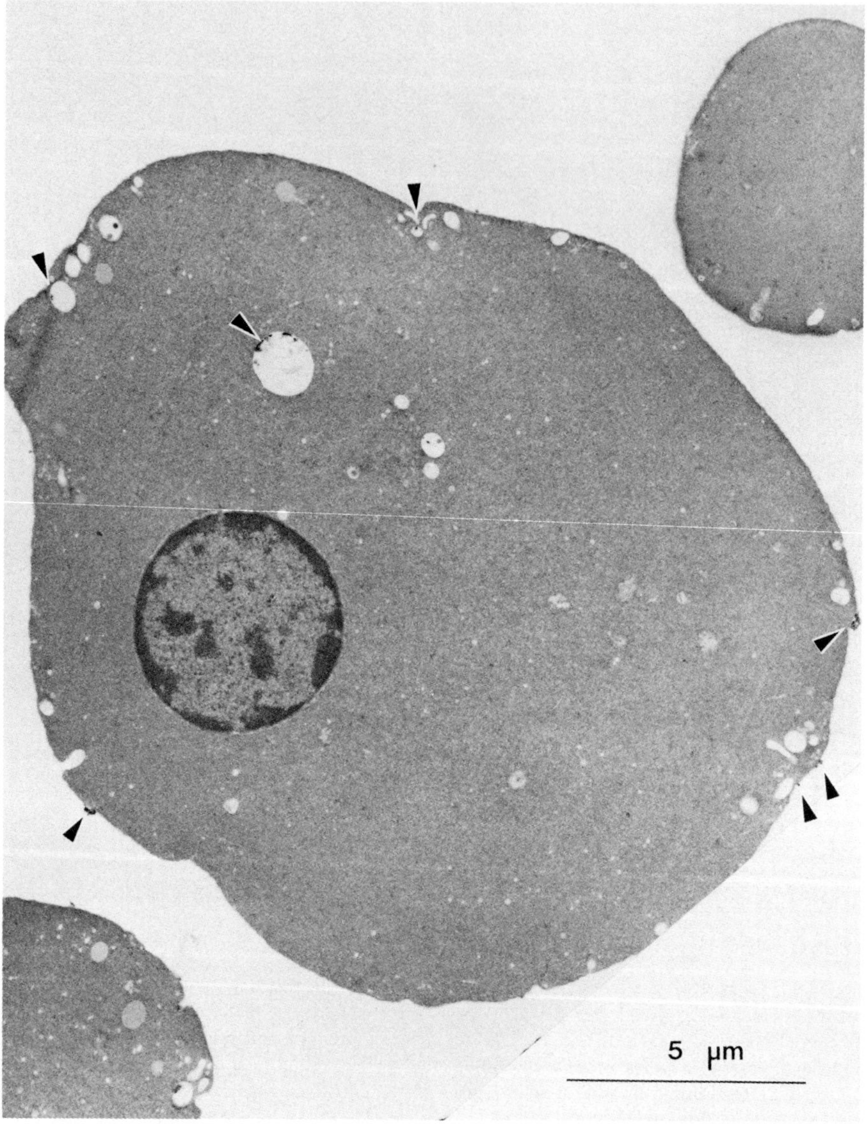

Fig. 5. Pinocytosis of ferritin by *Glycera* red coelomocytes. The cells were incubated in cationized ferritin for 15 min at 20° C. Ferritin deposits are clearly seen along the surface membrane as well as inside the cell (arrowheads).

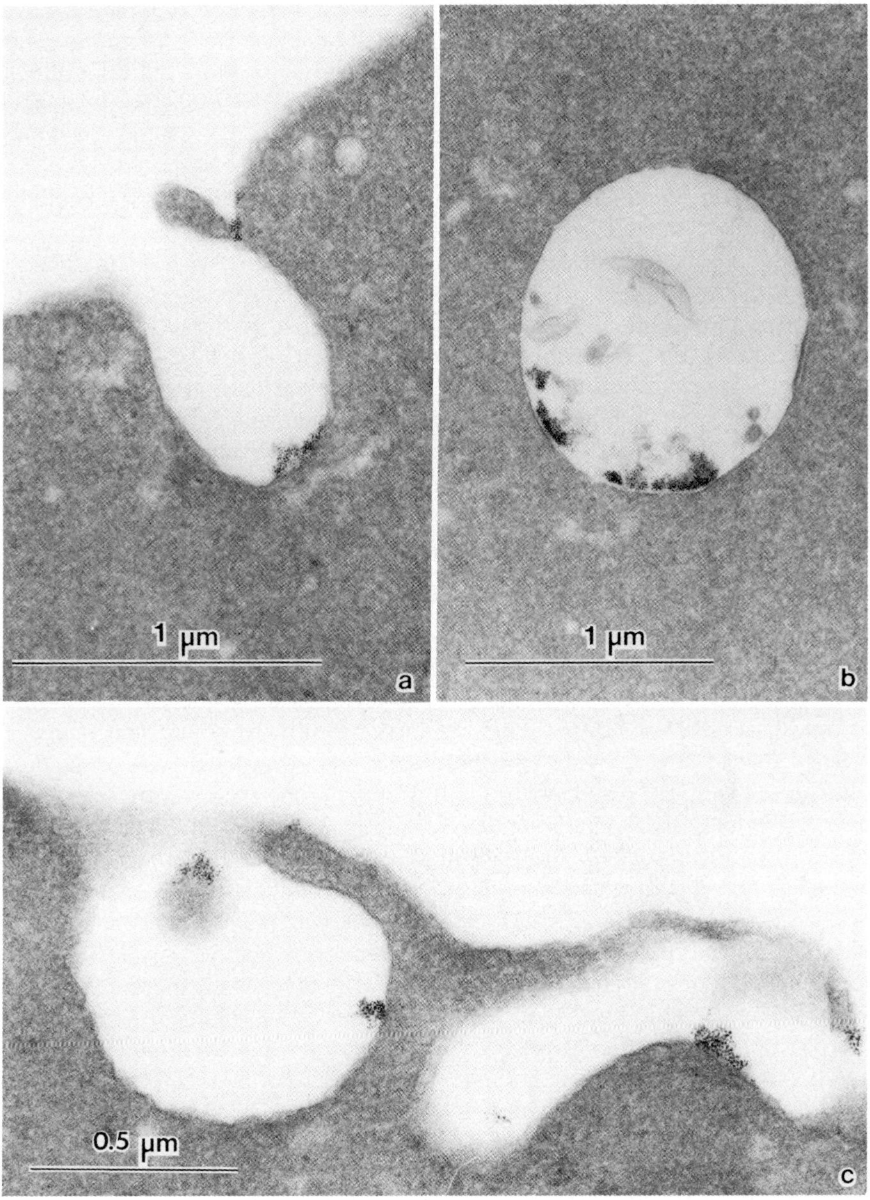

Fig. 6. High-magnification micrographs (a–c) show both vacuoles forming around surface ferritin deposits as well as the details of a ferritin containing vacuole within the cytoplasm (b).

Schumacher, 1972]. That experiment was done at 4°C, however, so we have reexamined the question. The cells will rapidly enclose ferritin into the clear vacuoles at 20°C (Figs. 5,6). However, in preliminary tests, the cells do not seem to take up india ink or colloidal thorium. We are working on the details of these experiments at present, but it is possible that the coelomocytes are conserving heme iron from the coelomic fluid with some degree of specificity. In any case, the ferritin experiments clearly indicate that the red coelomocytes are quite capable of pinocytosis.

Finally, the source of the red coelomocytes is unknown. The earliest studies of hematopoiesis indicated that the amoeboid cells might differentiate into red coelomcytes [Goodrich, 1899]. Goodrich also reported amitotic division among the red coelomocytes. Subsequent studies failed to confirm these early observations, but they have also failed to find the site of red coelomocyte production [Cowden, 1966; Seamonds and Schumacher, 1972; reviewed by Dales and Dixon, 1981]. In other polychaete genera the coelomocytes arise from specialized patches in the peritoneum or from the blood vessel epithelial layer [Dales and Dixon, 1981].

NOETIA PONDEROSA RED BLOOD CELLS

The hemoglobin-containing blood cells of *N. ponderosa* are probably less well known than the *Glycera* red coelomocytes, although the red blood cells of other Arcidae and Glycymerididae have received some attention from time to time [Sato, 1931; Dawson, 1933; Ohuye, 1938]. There are two types of cells in *Noetia* blood: white amoeboid cells and corpuscular red cells (Fig. 7). The red cells are reasonably plentiful in the blood (hematocrit = 6–7%), have a diameter of 15–17 μm, and are easily isolated by centrifugation. They have a prominent nucleus, but other than a few scattered vacuoles and some endoplasmic reticulum, the cytoplasmic portions of the cell essentially contain no other organelles (Fig. 8). We have not yet found mitochondria with the electron microscope, but succinate c reductase activity is abundant. A marginal band of microtubules is associated with the surface membrane (Fig. 9) (see Chapter One by Cohen and Nemhauser, this volume). There is no morphological indication of phagocytic activity nor amoeboid movements.

The site of erythropoiesis in *Noetia* or any bivalve is unknown, although speculations are frequent. Most attention has been focused on the amoeboid cells in this regard. In his review Cheng [1981] indicates that it is generally held that connective tissue is the hematopoietic site, but there is scant evidence. Other studies suggest that the epithelial cell layer of the digestive tubules may be the source of some of the blood amoebocytes [Morton, 1969] and still others find amoeboid blood cells appearing out of tissue (usually heart) explants [Perkins and Menzel, 1964; Tripp et al., 1966; Li et al., 1966;

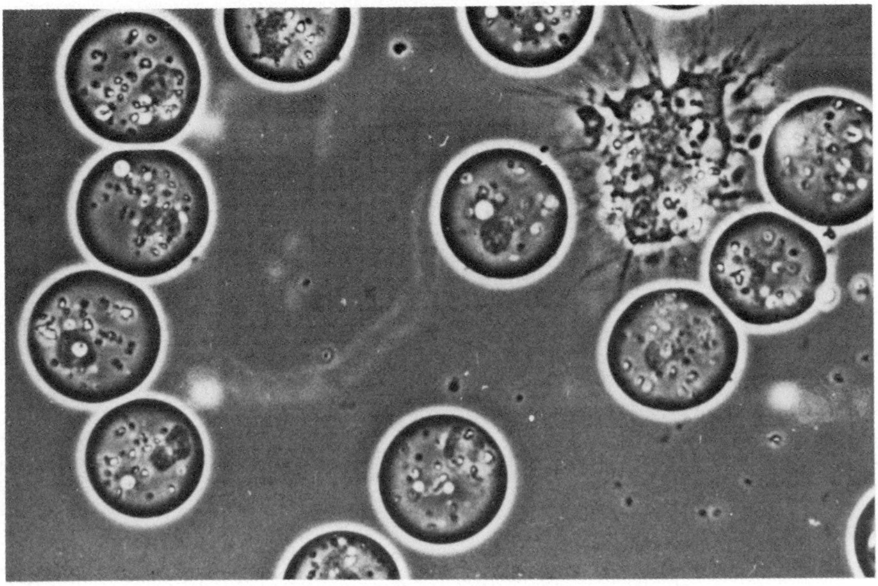

Fig. 7. Light micrograph of unfixed *Noetia ponderosa* blood cells. A single amoebocyte is present surrounded by hemoglobin-containing, nucleated blood cells. The cells are 15–17 μm in diameter. Photo by L.M. Amende.

Narain, 1973]. None of these comments on bivalve erythropoiesis contain experimental validation of the speculations. The only blood cell type whose source seems well established is the rather specialized serous cell that is a product of the pericardial glands (see, for example, Cheng and Burton [1966] or Cheng [1981]). Finally, the lifespan of the *Noetia* red cell is unknown. There is no convincing evidence of cell division occurring once the cells are in the plasma, although the red cells of both *Arca inflata* and *Glycimeris vestitus* frequently have multiple nuclei, suggesting amitotic division [Ohuye, 1938]. However the *Noetia* cells do not usually have more than one nucleus per cell, although we have not looked at that particular characteristic systematically.

Thus, other than the oxygen transport properties of the hemoglobin [Freadman and Mangum, 1976] (see also Nagel, this volume) and some studies on the marginal band of microtubules, little is known about the function of the *Noetia* red blood cell, except for the mechanism of cellular water balance.

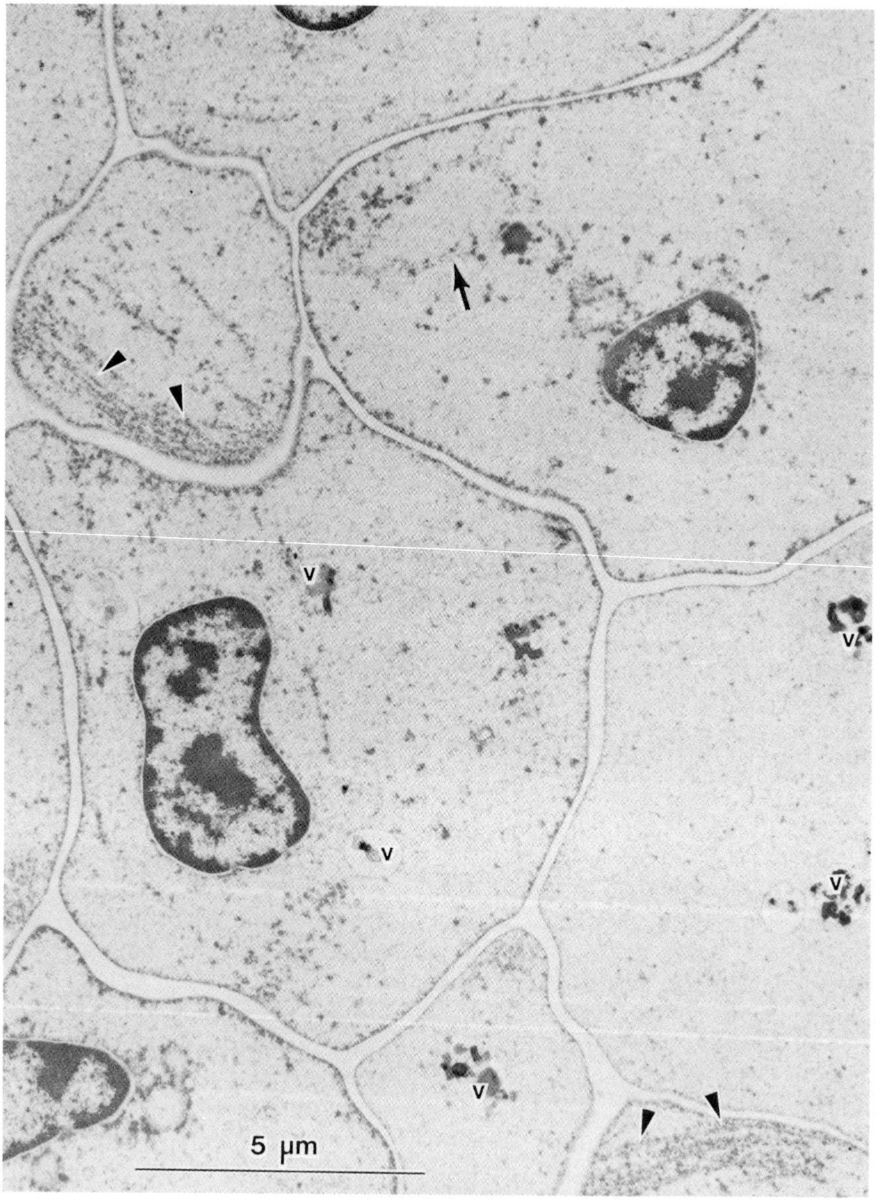

Fig. 8. Electron micrograph of a sectioned pellet of *Noetia* red blood cells. Nuclei and microtubules associated with the marginal band (arrowheads) are visible. Occasional profiles of endoplasmic reticulum are found in most of the cells (arrow). Vacuoles containing dense material reminiscent of heme iron deposits (v) are also found in these cells.

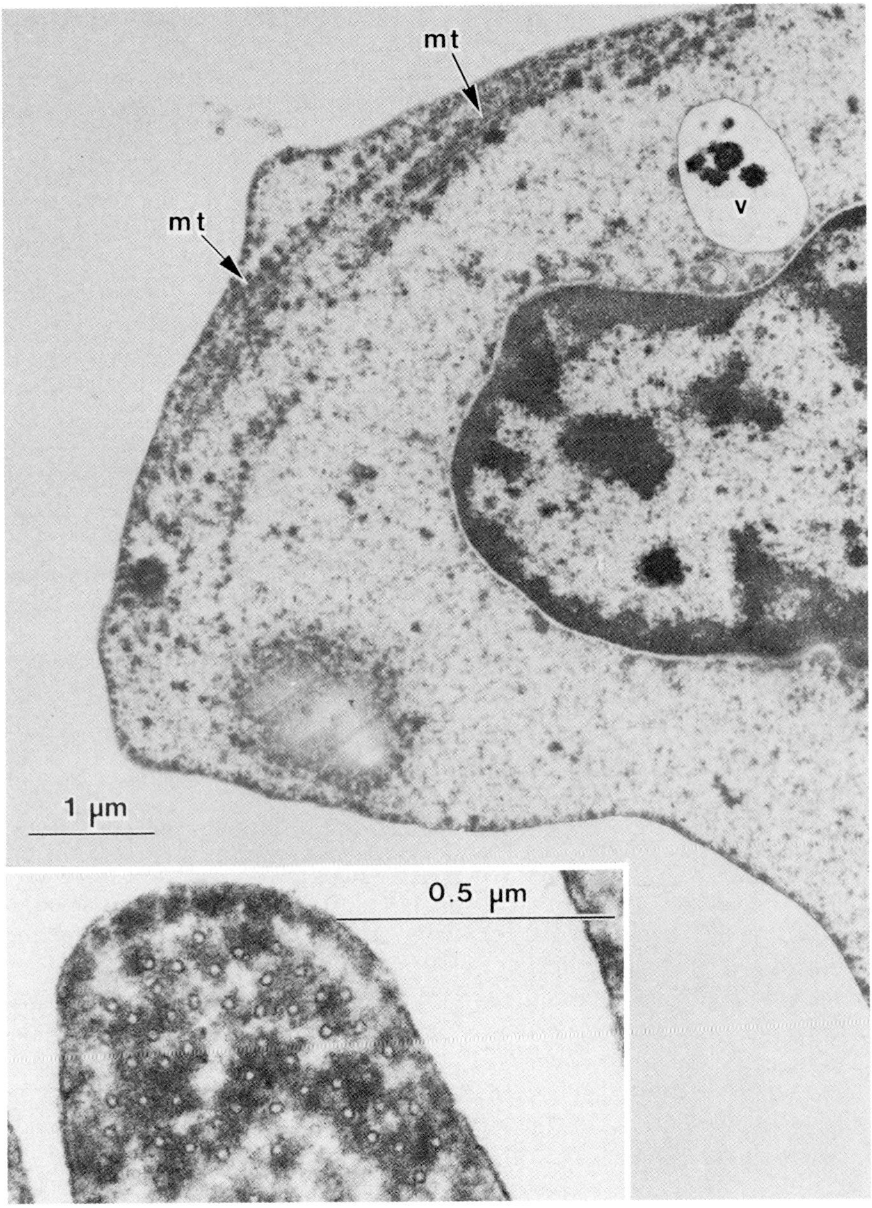

Fig. 9. High-magnification micrograph of a portion of a single *Noetia* red cell showing details of the obliquely sectioned marginal band of microtubules (mt), nucleus, and vacuole (v). Cross-sectioned microtubules of the marginal band appear in the inset.

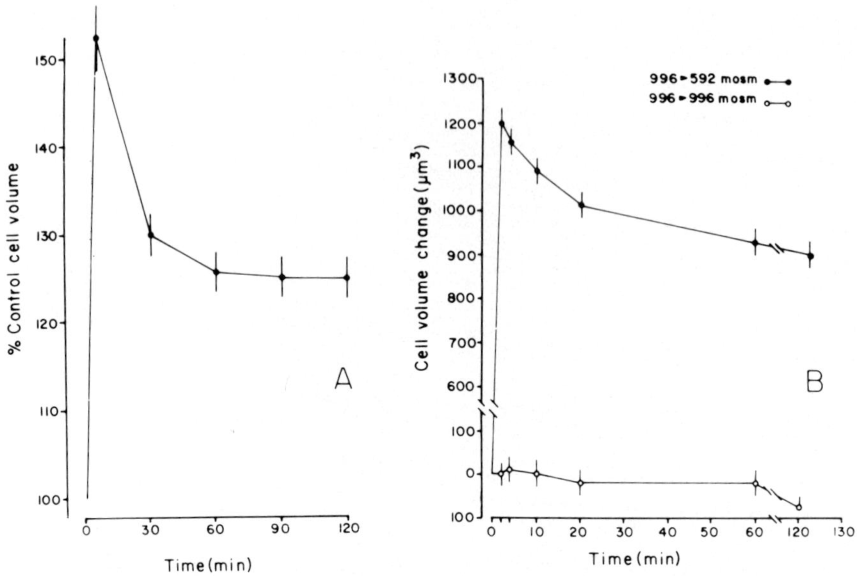

Fig. 10. A. Pattern of volume regulation by red blood cells isolated from *Noetia ponderosa* adapted to full strength seawater and exposed to 50% seawater at time 0. Cell volume was determined as packed cell hematocrits. Data from Amende and Pierce [1980b]. B. Pattern of volume regulation by red coelomocytes isolated from *Glycera dibranchiata* adapted to 996 mosm and then exposed to the osmotic concentration indicated at time 0. Cell volume was measured with a Coulter counter. Data from Costa et al. [1980].

VOLUME REGULATION BY *GLYCERA* AND *NOETIA* CELLS—TIME COURSE AND SOLUTES

The isolated red cells of both *Glycera* and *Noetia* swell when exposed to a hypoosmotic stress and then partially recover the original cell volume [Costa et al., 1980; Amende and Pierce, 1980a] (Fig. 10). The time courses of the volume regulation of the two cell types are rather similar. The *Noetia* cells do not swell as much as the red coelomocytes and the volume recovery is more complete in the *Noetia* cells (compare panels A and B of Fig. 10). Both cell types effuse intracellular free amino acids during the period of volume recovery (Table I). The efflux from *Noetia* cells contains amino acids in approximate proportion to the concentration of the amino acids in the intracellular pool and is reasonably large relative to the total pool size [Amende and Pierce, 1980a]. The amino acid efflux from the worm red coelomocytes is quite different in relative amounts from the intracellular pool and quite small in comparison to the total pool [Costa et al., 1980] (Table I). The significance of the difference in efflux patterns is unclear at present, but

TABLE I. Intracellular Free Amino Acid Pool Composition in *Noetia* and *Glycera* Red Cells Taken From Animals Adapted to 100% Seawater and Amino Acid Efflux Composition From Salinity-Stressed Cells

	Noetia			*Glycera*	
Amino acid	Cell[a]	Efflux[b]	Amino acid	Cell[c]	Efflux[d]
Taurine	48.6[e]	13.8	Taurine	230[e]	6
Hypotaurine	3.7	0.8	Proline	170	18
Aspartate	14.5	1.6	Asparagine	105	8
Threonine	2.7	0.6	Alanine	98	2
Serine	5.9	1.2	Glutamine	80	4
Asparagine	2.1	0.5	Serine	30	not present
Glutamate	6.5	0.5			
Glutamine	3.1	0.5			
Glycine	1.4	0.3			
Alanine	1.9	0.4			

Data from Amende and Pierce [1980a] and from Costa et al. [1980]. Only the major amino acids are reported.
[a]Cells from animals adapted to 1,056 mosm seawater.
[b]Cells exposed to 527 mosm seawater for 2 hr.
[c]Cells from animals adapted to 1,001 mosm seawater.
[d]Cells exposed to 592 mosm seawater for 40 min.
[e]nmoles per 10^6 cells.

these results indicate that these two cells types are typical of the classical pattern of volume regulation by invertebrate cells (reviewed by Pierce [1982]).

In addition to the amino acid solute, the volume regulating process in the *Glycera* coelomocytes has an inorganic ion component. Following exposure of these cells to a hypoosmotic stress, a very rapid decrease in intracellular K^+ occurs [Costa and Pierce, 1983]. This decrease is unaffected by ouabain, but is potentiated by 2,4-dinitrophenol (DNP). The utilization of K^+ for volume control is only transient, however. There is no difference in K^+ content of red coelomocytes taken from worms adapted to various salinities [Costa and Pierce, 1983]. The utilization of two solute types of the red coelomocytes is similar to the mechanism of cell volume control in the *Limulus* myocardium [Warren and Pierce, 1982] and, probably, of most other cell types, including those of the vertebrates where organic solute components of volume regulation complementary to the usual inorganic solutes have recently been discovered (see Pierce [1982] for a review). We are only just now measuring Na^+ changes in the *Glycera* cells and looking for an ionic component to volume control in the *Noetia* red cells; it is premature to present those data here. However, there is some additional information available concerning the mechanism of solute regulation by both the *Glycera* coelomocyte and the *Noetia* blood cell.

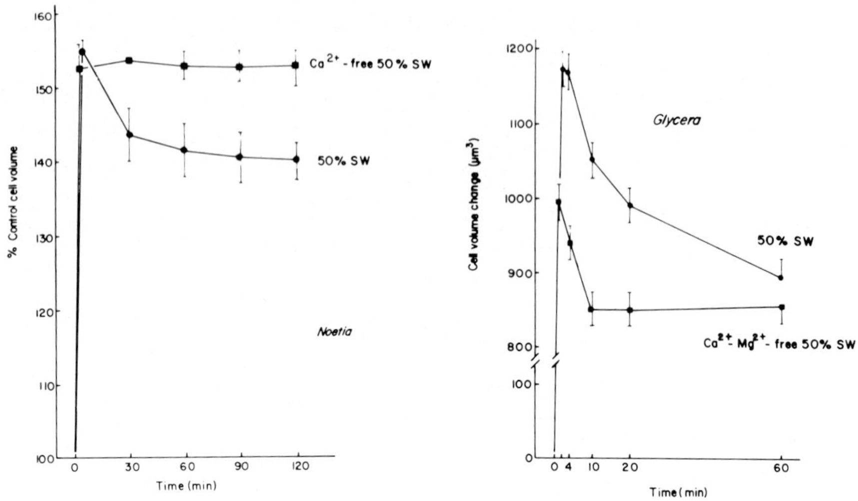

Fig. 11. The effects of the removal of divalent cations on the response of *Noetia* red blood cells and *Glycera* red coelomocytes to hypoosmotic stress. The *Noetia* cells were taken from clams adapted to full strength seawater and then exposed to either 50% seawater or Ca^{2+}-free 50% seawater. Cell volume was measured as packed cell hematocrits. Removal of Mg^{2+} had no effect on either the response to 50% seawater or Ca^{2+}-free 50% seawater. Data from Amende and Pierce [1980b]. The *Glycera* cells were taken from seawater adapted worms and exposed to either 50% seawater or $Ca^{2+}-Mg^{2+}$-free 50% seawater. Cell volume was determined with a Coulter counter. Data from Costa and Pierce [1983].

Control of Solute Efflux by Divalent Cations and ATP

When it has been tested, almost all cell volume regulating systems respond to changes in external Ca^{2+} concentration. On occasion, some cells also are affected by Mg^{2+} change and/or simultaneous variation of Ca^{2+} and Mg^{2+} (reviewed by Pierce [1982]). The worm red coelomocyte and bivalve red blood cell are quite typical in this regard, although the details of the response of each cell type are slightly different.

Deletion of Ca^{2+} blocks both the volume regulating response and the amino acid efflux from hypoosmotically stressed *Noetia* red blood cells (Fig. 11 and Table II) [Amende and Pierce, 1980b]. In contrast, $Ca^{2+}-Mg^{2+}$-free conditions potentiate the amino acid efflux from hypoosmotically stressed *Glycera* red coelomocytes, causing a larger volume recovery (Fig. 11 and 12). However, if either Ca^{2+} or Mg^{2+} is present the response of the worm cells to the hypoosmotic stress is normal [Costa and Pierce, 1983]. None of these responses are affected by alterations in Na^+, K^+, or Cl^-. Further, they are not modified by ouabain [Amende and Pierce, 1980a,b; Costa and Pierce, 1983]. While the sodium pump does not seem to be a part of the volume regulating responses to hypoosmotic stress by these two cell types,

TABLE II. Effect of Divalent Cation Deletion on the Free Amino Acid Efflux from *N. ponderosa* Red Blood Cells

Treatment	Total efflux[a] in 50% ASW	Total efflux[a] in 100% ASW
ASW	21.4 (0.65)*	0.46 (0.004)*
Mg^{2+}-free	21.2 (0.14)*	0.40 (0.024)*
Ca^{2+}-free	14.7 (0.71)*	0.54 (0.027)*
Ca^{2+}-Mg^{2+}-free	15.5 (0.08)**	0.73 (0.73)**

Data from Amende and Pierce [1980b].
ASW = artificial seawater.
[a]nmoles per 10^6 cells (+ SE).
*,**Values that do not have common superscripts are significantly different ($P < 0.05$).

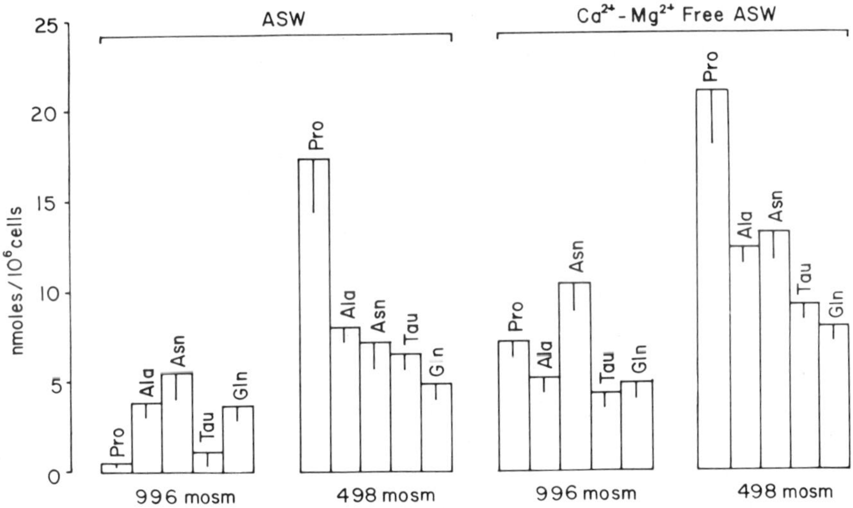

Fig. 12. Effect of hypoosmotic stress with and without Ca^{2+} and Mg^{2+} on the amino acid efflux from *Glycera* red coelomocytes. Cells were taken from animals adapted to seawater (996 mosm), then exposed to the osmotic concentrations indicated for 60 min. ASW = artificial seawater. Data from Costa and Pierce [1983].

or any other cell for that matter [Pierce 1982], ATP seems to be involved.

DNP inhibits volume regulation and amino acid efflux from the *Noetia* cells, an effect similar to Ca^{2+} deletion [Amende and Pierce, 1980b]. The effect of DNP on the volume response of the *Glycera* red coelomocyte to hypoosmotic stress is also similar to Ca^{2+}-Mg^{2+} deletion—namely, a reduced initial swelling occurs followed by a more complete volume recovery. However, the amino acid efflux from *Glycera* cells is unaltered by the DNP

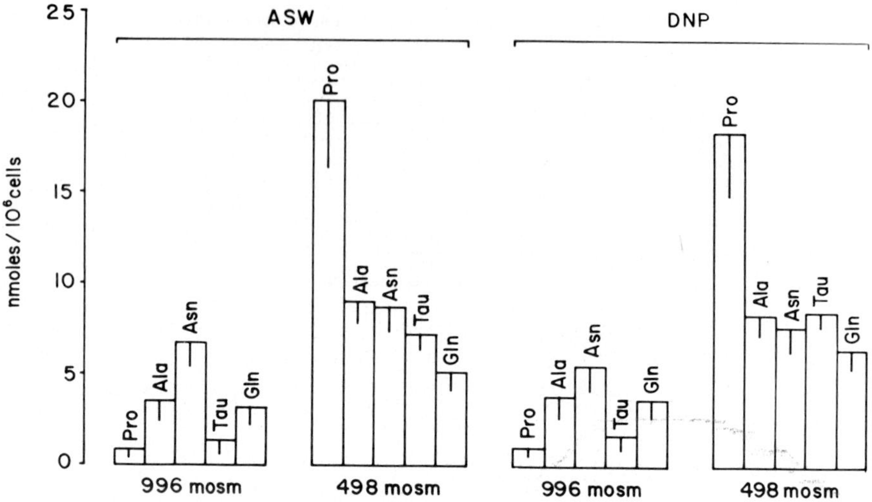

Fig. 13. Effect of 1 mM DNP on the amino acid efflux from *Glycera* red coelomocytes exposed to either isosmotic (996 mosm) or hypoosmotic (498 mosm). DNP was without effect on the efflux. ASW = artificial seawater. Data from Costa and Pierce [1983].

(Fig. 13). Instead, intracellular K^+ content is decreased below control levels in the presence of the inhibitor (Fig. 14) [Costa and Pierce, 1983]. The mechanism by which DNP exerts these differential effects is not yet clear, nor is it assured that the DNP is affecting similar processes by the same mechanism in both cell types. However, these results do suggest that ATP is necessary for normal cell volume regulation in both cell types. Importantly, the DNP results also clearly demonstrate that volume regulation in the *Glycera* coelomocytes at least is accomplished by means of two permeability control systems that can act independently of each other: the amino acid system (unaffected by DNP), which seems relatively slow to respond to the osmotic stress and is used for long-term adaptation, and the K^+ system (sensitive to DNP), which responds relatively fast and is used transiently. External Ca^{2+} concentrations also affect the intracellular K^+ content of the *Glycera* red coelomocyte. K^+ content is reduced by exposure to $Ca^{2+}-Mg^{2+}$-free seawater and the coelomocytes continue to leak K^+ regardless of the external osmotic concentration [Costa and Pierce, 1983]. Thus, Ca^{2+} appears to be involved in the permeability control mechanisms in both solute types and may in some manner control the two mechanisms, although there is no evidence for that at present. There are also no comparable data on the *Noetia* red cell, but it is a matter that is currently being investigated in our laboratory.

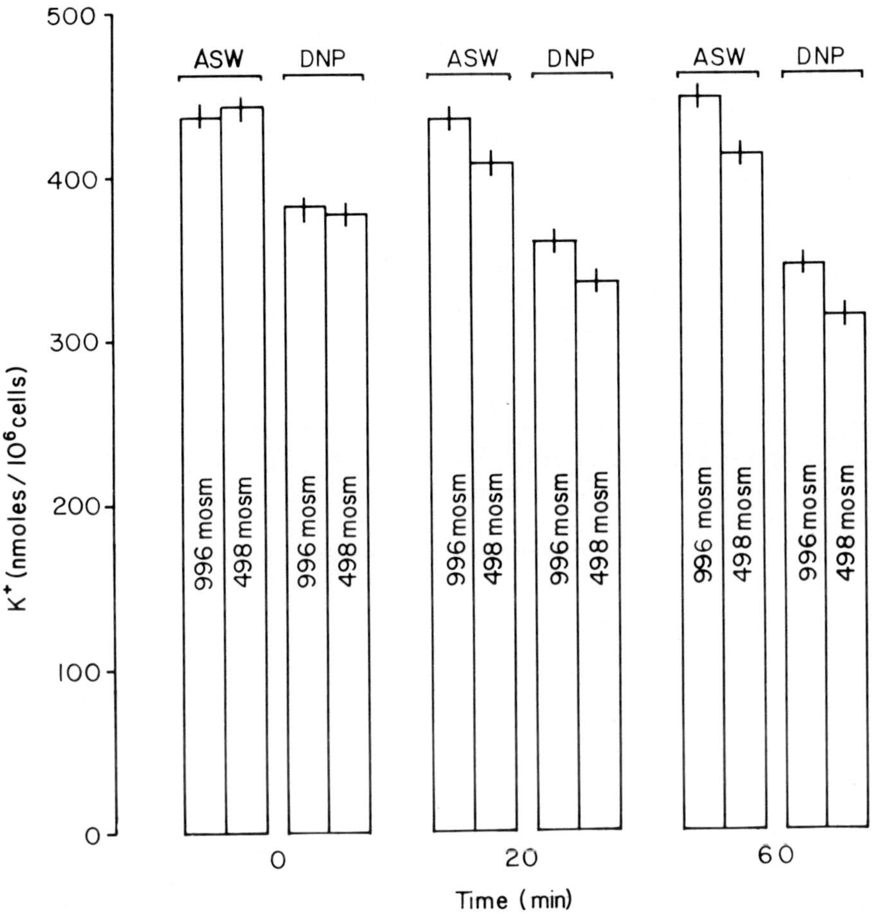

Fig. 14. Effect of 1mM DNP on the intracellular K^+ content of *Glycera* red coelomocytes in both isosmotic (996 mosm) and hypoosmotic (448 mosm) conditions. DNP clearly depletes intracellular K^+. ASW = artificial seawater; DNP = 2,4-dinitrophenol. Data from Costa and Pierce [1983].

Although the nature of the permeability systems that control the volume-regulating solute are still elusive, a few additional pieces of evidence are available.

Permeability Control System—Some Possibilities

The similarities between the requirements of the volume regulating systems in many of the invertebrate cell types and the mammalian red blood cell (specifically Ca^{2+} and ATP) led to the hypothesis that similar permeability control systems were involved. A rather aging literature indicates that the passive permeability and osmotic properties of mammalian red cell ghost membranes are regulated by a surface membrane associated, divalent cation requiring ATPase (reviewed by Pierce and Amende [1981]). A similar enzyme occurs in isolated membranes of bivalve (*Modiolus demissus*) myocardial cells, and alterations in the activity of that ATPase produces a concomitant alteration in the response of the cells to osmotic stress [Watts and Pierce, 1978a,b]. This type of enzymology has not yet been done on either the *Glycera* or *Noetia* red cells. Furthermore, while the control of permeability during volume regulation by a divalent cation-activated ATPase (in some unspecified manner) is still a viable hypothesis for these two cell types, some additional possibilities have appeared. For example, some of the effects of divalent cations on volume regulation of the *Glycera* red coelomocyte suggest that surface membrane binding of Ca^{2+} and Mg^{2+} rather than an ATPase may be the mechanism of efflux control [Costa and Pierce, 1983]. Either Ca^{2+} or Mg^{2+} will suffice to maintain normal permeability of the worm cells. Ca^{2+} is more effective than Mg^{2+}, but that may reflect the usual difference in binding affinities for these ions to both protein and phospholipid [Hauser et al., 1976].

There is also some evidence that actin polymerization is involved in the recovery of normal permeability in the *Noetia* cells following hypoosmotic stress. Cytochalasin D, which inhibits actin polymerization, causes increased volume recovery by the salinity stressed clam red blood cells. The potentiated volume response is produced by an increased taurine efflux [Smith and Pierce, 1983]. These results implicate cytoskeletal actin in the restoration of low membrane permeability to at least taurine during volume regulation, but additional experiments are required to clarify the situation.

Taken together, the results of experiments on the worm and bivalve red cells have uncovered much about the mechanism of cell volume control in response to a hypoosmotic stress. It seems a bit too early to generalize these mechanisms to all cell types. Indeed, as we have pointed out above, some differences of yet unknown significance exist between the water balance systems of the *Glycera* and *Noetia* cells. Nonetheless, there seems to be a growing list of similarities between the cell volume regulating systems of most cell types, including the categories of intracellular solutes utilized and the permeability control systems involved. If future research bears these similarities out, invertebrate blood cells may prove to be very useful models not only of cellular water balance, but also of membrane permeability control mechanisms.

ACKNOWLEDGMENTS

We thank C.J. Costa and L.M. Amende for providing the light micrographs of the *Glycera* and *Noetia* cells, respectively. A. Politis assisted with the pinocytosis experiments. Several of the studies reported in this paper were supported by National Institutes of Health grant GM 23731. This is contribution No. 223 from the Tallahassee, Sopchoppy & Gulf Coast Marine Biological Association, Inc and Contribution No. 40 from the Laboratory of Ultrastructure Research.

REFERENCES

Amende LM, Pierce SK (1980a): Cellular volume regulation in salinity stressed molluscs: The response of *Noetia ponderosa* (Arcidae) red blood cells to osmotic variation. J Comp Physiol 138:283–289.

Amende LM, Pierce SK (1980b): Free amino acid mediated volume regulation of isolated *Noetia ponderosa* red cells: Control by Ca^{2+} and ATP. J Comp Physiol 138:291–298.

Ben-Sasson S, Shaviv R, Bentwich Z, Salvin S, Doljanski F (1975): Osmotic behavior of normal and leukemic lymphocytes. Blood 46:891–899.

Buckhold B, Adams RB, Gregg EC (1965): Osmotic adaptation of mouse lymphoblasts. Biochim Biophys Acta 102:600–608.

Bui AH, Wiley JS (1981): Cation fluxes and volume regulation by human lymphocytes. J Cell Physiol 108:47–54.

Cala PM (1977a) Volume regulation by flounder red cells: The role of the membrane potential. J Exp Zool 199:339–344.

Cala PM (1977b): Volume regulation by flounder red blood cells in anisotonic media. J Gen Physiol 69:537–552.

TC (1981): Bivalves. In Ratcliffe NA, Rowley AF (eds): "Invertebrate Blood Cells, I." New York: Academic, pp 233-300.

Cheng TC, Burton RW (1966): Relationships between *Bucephalis* sp. and *Crassostrea virginica*: A histochemical study of some carbohydrates and carbohydrate complexes occurring in the host and parasite. Parasitology 6:111–122.

Costa CJ, Pierce SK (1983): Volume regulation in the red coelomocytes of *Glycera dibranchiata:* An interaction of amino acid and K^+ effluxes. J Comp Physiol 151:133–144.

Costa CJ, Pierce SK, Warren MK (1980): The intracellular mechanism of salinity tolerance in polychaetes: Volume regulation by isolated *Glycera dibranchiata* red coelomocytes. Biol Bull 159:626–638.

Cowden RR (1966): A cytochemical study of the nucleated, hemoglobin-containing erythrocytes of *Glycera americana*. Trans Am Microsc Soc 85:45–53.

Dales RP, Dixon LRS (1981): Polychaetes. In Ratcliffe NA, Rowley AF (eds): "Invertebrate Blood Cells, I." New York: Academic, pp 35–74.

Dawson AB (1933): Supravital studies on the colored corpuscles of several marine invertebrates. Biol. Bull 64:233–242.

Freadman MA, Mangum CP (1976): The function of hemoglobin in the arcid clam, *Noetia ponderosa*. I. Oxygenation *in vitro* and *in vivo*. Comp Biochem Physiol 53A:173–179.

Fugelli K (1967): Regulation of cell volume in flounder (*Pleuronectes flesus*) erythrocytes accompanying a decrease in plasma osmolarity. Comp Biochem Physiol 22:253–260.

Goodrich ES (1899): On the nephrida of the Polychaeta. Part II. *Glycera* and *Goniada*. J Microsc Sci 41:263–302.

Hauser HB, Levine BA, Williams RJP (1976): Interactions of ions with membranes. Trends Biochem Sci 1:278–281.

Hempling HG, Thompson S, DuPre A (1977): Osmotic properties of human lymphocyte. J Cell Physiol 93:293–302.

Hempling HG, Cicoria AD, DuPre AM, Thompson S (1981): State of water and electrolytes in mammalian cells during maturation and division. J Exp Zool 215:259–276.

Hendil K, Hoffmann EK (1974): Cell volume regulation in Erlich ascites tumor cells. J Cell Physiol 84:115–126.

Hoffman EK (1980): Cell volume regulation in mammalian cells. In Gilles R (ed): "Animals and Environmental Fitness." Oxford: Pergamon, pp 43–59.

Hoffmann EK, Hendil K (1976): The role of amino acids and taurine in isosmotic intracellular regulation in Erlich ascites mouse tumor cells. J Comp Physiol 108:279–286.

Hoffmann R, Mangum CP (1970): The function of coelomic cell hemoglobin in the polychaete *Glycera dibranchiata*. Comp Biochem Phsyiol 36:211–288.

Kregenow FM (1971): The response of duck erythrocytes to nonhemolytic hypotonic media. J Gen Physiol 58:372–412.

Lambert I, Hoffmann EK (1982): Amino acid metabolism and protein turnover under different osmotic conditions in Erlich ascites tumor cells. Mol Physiol 2:273–286.

Li MF, Stewart JE, Drinnan RE (1966): *In vitro* cultivation of cells of the oyster *Crassostrea virginica*. J Fish Res Bd Can 23:595–599.

Morton B (1969): Studies of the biology of *Dreissena polymorpha* Pall. II. Correlation of the rhythms of adductor activity, feeding, digestion and excretion. Proc Malacol Soc London 38:401–414.

Narain AS (1973): The amoebocytes of lamellibranch molluscs, with special reference to the circulating amoebocytes. Malacol Rev 6:1–12.

Negendank W (1982): Studies of ions and water in human lymphocytes. Biochim Biophys Acta 694:123–161.

Ohuye T (1938): On the coelomic corpuscles in the body fluids of some invertebrates. VII. On the formed elements in the body fluids of some marine invertebrates which possess the red blood corpuscles. Sci Rep Tohoku Imp Univ Ser 4 12:203–239.

Parker JC, Gitelman HJ, Glosson PS, Leonard DL (1975): Role of calcium in volume regulation by dog red blood cells. J Gen Physiol 65:84–96.

Parker JC, Castranova V, Goldinger JM (1977): Dog red blood cells: Na^+ and K^+ diffusion potentials with intracellular ATP. J Gen Physiol 69:417–430.

Perkins FO, Menzel RW (1964): Maintenance of oyster cells *in vitro*. Nature 204:1106–1107.

Pierce SK (1982): Invertebrate cell volume control mechanisms: A coordinated use of intracellular amino acids inorganic ions as osmotic solute. Biol Bull 163:405–419.

Pierce SK, Amende LM (1981): Control mechanisms of amino acid mediated cell volume regulation in salinity stressed molluscs. J Exp Zool 215:247–257.

Romieu M (1923): Recherches histophysiologiques sur le sang et sur le corps cardiaque des annelides polychetes. Arch Morphol Gen Exp 17:1–339.

Sato T (1931): Untersuchungen am Blut der gemeinen japanischen Archemuschel (*Arca inflata* Rve.). Zeit Vergl Physiol 14:763–783.

Seamonds B, Schumacher HR Jr (1972): Fine structure of erythrocytes of the common bloodworm *Glycera dibranchiata*. Cytologia 37:359–363.

Smith LH, Pierce SK (1983): Actin may control membrane permeability to osmotic solute during volume regulation in clam erythrocytes. Proc Int Union Physiol Sci 15:215.

Spring KR, Ericson A-C (1982): Epithelial cell volume modulation and regulation. J Membrane Biol 69:167–176.

Tripp MR, Bisignani LA, Kenny MT (1966): Oyster amoebocytes *in vitro*. J Invert Pathol 8:137–140.

Warren MK, Pierce SK (1982): Two cell volume regulatory systems in the *Limulus* myocardium: An interaction of ions and quaternary ammonium compounds. Biol Bull 163:504–516.

Watts JA, Pierce SK (1978a): Characterization of the divalent cation activated adenosine triphosphatase from the membrane of the cardiac cell of *Modiolus demissus demissus*. J Exp Zool 204:43–48.

Watts JA, Pierce SK (1978b): A correlation between the activity of divalent cation activated adenosine triphosphatase in the cell membrane and low salinity tolerance of the ribbed mussel *Modiolus demissus demissus*. J Exp Zool 204:49–56.

INTRACELLULAR RESPIRATORY PROTEINS

Blood Cells of Marine Invertebrates: Experimental Systems in Cell Biology and Comparative Physiology, pages 193–225

Chapter Seven
Intracellular Respiratory Proteins of Sipuncula, Echiura, and Annelida

Nora B. Terwilliger, Robert C. Terwilliger, and Eric Schabtach
Oregon Institute of Marine Biology, University of Oregon, Charleston, Oregon 97420 (N.B.T., R.C.T.) and Department of Biology, University of Oregon, Eugene, Oregon 97403 (N.B.T., R.C.T., E.S.)

INTRODUCTION

Several kinds of respiratory proteins with remarkable structures and a wide range of oxygen-binding abilities are found among the invertebrates. Very large (4.3×10^5 to 8×10^6 daltons) extracellular hemoglobins, with subunits that are probably homologous to the globin chain of vertebrate hemoglobin, are present in certain annelids, crustaceans, and molluscs [Terwilliger, 1980; Terwilliger and Terwilliger, 1983]. A large red-green dichroic protein, chlorocruorin, whose prosthetic group differs only slightly from the heme of hemoglobin, occurs as an extracellular oxygen transport molecule in four families of polychaetes [Fox, 1949]; this protein is similar structurally to the extracellular annelid hemoglobins [Terwilliger et al., 1976]. A third iron-containing respiratory protein, but one without a heme group, hemerythrin, is found within cells of four different phyla: Sipuncula, Priapula, Brachiopoda, and one genus of annelid polychaete [Manwell, 1964]. Hemocyanin is a blue extracellular copper-containing respiratory protein that is found in the hemolymph of many arthropods and molluscs [Van Holde and Miller, 1982]. Oxygen-binding properties of these invertebrate respiratory proteins are as diverse as their structures, ranging from simple hyperbolic curves that are independent of effectors to some of the most highly cooperative O_2-binding curves known [Weber, 1980].

Most vertebrates, on the other hand, utilize a relatively low molecular weight (M_r = 65,000) hemoglobin as an oxygen transport molecule. Vertebrate hemoglobin is always contained within an erythrocyte. Several invertebrates also contain hemoglobin or hemerythrin within cells. In contrast to the vertebrate cells, these cells are usually not found in a well-defined vascular system, and in most invertebrates the cells are morphologically more complex than the extensively studied mammalian red cell. In this chapter we will describe some invertebrate iron-containing respiratory proteins and the cells in which they are found. We will discuss the hematology and cytology of the cells together with the structure and function of the respiratory proteins. Some examples that have been studied in our laboratory will be described together with those found in the literature.

SIPUNCULANS

The erratic distribution of the respiratory protein hemerythrin in only four invertebrate phyla is intriguing. Purple-colored oxyhemerythrin is found in members of the phyla Sipuncula, and Priapulida, two ecardine Brachiopoda, and one polychaete Annelida, *Magelona* [Manwell, 1964; Wells and Dales, 1974]. Hemerythrin does not occur free in solution but rather is enclosed within cells variously designated as red corpuscles, erythrocytes, hemocytes, and hemerythrocytes. In *Magelona,* the hemerythrin-containing cells circulate in blood vessels; however, the sipunculans, priapulids, and brachiopods lack a vascular system and the cells are found elsewhere [Dehorne, 1949; Wells and Dales, 1974]. A myohemerythrin is found in the retractor muscles of some sipunculans [Manwell, 1960b].

In sipunculans, hemerythrin-containing cells circulate throughout the large coelomic cavity; they are also present within the lumen of the tentacles that connect to one or two blind-ended tubular sacs or contractile vessels (the "compensation sac" of Hyman [1959]). In some species, the contractile vessels exhibit extensive branching. These thin-walled contractile vessels extend into the coelom and are bathed by coelomic fluid. However, the tentacular-contractile vessel lumen is not continuous with that of the coelom [Hyman, 1959]. In certain species, the two compartments reportedly contain two structurally different hemerythrins [Manwell, 1960b, 1963; Klippenstein et al., 1972], which suggests that the two proteins and probably the two cell populations have different origins. Other cells, including gametes, are also present in the coelom of sipunculans and are described elsewhere (cf. [Hyman, 1959; Dybas, 1981]). In this chapter we will limit our discussion to coelomic and contractile vessel cells containing hemerythrin.

Hematology

The hemerythrin-containing cells constitute about 90% of the total coelomic cells in some species *(Phascolosoma agassizii* [Dybas, 1975]; *Sipunculus nudus* [Valembois and Boiledieu, 1980]). Mangum and Kondon [1975] report that *Phascolopsis gouldii* coelomic fluid has a hematocrit of 11.2% with a hemerythrin content of about 1.23–2.31 gm/100 ml. The volume of coelomic fluid in *P. gouldii* is about 2 ml; thus, each animal contains about 40 mg of hemerythrin. We have found the hematocrit for *Themiste dyscrita* coelomic fluid (five animals of about 2.3–4.5 gm wet weight) to be 33%. The average hemerythrin content of *T. dyscrita* is 1.94 gm/100 ml, and the average total volume of coelomic fluid is 1.2 ml. Thus, approximately 23 mg of hemerythrin can be obtained from a 4-gm *T. dyscrita*.

Morphology

The hemerythrin-containing cells of sipunculans vary in size from about 6 μm to 32 μm in diameter, depending on the species [Hyman, 1959]. The size variation may also be due to the way that the cells were handled for analysis [Dybas, 1981]. The cells have been described as circular, biconvex or biconcave disks or ellipses [Ohuye, 1937; Hyman, 1959; Ochi and Ohnishi, 1971; Valembois and Boiledieu, 1980; Nemhauser et al., 1980].

The coelomic hemerythrin-containing cells of *Themiste dyscrita* are shown in Figure 1. The cells have an average diameter of 27 μm, although the size ranges from 19 μm to 34 μm. When the cells are examined in coelomic fluid immediately upon removal from the animal, their shapes vary from disks to spheres. The cells are easily temporarily deformed as they float past one another on a slide. Some of the cells appear indented or lumpy (Fig. 1A). Within minutes, all of the cells undergo a shape change involving more indentations and surface wrinkles. Neither dilution into filtered 100% sea-water nor low temperature inhibit the shape change, but salinity extremes do affect the extent of shape change. In both bright-field and Nomarski phase-interference optics, the nucleus is barely visible unless vitally stained; it is small (2.5 μm) and eccentrically located. A vacuole about twice as large as the nucleus is usually present and clearly visible, as are several smaller vesicles. The indented shape and smooth surface of a cell are evident in the scanning electron micrograph (Fig. 1B). Figure 2 is a transmission electron micrograph of a coelomic cell; patchy electron-dense cytoplasm containing both presumptive hemerythrin and glycogen rosettes, a small nucleus, a few lysosome-like vacuoles, lipid droplets, and mitochondria are typically pres-ent. Of interest is the presence of numerous membranous lamellae, which resemble hollow tubules in cross section (Figs. 2–4). The few mitochondria found in these cells are generally closely associated with the tubule clusters (Fig.3). What these membranous structures represent is not known at present. They may correspond to the bands or "ribs" of dark material described in the cytoplasm of *Sipunculus nudus* cells by Valembois and Boiledieu [1980]. Although marginal band microtubules were not observed in *T. dyscrita* cells, they have been reported in *P. gouldii* cells [Nemhauser et al., 1980 as

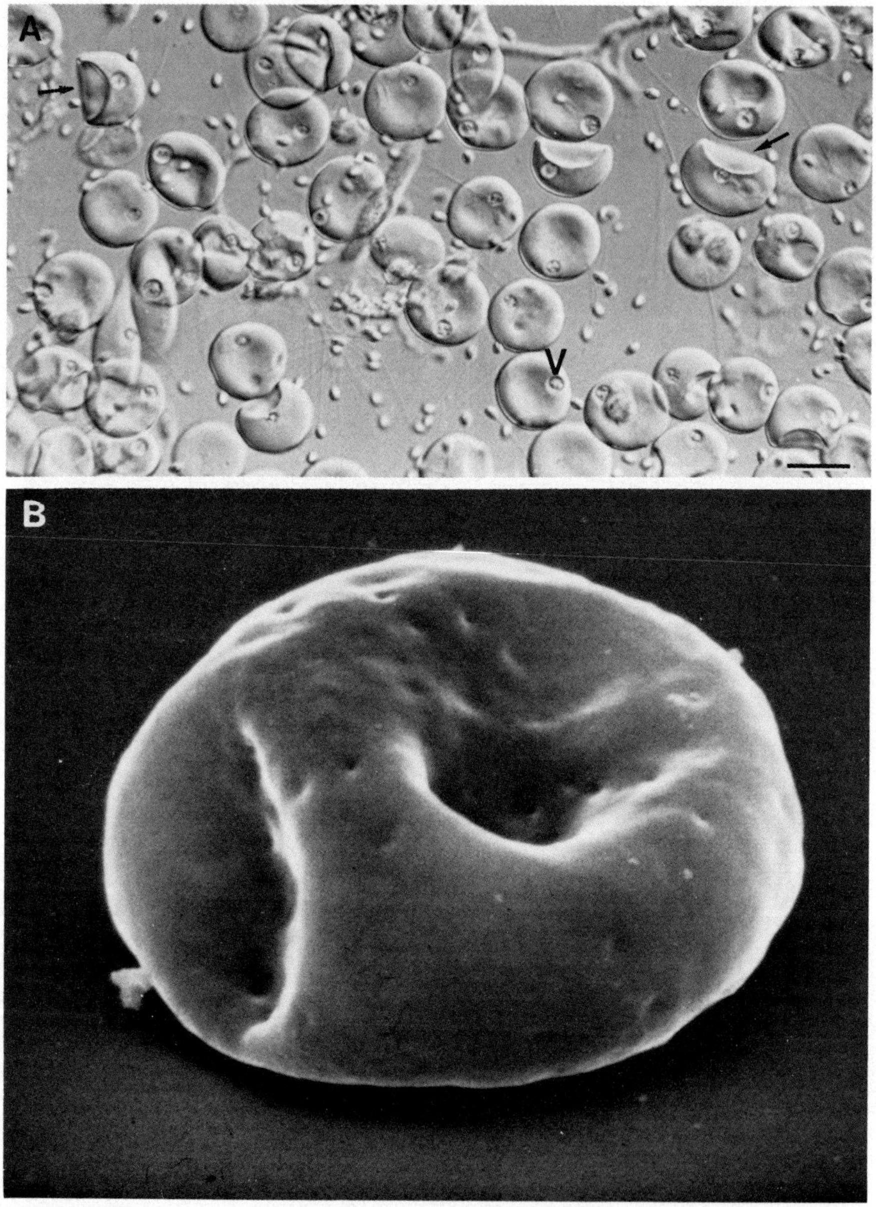

Fig. 1. *Themiste dyscrita* coelomic hemerythrin-containing cells. A. Living cells in fresh coelomic fluid photographed by Nomarski differential interference. Cell shape and size are variable (diameter 19–34 μm). Vacuoles (V) and indentations (arrows) are visible. Spermatozoa are also present in coelomic fluid. Bar = 30 μm. B. SEM of fixed, critical-point-dried cells showing a relatively smooth surface and major indentations. Considerable shrinkage occurs during this preparation process; therefore scale bars have not been included in the SEM micrographs.

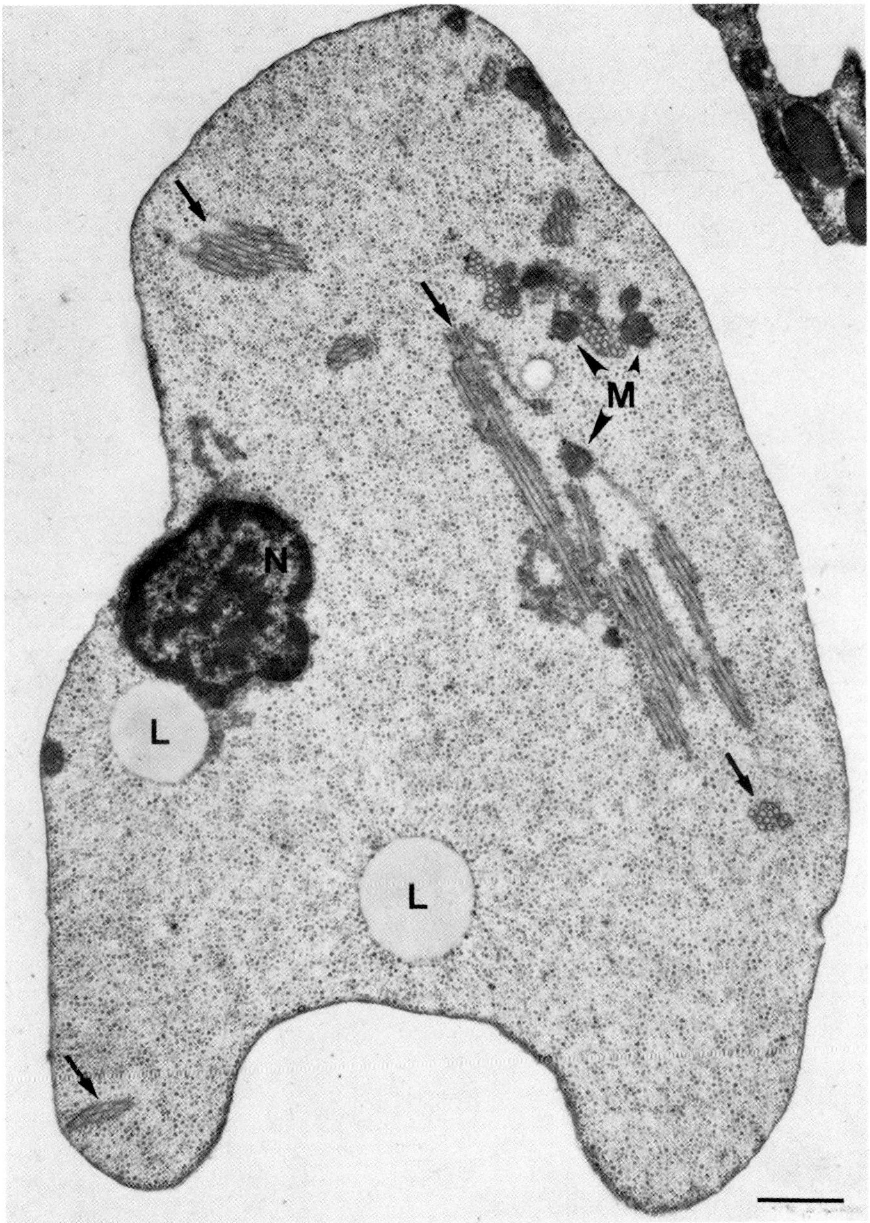

Fig. 2. Low-magnification view of thin section of *Themiste dyscrita* coelomic hemerythrin-containing cells. Eccentric nucleus (N), lipid (L), and mitochondria (M) are present. Some of the areas of membranous tubules, both parallel and perpendicular to the plane of section, are indicated by arrows. The large vacuole is not included in this section. Background cytoplasm contains glycogen rosettes and electron-dense cytoplasm presumably corresponding to hemerythrin. TEM. Bar = 1 μm.

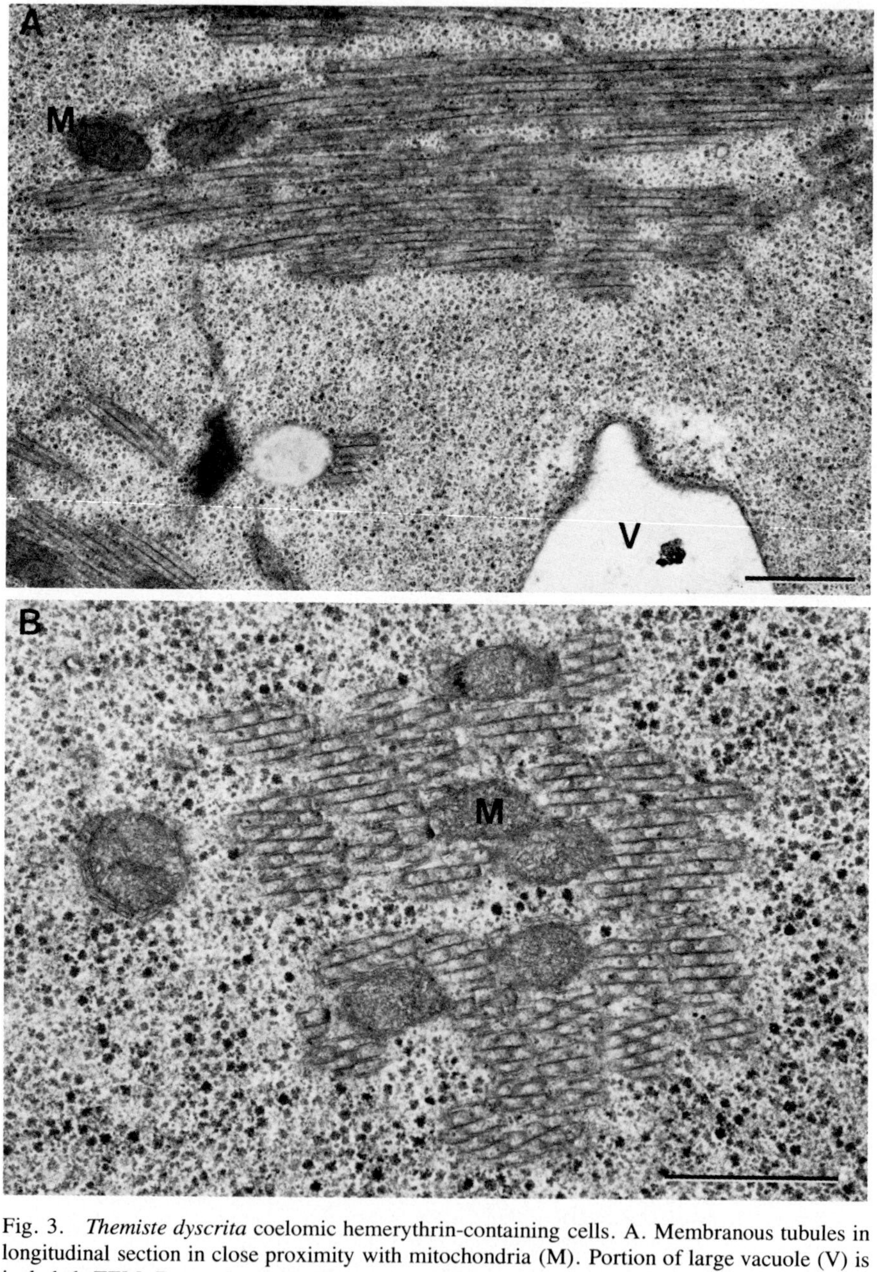

Fig. 3. *Themiste dyscrita* coelomic hemerythrin-containing cells. A. Membranous tubules in longitudinal section in close proximity with mitochondria (M). Portion of large vacuole (V) is included. TEM. Bar = 1 μm. B. Higher magnification of membranous tubules and mitochondria. Bar = 1 μm.

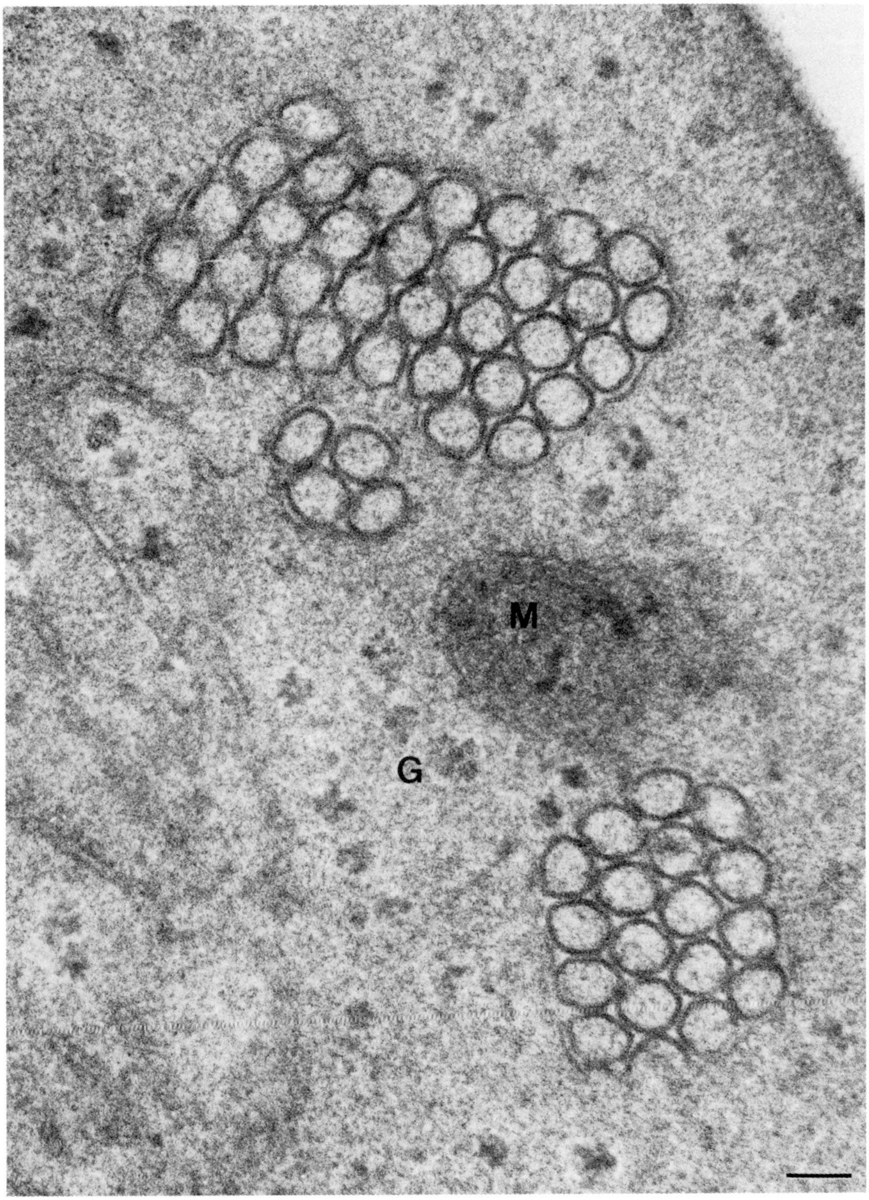

Fig. 4. *Themiste dyscrita* coelomic hemerythrin-containing cell. Cross section of membranous tubules. Mitochondrion (M) and glycogen rosettes (G) are present. Bar = 0.1 μm.

Golfingia gouldii] (see chapter by Cohen and Nemhauser, this volume). The general cytology of *T. dyscrita* hemerythrin-containing coelomic cells resembles that reported for other sipunculans; that is, they are nucleated cells with a limited number of organelles [Ochi and Ohnishi, 1971; Valembois and Boiledieu, 1980; Dybas, 1981].

Hemerythrin-containing cells are also found within the contractile vessels of *T. dyscrita,* a species with a well-developed system of contractile vessel branchings. The contractile vessel cells are smaller (19 $\pm$ 3.5 μm) and more uniform in size than the coelomic cells. Cells observed while still within the lumen of the contractile vessel are exceedingly plastic, changing shape as they tumble against one another. When removed from the vessel, the cells quickly assume a cup-shaped appearance (Fig. 5A,C) and tend to settle onto the slide with the cupped surface down. Neither coelomic nor contractile vessel hemerythrin-containing cells of *T. dyscrita* appear to aggregate upon removal from the animal. Contractile vessel cells contain many more small vacuoles than do the coelomic cells (Figs. 5B, 6). The membranous lamellae and tubules seen in the *T. dyscrita* coelomic cells are absent in contractile vessel cells. Several mitochondria and a small nucleus are present (Figs. 6, 7); the cell surface, like that of the coelomic cells, is relatively smooth (Fig. 5C). The cytoplasm appears more electron-dense than that of the coelomic cells.

The contractile vessel cells of the sipunculan *T. zostericola* are also smaller than its coelomic cells (discussed in Manwell [1960] as *Dendrostomum zostericolum).* The polymorphism in cell size observed in the two species *T. zostericola* and *T. dyscrita*, and the polymorphism in hemerythrin structure reported by Manwell [1963] and Klippenstein et al. [1972], suggest two possible scenarios. The first is that two different cell populations, coelomic and contractile vessel, may be synthesizing and may contain different hemerythrins. Conversely, different hemerythrins may be synthesized or modified during the course of differentiation of a single cell population. Valembois and Boiledieu [1980] have described cells that they presume are hemerythrin-containing stem cells. These "hemerythroblasts" are relatively small (approx. 8 μm in diameter), with a large nucleus, large tubular mitochondria, well-developed Golgi structure, and free ribosomes. They also find "transitional cells," relatively large (10–20 μm in diameter) with large mitochondria at the pole of the cell and nuclei that are larger than the nuclei present in mature cells. It is not known whether these hemerythroblasts and transitional cells contain different hemerythrins. It has been observed that "coelomocytes" can pass through the wall of the contractile vessel [Metalnikoff, 1900; Rice, 1975]. Thus the possibility exists that hemerythrin-containing cells originate and differentiate in the coelom and upon maturity pass into the contractile vessels or vice versa. Little is known about the site or process of hemerythrin synthesis. Do hemerythrin-containing cells mature in a manner

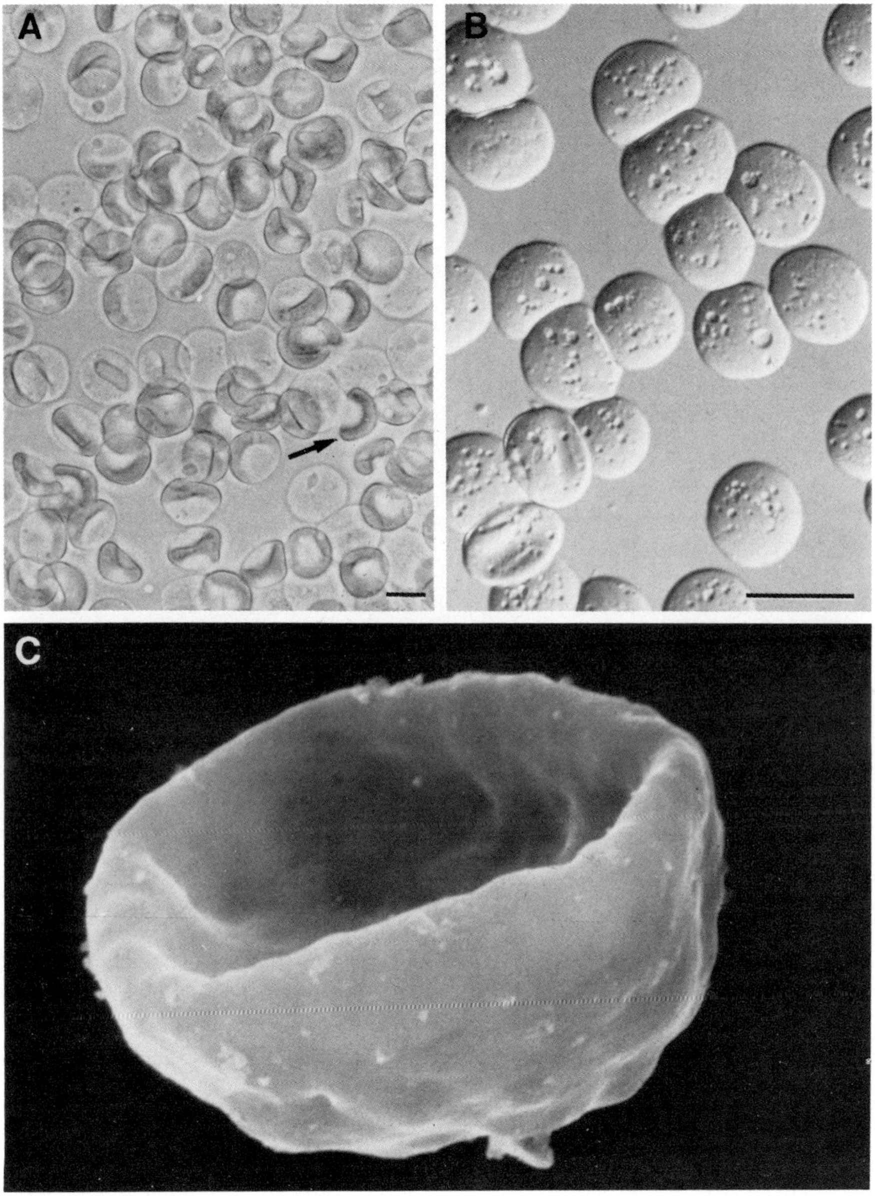

Fig. 5. *Themiste dyscrita* contractile vessel hemerythrin-containing cells. A. Living cells, some of which have already assumed a cupped shape (arrow). Bright-field light micrograph. Bar = 20 μm. B. Similar sample photographed by Nomarski differential interference. Many vacuoles are present in the cytoplasm. Bar = 20 μm. C. SEM showing smooth surface and cupped shape of the cell.

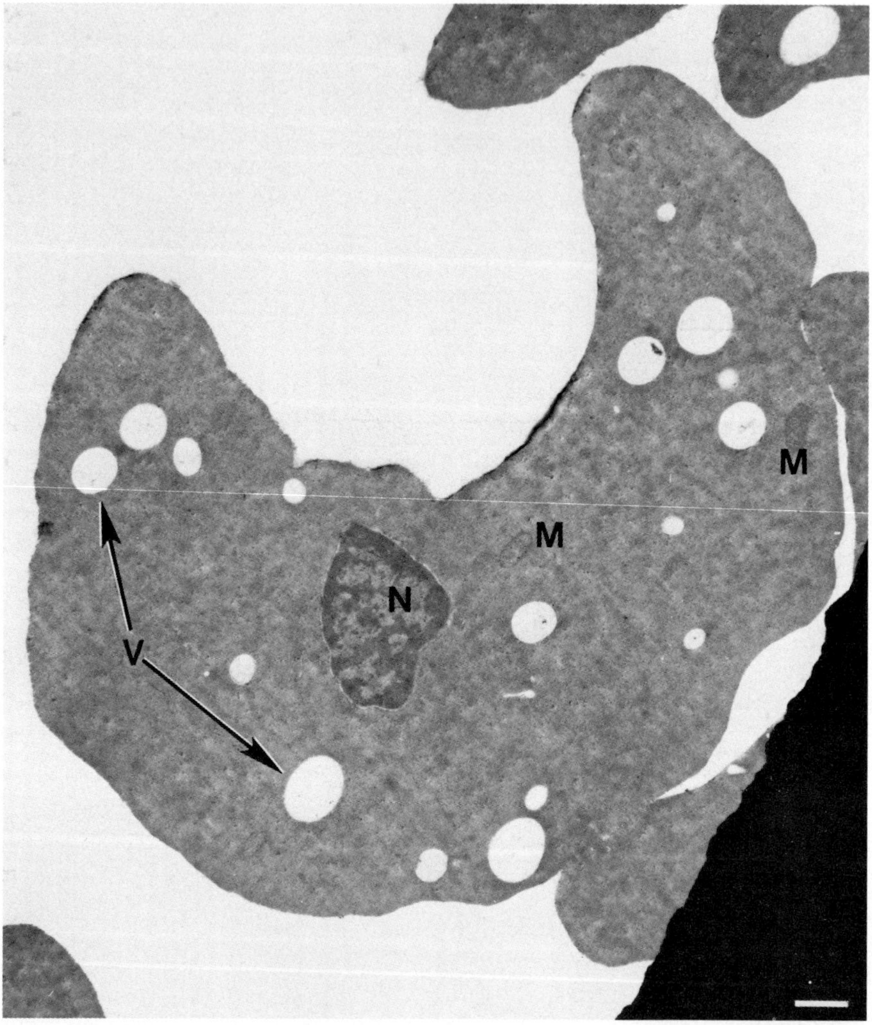

Fig. 6. *Themiste dyscrita* contractile vessel hemerythrin-containing cell. Low-magnification TEM of thin section. A nucleus (N), several mitochondria (M), and many vacuoles (V) are present, and the cytoplasm appears more electron-dense than in the coelomic cells (Fig. 2). Membranous lamellae are conspicuously absent. Bar = 1 μm.

similar to that of vertebrate erythrocytes? What is the cell's role in incorporating iron into the protein? The question of whether the coelomic and contractile vessel hemerythrin-containing cells belong to genetically or chronologically separate populations is certainly worthy of further investigation.

Hemerythrin

The major constituent of the hemerythrin-containing cells is the protein hemerythrin. Our understanding of this protein's structure in a number of species is almost as refined as that of vertebrate hemoglobin [Klotz et al., 1976; Loehr and Loehr, 1979; Klippenstein, 1980]. Hemerythrins do not resemble structurally either the hemoglobins or the hemocyanins. Most hemerythrins, including that of *T. dyscrita,* have a M_r of 100,000–110,000 and are composed of eight identical subunits, each with two iron atoms. Hemerythrin is an apparent tetramer (M_r = 60,700) in *P. lurco* (syn *P. arcuatum)* [Manwell, 1977]. Trimeric hemerythrins (M_r = 40,000) occur in the sipunculans *Phascolosoma agassazii* [Liberatore et al., 1974], *Siphonosoma* sp (discussed in Addison and Bruce [1977] as *Phascolosoma lurco)* and *Siphonosoma cumanense* [Addison and Dougherty, 1982]. A trimeric hemerythrin is unusual, since relatively few proteins show a trimeric subunit arrangement. A description of the mode of association of *Siphonosoma* trimeric hemerythrin based on X-ray crystallography has recently been published [Smith et al., 1983]. Myohemerythrin, found in the muscles of sipunculans, is monomeric (M_r = 13,900) [Klippenstein et al., 1972]. Amino acid sequence data are available for *T. dyscrita* [Loehr et al., 1978] and *P. gouldii* (discussed in Klippenstein, et al. [1968] as *Golfingia gouldii),* hemerythrins and the myohemerythrin of *T. zostericola* [Klippenstein et al., 1976]. A comparison of the coelomic cell hemerythrin sequences from the two species *T. dyscrita* and *P. gouldii* show a high degree of homology with 79% identical amino acids. The homology is lower, 42%, when coelomic cell hemerythrin from either species is compared with myohemerythrin from *T. zostericola* [Klippenstein, 1980]. With 70% of the polypeptide chain in an α-helix, the conformation of the hemerythrin has been readily resolved by X-ray crystallography to follow a "hemerythrin fold" that is present in all hemerythrins and myohemerythrins so far investigated [Hendrickson et al., 1975; Ward et al., 1975; Stenkamp et al. 1976, 1978]. A well-refined picture of the active site that includes the two iron atoms as well as some conservative amino acid sequences is currently being worked out [Loehr and Loehr, 1979; Elam et al., 1982; Hendrickson et al., 1982].

Why is hemerythrin contained within cells? The complex polymeric structure of hemerythrin strongly suggests that it might be modulated by allosteric effectors and that it might show homotropic interactions among the individual subunits. Furthermore, the inclusion of this protein in cells that appear to be capable of aerobic [Mangum and Kondon, 1975] as well as anaerobic respiration suggests that a metabolite would be present that could affect the oxygen affinity of hemerythrin in a manner similar to that observed for organic phosphate regulation of hemoglobin function. In our laboratory we have carried out some oxygen-binding experiments on *T. dyscrita* coelomic hemerythrin that had been stripped of allosteric modulators. Our results indicate

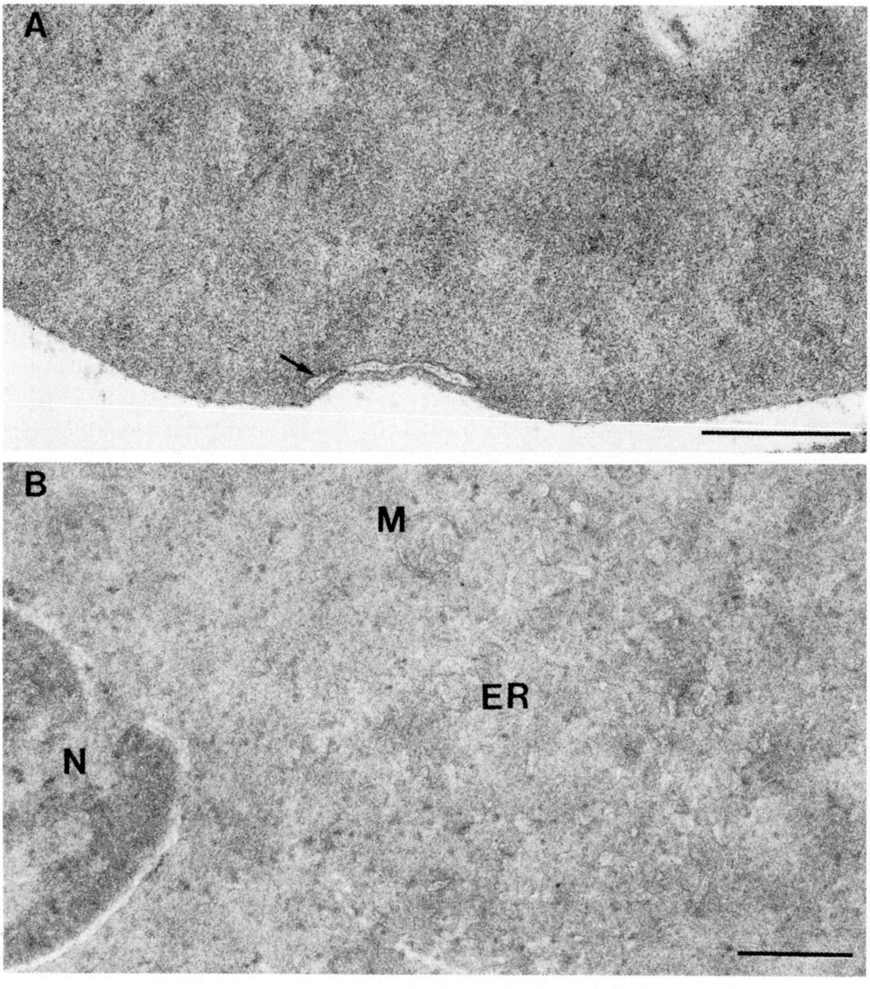

Fig. 7. *Themiste dyscrita* contractile vessel hemerythrin-containing cells. A. The cell surface appears smooth, except for an occasional flattened membranous vesicle just beneath the surface (arrow). Note background density and absence of other organelles. TEM. Bar = 0.4 μm. B. A cluster of smooth membranes, probably smooth endoplasmic reticulum (ER), a mitochondrion (M), and the nucleus (N) are present in this higher-magnification view (low contrast of membranes vs. background density makes them difficult to see). Bar = 0.4 μm.

that this octomeric hemerythrin is unaffected by a variety of metabolites such as D- and L-lactate, ATP, and hydrogen ions. Furthermore, the protein shows little evidence of cooperativity. Oxygen-binding studies have been carried out on numerous other hemerythrins [cf Klippenstein, 1980]. The P_{50} values range from to 1 to 15 mmHg for sipunculan hemerythrins. So far, no modulator that might be important physiologically has been demonstrated; this includes H^+ ions, and thus hemerythrin lacks a Bohr effect. Furthermore, even homotropic interactions appear to be lacking under the experimental conditions employed; n_H values range from 0.92 to 1.3. The one exception may be the hemerythrin of *Xenosiphon mundanus* [Wells, 1982]. Hemoglobins that are affected by allosteric modulators do show cooperative oxygen-binding properties.

Although we have not yet demonstrated an allosteric effector of hemerythrin function, the list of possible effectors has not been exhausted. Furthermore, hemerythrin removed from the cells of *Phascolopsis gouldii* shows a P_{50} that is half the value for the protein within the cell [Mangum and Kondon, 1975]. An explanation of this finding is not known.

Another reason for packaging hemerythrin in cells may be related to the finding that hemerythrin-containing cells of numerous species of sipunculans contain superoxide dismutase. It may be that the cell helps to enzymatically maintain hemerythrin in the reduced form that is necessary for reversible oxygen binding [Manwell, 1977]. An additional possibility is that the cell requires hemerythrin in order to provide oxygen for its own aerobic metabolism.

Although the main function of these cells may be to provide the proper environment for the respiratory protein hemerythrin so that it can bind with and transport oxygen, other functions are possible as well. One such function could be glycogen storage and transport. Recent studies on *T. dyscrita* coelomic hemerythrin-containing cells indicate that the cells contain an L-glucose stereospecific transport system (Ingermann R., unpublished). The cells undergo a very rapid rate of glucose uptake at 10°C with a half-time equilibrium of less than a minute. At the same time, the concentration of glucose in the coelomic fluid is about 1 mM, a threefold concentration over that of seawater. The abundance of intracellular glycogen and the periodic exposure of sipunculans to anaerobic conditions lend further credence to the possibility that the hemerythrin-containing cells also serve as a glycogen depot. The sipunculan coelomic cells may also be implicated in steroid hormone synthesis. A membranous array similar to that described here in *T. dyscrita* coelomic hemerythrin-containing cells has been reported in several mammalian cholesterol/steroid-synthesizing cells [Block, 1972; Anderson et al., 1983].

Why do the hemerythrins show such complex quaternary structure? A possible answer to this question may be evident when we know more about the protein's ancestry. It is not yet certain to what other protein hemerythrin might be related. Such information may in turn shed light on the evolution of the hemerythrin-containing cells.

ECHIURANS

Many echiurans have a closed circulatory system, but there are no respiratory proteins in the blood of those specimens that have been examined. Hemoglobin, however, is present in coelomic cells, coelomic epithelium, body wall muscles, gut wall, fat cells, nerve cord, anal vesicles, and eggs of various species [Lankester, 1881; Fox and Vevers, 1960]. Echiuran coelomic cells and their hemoglobins will be the subject of the following discussion.

Hematology

Hemoglobin-containing cells are abundant in the coelomic fluid of *Urechis caupo,* an echiuran with a degenerate vascular system. The cells make up 18–40% of the total volume of the coelomic fluid, which has an oxygen capacity of 2.66–7.22 ml O_2 per 100 ml [Redfield and Florkin, 1931] or 1.6–5 gm hemoglobin per 100 ml. The size of the cells and their contents vary with the apparent age of the animal as well as with its sex [Baumberger and Michaelis, 1931]; thus, it is likely that sex and age differences in hematocrit and hemoglobin concentration will be evident as well. Comparable measurements of volume and hematocrit were carried out by Ditadi [1975] on *Lissomyema exilii,* an echiuran obtained in Brazil. The mean hematocrit of 66% for this species is higher than that for *U. caupo;* no hemoglobin concentration was reported.

Morphology

We have examined the hemoglobin-containing cells of *U. caupo* by light microscopy, scanning electron microscopy (SEM) and transmission electron microscopy (TEM). As seen in Figure 8, *U. caupo* cells are spherical, ranging in diameter from 30 μm to 45 μm. The shape is quite stable in either coelomic fluid or seawater. With bright-field and Nomarski interference optics, numerous granules of varying densities are visible (Fig. 8A,B). The spherical cell shape is also apparent by SEM; the cell surface appears somewhat irregular, with both pits and protrusions (Fig. 8C). By transmission electron microscopy, shown in Figure 9, the typical small nucleus of the hemoglobin-containing cell is visible. A distinct nucleolus is often present (Fig. 10). The cytoplasm contains electron-dense areas presumably filled with hemoglobin, interspersed with large spaces containing glycogen rosettes (Figs. 9, 10). Numerous other organelles and inclusions are present, includ-

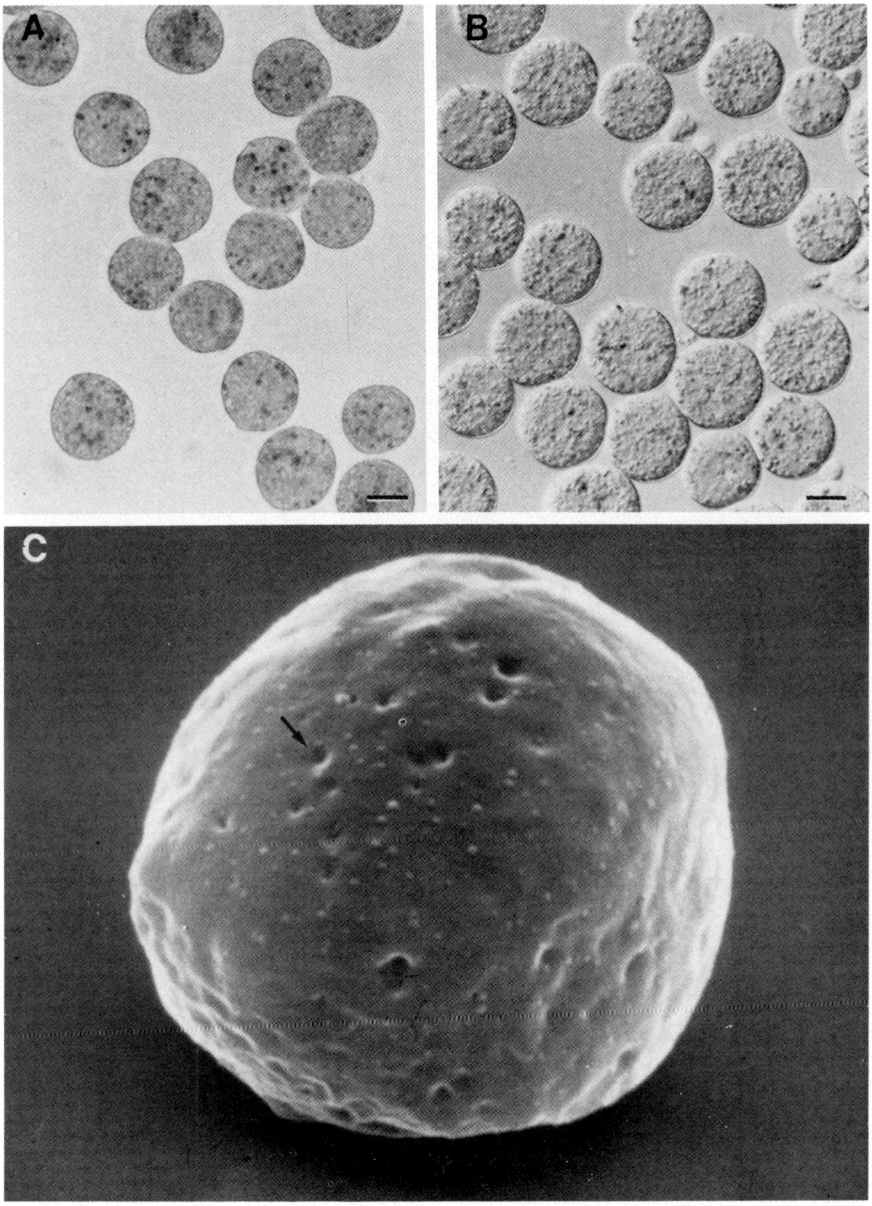

Fig. 8. *Urechis caupo* coelomic hemoglobin-containing cells. A. Living cells in coelomic fluid. Numerous granules are present in the spherical cells.Bright-field light micrograph. Bar = 20 μm. B. Living cells, Nomarski differential interference. Bar = 20 μm. C. SEM showing the presence of pits (arrow) and small protrusions on cell surface.

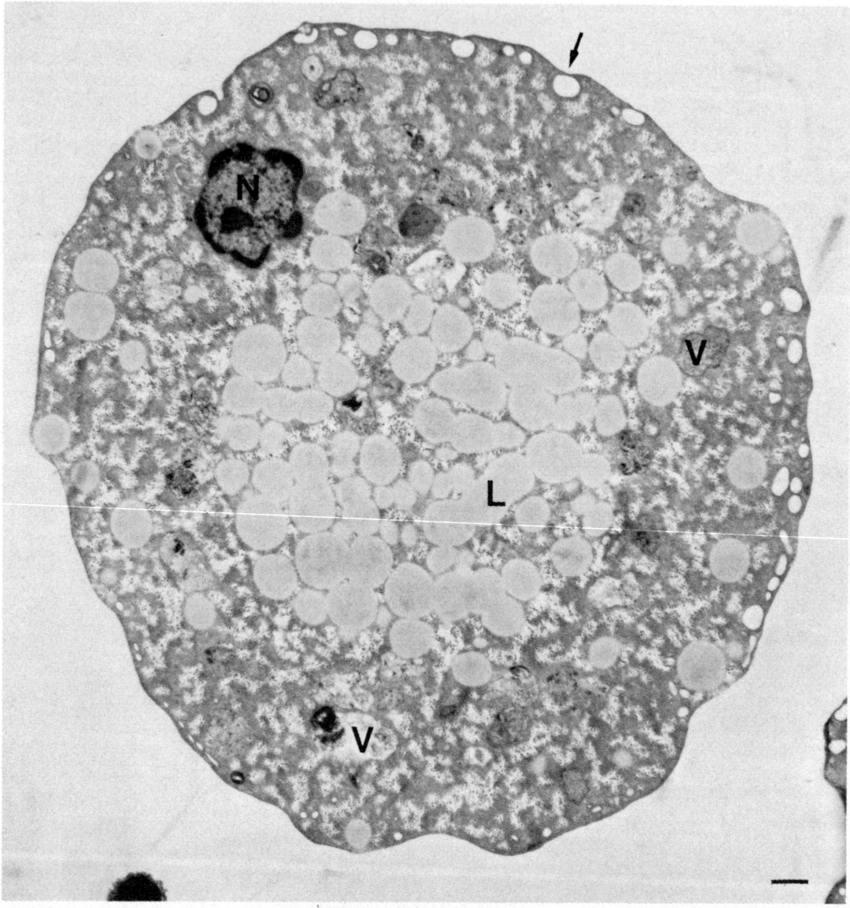

Fig. 9. *Urechis caupo* coelomic hemoglobin-containing cell. Low-magnification TEM showing the single eccentric nucleus (N) and numerous lipid droplets (L). Lysosome-like vacuoles (V) containing variable amounts of electron-dense material are scattered throughout the cytoplasm. The cell periphery contains many moderately sized vesicles (arrow). Bar = 1 μm.

ing lipid droplets, lysosome-like vacuoles, and mitochondria. The cortical region contains moderately sized vesicles, suggesting active uptake or transport of substances.

The color of the coelomic fluid of *U. caupo* varies from bright red (characteristic of oxyhemoglobin) to dark brown-black, even when the blood is saturated with oxygen [Baumberger and Michaelis, 1931; personal observation]. Most *U. caupo* have dark coelomic fluid. It has been reported by a number of workers that the coelomic fluid color is a function of granules in

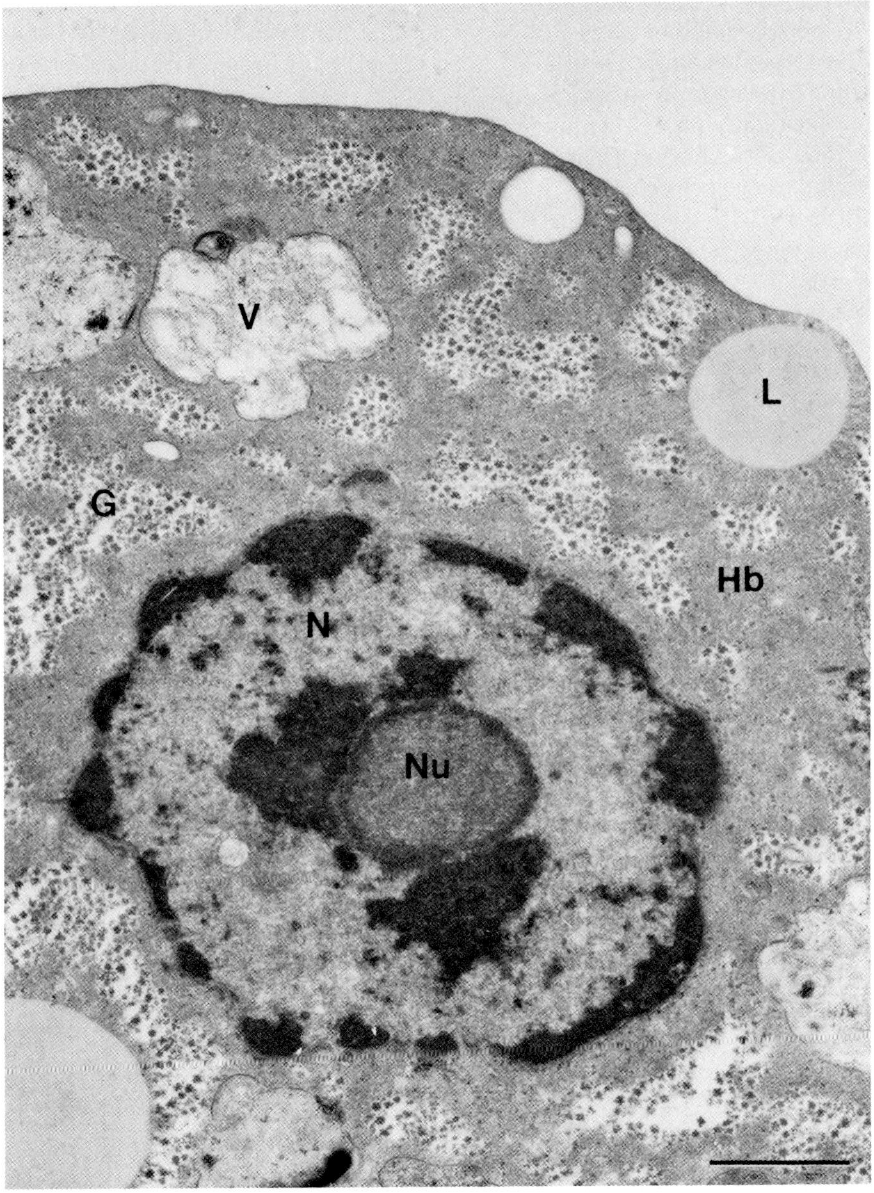

Fig. 10. *Urechis caupo* coelomic hemoglobin-containing cell. Higher-magnification view of nucleus (N) and nucleolus (Nu), lipid (L), and lysosome-like vacuole (V). The cytoplasm also contains patches of glycogen rosettes (G) interspersed with electron-dense regions presumably corresponding to hemoglobin (Hb). Bar = 1 μm.

the hemoglobin-containing cells. According to Baumberger and Michaelis [1931], some animals, presumed to be young, have bright red spherical cells about 10-15 μm in diameter. They show by light microscopy that the cells appear tightly packed with colorless spherical granules approximately 1 μm in diameter containing material with a high refractive index. In other animals with darker coelomic fluid, the granules are no longer colorless but appear filled with a brown pigment, which was identified spectrophotometrically as hematin. In sexually mature *U. caupo,* the hemoglobin-containing cells are larger, up to 35 μm in diameter. In mature male *U. caupo* the brown pigment is not only within the granules but also homogeneously scattered throughout the cytoplasm. Very small, spherical, black pigment-filled granules appear as well. The brown pigment in hemoglobin-containing cells of mature female *U. caupo* also is more scattered; however, none of the small black pigment granules are present. Baumberger and Michaelis [1931] proposed that small black pigment granules, identified as a hemochrome [Horowitz and Baumberger, 1941] in the eggs of *U. caupo,* are derived from the brown hematin pigments in the hemoglobin-containing cells of the female. The relationship, if any, between the coelomic cell pigments and the egg pigments remains to be shown.

The only other echiuran red cells that have been described in detail are those from *Urechis unicinctus* and *Ikedosoma gogoshimense* [Ohuye, 1937; Ochi, 1969, 1975]. As in *U. caupo,* the hemoglobin-containing coelomic cells of *U. unicinctus* are large spherical cells (approx. 30–50 μm in diam.) that contribute either a bright red, brown, or black color to the coelomic fluid. The cells contain abundant lipid granules, glycogen, mitochondria surrounding the nucleus, and in larger mature worms iron-containing granules or lysosomes. The lysosomes are larger and more numerous in cells taken from the darker coelomic fluid of older worms. Cells from both sexes appeared to have similar morphology. Ochi [1969, 1975] suggests that *U. unicinctus* cells respire by utilizing their intracellular glycogen or lipid as a metabolite. The cells of *I. gogoshimense* are smaller than *U. unicinctus* cells (10–30 μm in diameter), and although they are spherical, their cell margins appear to be strikingly irregular.

More recent studies of *U. caupo* red cells were presented by Dybas [1981]. Hemoglobin crystals as well as lipid granules were recognized in air-dried whole red cells as suggested earlier [Baumberger and Michaelis, 1931]. In agreement with Redfield and Florkin [1931], Dybas [1981] and we note that the cells do not clot or aggregate.

Hemoglobin

The coelomic cells of echiurans do contain hemoglobin as first described by Lankester [1881]. *U. caupo* hemoglobin has been investigated by several laboratories, including ours. The hemoglobin is a tetrameric protein, $S_{20,w} = 4S$ in both the oxy and deoxy state, with a $M_r = 57{,}000–60{,}000$ and a subunit of $M_r = 14{,}000–15{,}000$ [Bonaventura and Kitto, 1973; Hall et al., 1981; Garey and Riggs, 1982]. *U. caupo* hemoglobin appears to consist of more than one tetramer [Hall et al., 1981; Garey and Riggs, 1982]. The most abundant tetramer seems to be composed of a single polypeptide chain whose partial sequence suggests homology with other hemoglobins [Garey and Riggs, 1982]. The c-DNA from *Urechis* red cell RNA is being prepared [Garey and Riggs, 1983]. The hemoglobins of *U. unicinctus* and *I. gogoshimense* are also electrophoretically heterogeneous, consisting of one major and one minor component in *U. unicinctus* and two or three components in *I. gogoshimense* [Ochi, 1969].

The bright red color of coelomic cells from some echiurans immediately captures the attention of the respiratory physiologist. What is the role of these cells in oxygen transport or storage? Early O_2 binding measurements indicated that intact coelomic cells, presumably from normoxic animals, have a relatively low O_2 affinity ($P_{50} = 10–12$ mmHg at 10°C) and that they lack a Bohr effect [Redfield and Florkin, 1931]. More recently, it was suggested that the O_2 affinity of *U. caupo* hemoglobin increases during hypoxic exposure of the animals [Garey and Davis, 1978]. However, it was concluded that ATP does not appear to influence O_2 binding of *U. caupo* hemoglobin [Garey and Riggs, 1982]. In our laboratory, we have found that O_2 affinities of intact coelomic cells are the same in both hypoxic and normoxic animals [Mangum et al., 1983]. Furthermore, the oxygen affinity of intact cells is the same as that of stripped hemoglobin. Stripped hemoglobin appears to be insensitive to ATP, IHP, or hydrogen ions between pH 6.8 and 8.0, and there is no evidence for cooperativity under these conditions [Mangum et al., 1983]. Thus, although *U. caupo* hemoglobin is tetrameric and contained within cells, it apparently exhibits neither heterotropic nor homotropic interactions.

The hemoglobin-containing cells of *U. caupo* function to transport O_2 [Redfield and Florkin, 1931; Pritchard and White, 1981]. The thin-walled hind gut is periodically inflated with seawater. The coelomic fluid is then pressed between the inflated gut and the body wall, which contains monomeric myoglobin. One can observe convection of the coelomic fluid caused by peristaltic waves passing the length of the echiuran's body. It seems likely that transfer of O_2 can occur from coelomic cells to the myoglobin in the muscles used in burrow ventilation, especially since the myoglobin has a higher oxygen affinity than does the coelomic cell hemoglobin [Hall et al., 1981; Pritchard and White, 1981]. A different pathway of O_2 diffusion may exist in the relatively rare echiuran *Arhynchite pugettensis,* since the O_2 affinity of its body wall myoglobin is lower than that of its coelomic cell hemoglobin [Manwell, 1960a].

The number and variety of intracellular structures sets *U. caupo* hemoglobin-containing cells distinctly apart from the sipunculan hemerythrin-containing cells, as well as from nonmammalian vertebrate erythrocytes and many invertebrate hemoglobin-containing cells. The morphological complexity of the cells implies a more catholic function than just O_2 transport, perhaps functions similar to those of mammalian leukocytes as suggested by Ochi [1969, 1975]. Ochi [1975] examined the O_2 uptake in *U. unicinctus* cells and found that, like some vertebrate leukocytes, their metabolism was not stimulated by glucose but rather depended on glycogen or lipid metabolism. Functions of these cells might include active uptake and transport of nutrients to developing gametes in the coelom or scavenging and processing of coelomic detritus. A perplexing question concerns the variation in color of the hemoglobin-containing coelomic cells between different individuals. If the main role of these cells were to transport oxygen, one would expect bright red coelomic cells in mature animals whose coeloms are filled with developing gametes. Yet most echiurans contain dark coelomic cells. It is still not known whether adult echiurans have coelomic fluid with higher O_2 capacity than younger ones or if there is an inverse relationship between the presence of hematin and hemoglobin content of a cell. The dark hematin may be a waste product or may be used in some way not yet understood. It would be of great interest to know the lifespan of an echiuran red cell as well as to understand how these cells age or endure hypoxic conditions.

ANNELIDS

Annelid hemoglobins are found not only in coelomic cells and tissues such as muscle and nerve but also as extracellular proteins in vascular circulation. The vascular hemoglobins are giant molecules with $M_r = 3 \times 10^6$ to 4×10^6 [Weber, 1978; Terwilliger, 1980; Vinogradov et al., 1982] and a characteristic appearance in the electron microscope. An example of negatively stained extracellular hemoglobin of the terebellid polychaete *Pista pacifica* is shown in Figure 11. Low-molecular-weight (M_r = 15,000–125,000) intracellular hemoglobins are present in relatively few representatives of at least five polychaete families: the Capitellidae, Cirratulidae, Glyceridae, Opheliidae, and Terebellidae [Romieu, 1923; Weber, 1978; Dales and Dixon, 1981]. There is no record of intraerythrocytic hemoglobins in either oligochaetes or hirudineans. Annelid hemoglobin-containing cells are located exclusively in the coelom; they appear to belong to two general categories, depending on the worm species. In the cirratulids, opheliids, and terebellids, the hemoglobin-containing cells, sometimes referred to as "eleocytes," are relatively large, ~ 40 μm in diameter when mature, and contain abundant nutritive reserves, especially lipid. In the capitellids and glycerids, the hemoglobin-containing cells are quite different in appearance, showing few organelles and lipid inclusions [Dales and Dixon, 1981].

Hematology

The number of cells and their hemoglobin contents are variable. In *Pista pacifica,* we have recorded coelomic fluid hematocrit values ranging from 4.6 to 75.2% (avg. 40%, N = 10) with hemoglobin concentrations of 0.6–4.6 gm/100 ml (avg. 2.4, N = 8). The color of *P. pacifica* coelomic fluid can vary from red to black, similarly as described above for the echiuran *U. caupo.* Neither the Hct value nor hemoglobin concentration appeared to correspond to the size of *P. pacifica* or to the color of an individual worm's blood. Other polychaetes show comparable variations in their hematology. For example, in the glycerid *Glycera dibranchiata* the coelomic fluid Hct varies from 15.4 to 42 vol% with an average of 26.5 ± 10 SD vol %. The hemoglobin concentration is 3.54 ± 1.17 gm/100 ml for this species [Mangum and Carhart, 1972]. These values can be compared with a Hct of "cellular elements" of *Amphitrite ornata* coelomic fluid equal to 31.3% and a hemoglobin concentration of 0.045–0.45 gm/100 ml [Mangum et al.,

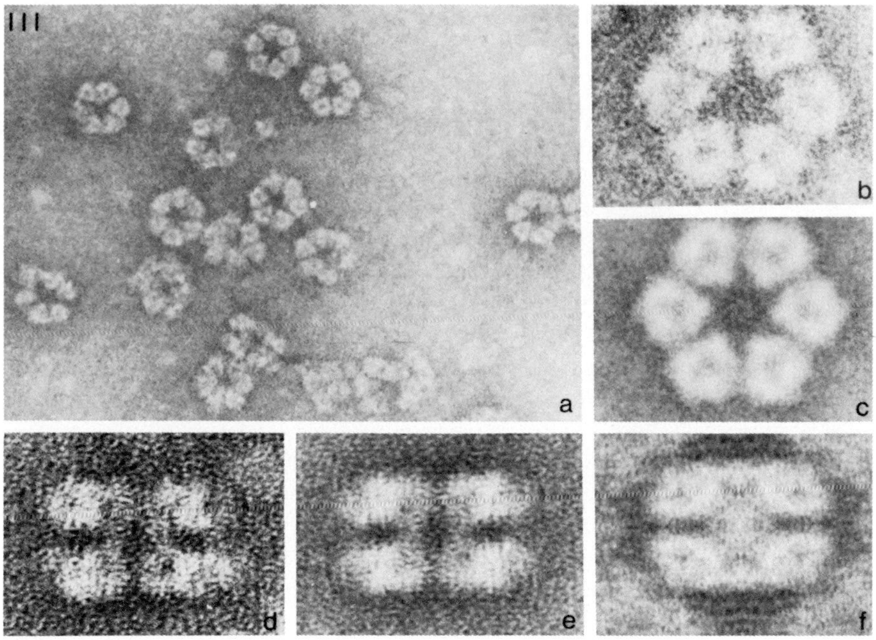

Fig. 11. TEM of *Pista pacifica* extracellular hemoglobin, M_r = 3.4 × 10^6, negatively stained with 1% ammonium molybdate. a,b. Face views. c. Sixfold optical rotation of b. d. Edge view. e. Fourfold optical rotation of d. f. Fourfold optical rotation of another edge view. Molecule is 25 ± 0.5 nm wide in face view and 17 ± 0.3 nm thick (edge view). From Terwilliger et al. [1976], with permission.

1975]. The same workers found that another terebellid, *Enoplobranchus sanguineus,* has a Hct of 30.6% and 2.75–8.4 gm hemoglobin per 100 ml blood. *Terebella lapidaria* has a Hct of 42% and a hemoglobin concentration of 4.2 gm/100 ml [Wells and Dales, 1975]. The variation in Hct and hemoglobin content may be related in part to the finding by Dales [1964] that the number of hemoglobin-containing coelomic cells in *A. johnstoni* increases during times of gamete production and decreases during gamete maturation. There could also be a fluctuation in hemoglobin concentration within individual cells, in a manner similar to *U. caupo* hemoglobin-containing cells, where hemoglobin is reported to be progressively converted to hematin [Baumberger and Michaelis, 1931]. On the basis of our preliminary studies, this does not appear to be true for *P. pacifica.* Using values in the literature to compute the amount of hemoglobin in the hemoglobin-containing cell (mean cell hemoglobin concentration, MCHC), we find levels varying from 0.1–1.4 gm/100 ml *(A. ornata)* to 8.8–27 gm/100 ml in *E. sanguineus. T. lapidaria* has a MCHC of 10 gm/100 ml; *G. dibranchiata* shows a similar MCHC value of 11.7 gm/100 ml and *P. pacifica,* 6 gm/100 ml.

Morphology

P. pacifica coelomic hemoglobin-containing cells are spherical (Fig. 12), ranging between 27 μm and 35 μm in diameter, and rapidly settle out of solution. The cells undergo no marked shape change except for a uniform swelling or shrinkage due to salinity changes in the suspension fluid. In the light microscope, the cytoplasm contains granules that when identified in the transmission electron microscope have the typical appearance of lipid droplets (Fig. 13). Electron-dense regions representing hemoglobin and patches of glycogen rosettes occupy most of the remaining cytoplasmic areas. A small eccentric nucleus is present. Mitochondria, endoplasmic reticulum, and a few lysosome-like structures containing electron-dense material are sparsely distributed. One of the more interesting features of these cells is that the periphery is packed with micropinocytotic vesicles, and a membrane system lies just beneath the periphery of the cell (Figs. 13, 14). This suggests that something is being transported across the cell membrane. The pinocytotic vesicles are apparent in the SEM as well (Fig. 12) (see also the *Glycera* red coelomocyte, especially Fig. 5, in chapter by Pierce and Maugal in this volume). It seems obvious that these cells are multifunctional, carrying not only oxygen but glycogen and lipid as well.

Dales [1964] studied the coelomocytes of the terebellid polychaete *Amphitrite johnstoni.* He described these cells as somewhat flattened, oval disks approximately 40 μm in diameter with a large nucleus and nucleolus. The small cells appear phagocytic; larger cells show pseudopodial entrapment of oil and other particles. The cells range in color from orange to dark brown, depending on the amount of β-carotene, hematin, and/or hemoglobin in the cells. An observed increase in polychaete coelomic hemoglobin-containing

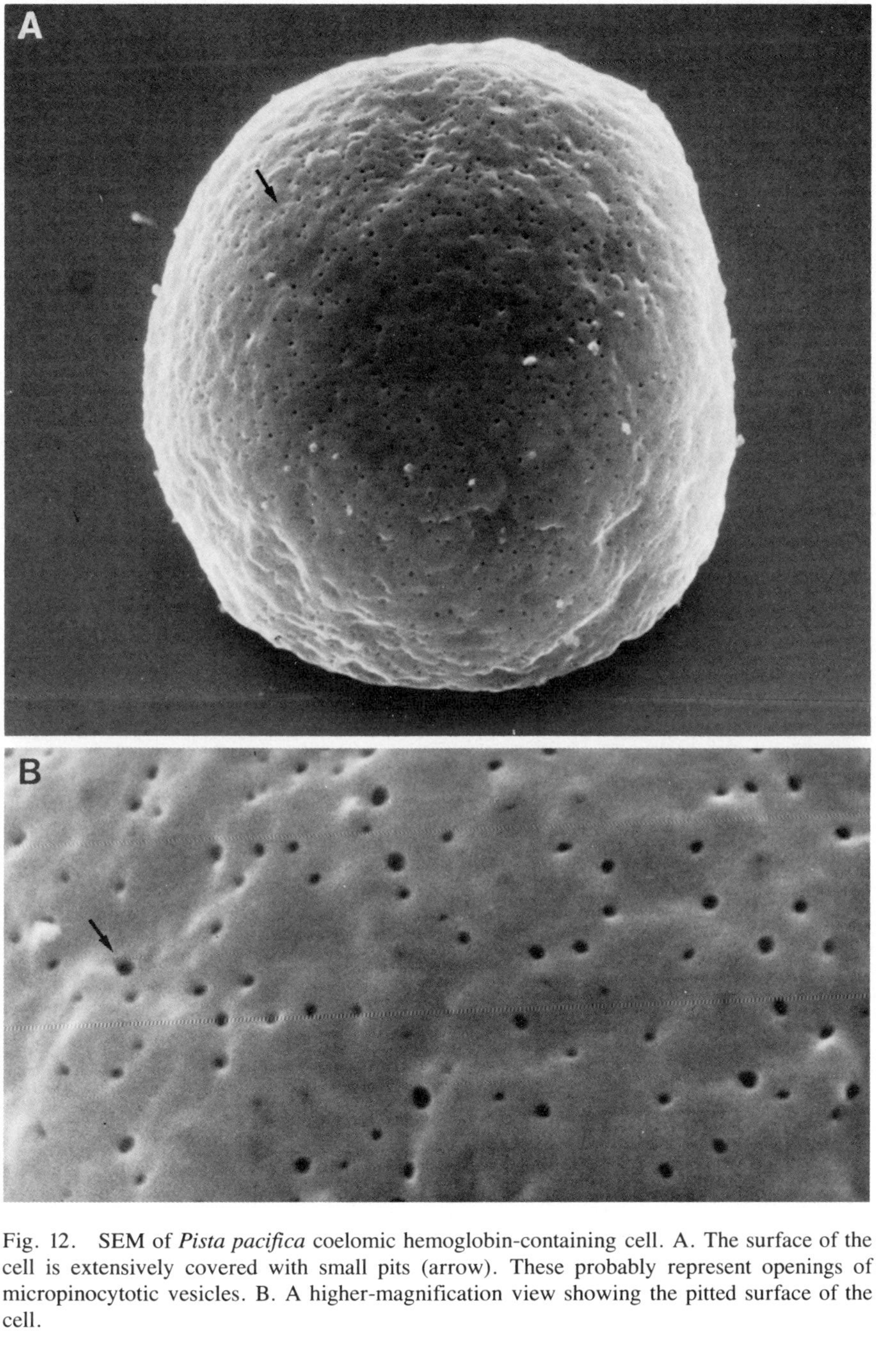

Fig. 12. SEM of *Pista pacifica* coelomic hemoglobin-containing cell. A. The surface of the cell is extensively covered with small pits (arrow). These probably represent openings of micropinocytotic vesicles. B. A higher-magnification view showing the pitted surface of the cell.

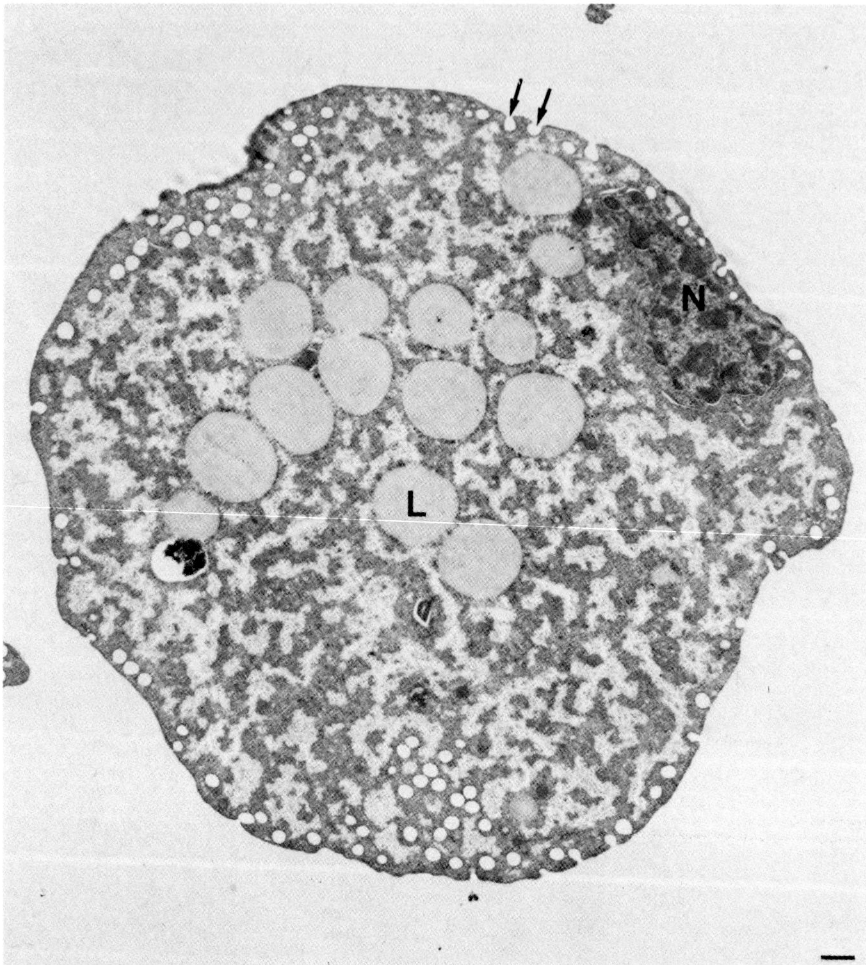

Fig. 13. *Pista pacifica* coelomic hemoglobin-containing cell. Low-magnification TEM view showing the nucleus (N), lipid (L), and numerous small pits (arrows) and vesicles, presumably engaged in micropinocytosis around the periphery of the cell. Bar = 1 μm.

cells, including those of *A. johnstoni,* during gametogenesis has led to the suggestion by a number of authors that the coelomic cells of some annelids supply nutrients to oocytes developing in the coelomic cavity (see Dales and Dixon [1981] for review). In support of this conjecture, there appears to be a selective uptake of β-carotene by *A. johnstoni* coelomocytes. A low concentration of the coelomocyte carotenoid is found within the eggs; astaxanthin-like material produced from a β-carotene precursor is present in eggs as

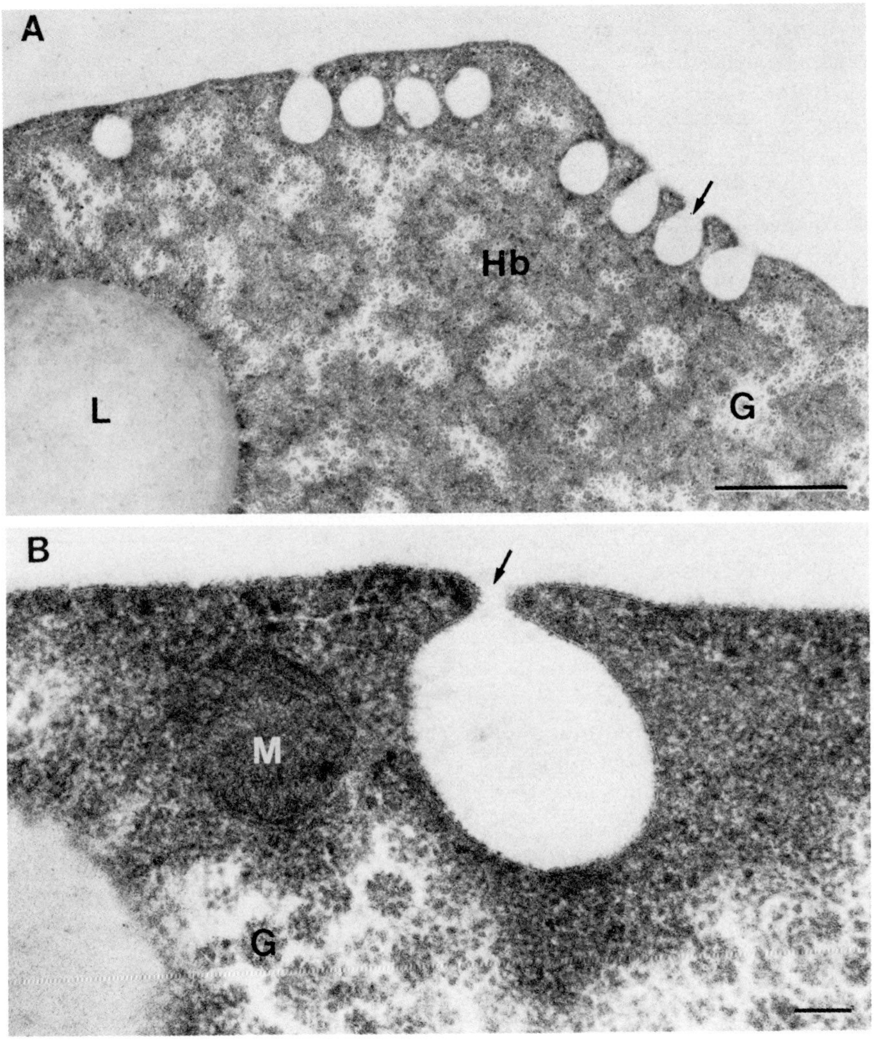

Fig. 14. *Pista pacifica* coelomic hemoglobin-containing cells. A. The surface pits (arrow) and vesicles are visible, as well as patches of glycogen (G) and electron-dense areas presumably corresponding to hemoglobin (Hb). TEM. Bar = 1 μm. B. A higher-magnification view of a membrane-bounded surface pit (arrow). Mitochondrion (M) and glycogen rosettes (G) are present. Bar = 0.1 μm.

well [Dales, 1964]. Coelomic hemoglobin-containing cells from the terebellid *Terebella ehrenbergi* are 30–70 μm in diameter and are described as oval cells with many large lipid granules and little hemoglobin [Ochi, 1969]. *T. ehrenbergi* cells, like those of *P. pacifica,* show electron-dense surface regions where small vesicles are found, irregularities in the cell surface, and inclusions such as membranous vesicles, lysosomes, and many glycogen particles. *A. ornata* has large cells, 17–35 μm in diameter, that are darkly granular and irregular in shape. *E. sanguineus* coelomic hemoglobin-containing cells are smaller, 11–14.5 μm [Mangum et al., 1975], which may account in part for their relatively high MCHC.

Few studies have been carried out on opheliid polychaete hemoglobin-containing cells. Those of *Travisia japonica* are oval, with a nucleus, mitochondria, lipid granules, and other granules [Ochi, 1969]. The cells, 30–45 μm in diameter, are larger in larger worms. Small and presumably young worms have red cells with few granules, whereas older larger worms have darker cells with an increased granule concentration especially in the males. The appearance of terebellid and opheliid hemoglobin-containing cells has led Ochi [1969] to describe them as "leukocytes with hemoglobin."

The glycerid and capitellid hemoglobin-containing cells appear to be more specialized [Weber, 1978; Dales and Dixon, 1981] or more highly evolved than the terebellid and opheliid cells [Ochi, 1969]. Studies of *G. americana* [Cowden, 1966], *G. decipiens* [Ochi, 1969], and *G. dibranchiata* [Seamonds and Schumacher, 1972] indicate that their coelomic cells are rounded or oval nucleated disks (20–70 μm in diameter). The hemoglobin is distributed throughout the cytoplasm. Glycerid cells, in contrast to terebellid cells, are notable for a paucity of lipid granules, glycogen, and organelles.

The hemoglobin-containing cells of the annelids show significant metabolic rates. For example, *E. sanguineus* cells respire at a rate of 455 μl O_2 gm^{-1} hr^{-1} and *A. ornata* cells at 677 μl O_2 gm^{-1} hr^{-1} [Mangum et al., 1975]. *T. lapidaria* coelomocytes show an O_2 consumption of 6.2 μl O_2 ml^{-1} hr^{-1} [Wells and Dales, 1975]. Metabolic rates of *G. dibranchiata* coelomocytes are slightly less than some of the terebellid cells with values = 289 μl O_2 gm^{-1} hr^{-1} [Mangum and Carhart, 1972]; however, metabolic rates of the *Glycera* cells are still considerably higher than those of vertebrate erythrocytes [Mangum, 1976]. Although some early studies (see, e.g., Cowden [1966]) suggested that hemoglobin synthesis did not occur continuously in *G. americana* coelomic cells, Shafie et al. [1976] showed that *G. dibranchiata* cells are capable of RNA and hemoglobin synthesis.

Hemoglobins

Annelid hemoglobins that occur in coelomic cells have relatively low molecular weights compared to the extracellular vascular hemoglobins. In the terebellid polychaetes (e.g., *P. pacifica, Thelepus crispus, A. ornata, E. sanguineus),* the coelomocytes contain monomeric hemoglobins with molecular weight of 15,000–17,500 [Terwilliger and Koppenheffer, 1973; Garlick and Terwilliger, 1974; Weber et al., 1977]. The one opheliid *(Travisia foetidae)* coelomic cell hemoglobin for which data are available shows a molecular weight of 34,000, a putative dimer [Terwilliger et al., 1980]. Capitellid hemoglobin *(Notomastus latericius)* also has a M_r = 36,400 [Svedberg and Eriksson-Quensel, 1934]. No data are available for cirratulid hemoglobins. The hemoglobins of numerous glycerids have been examined and show molecular weights ranging from a monomer (M_r = 15,000) to an octomer (M_r = 125,000) in *G. dibranchiata* [Hoffman and Mangum, 1970; Harrington et al., 1978]. The most thoroughly characterized annelid hemoglobin is an intracellular monomeric form of *G. dibranchiata.* This protein's sequence shows some homology to vertebrate hemoglobin and its tertiary structure resembles a typical vertebrate myoglobin-like fold [Padlan and Love, 1968]. Comparisons of amino acid compositions as well as some sequence data do not shed light on the relationships between these low-molecular-weight coelomic cell hemoglobins and the giant extracellular hemoglobins that often coexist within the same worm [Terwilliger et al., 1975; Weber et al., 1977; Garlick and Riggs, 1982].

The monomeric intracellular hemoglobins of the terebellid polychaetes show relatively simple O_2-binding characteristics, lacking both heterotropic and homotropic interactions [Garlick and Terwilliger, 1974; Mangum et al., 1975; Weber et al., 1977]. On the other hand, the dimeric intracellular hemoglobin of *T. foetidae* shows slight cooperativity [Terwilliger et al., 1980]. The glycerid polymeric intracellular hemoglobins in general have slightly lower oxygen affinities than those of the terebellids, with a small but distinct Bohr effect in some [Weber, 1978]. There is no effect of organic phosphate on hemoglobin oxygen binding in most annelid hemoglobins that have been examined [Mangum et al., 1975; Weber, et al., 1977; Harrington et al., 1978; Terwilliger and Garlick, 1978]. The sole exception is one of the *G. gigantea* intracellular hemoglobins in which ATP appears to slightly decrease the hemoglobin oxygen affinity [Weber, 1973]. There is some evidence of an effect of hemoglobin concentration on O_2 affinity in the hemoglobin-containing cells of *G. robusta* [Terwilliger and Garlick, 1978].

The presence of hemoglobin within cells in annelids cannot be explained, at least presently, as a way to modulate hemoglobin function. In contrast to the annelid intracellular hemoglobins, the oxygen-binding properties of the annelid extracellular hemoglobins show a remarkable range of homotropic and heterotropic modulation. Annelid extracellular hemoglobins can have highly cooperative oxygen binding with n_H values ranging as high as 6 or at the other end of the range may have hyperbolic binding curves. Many annelid extracellular hemoglobins have marked Bohr effects and some are sensitive to chloride or divalent cations [Antonini and Chiancone, 1977; Weber, 1978]. The presence of both intra- and extracellular hemoglobins within the same worm (certain terebellids and opheliids) or the co-occurrence of extracellular hemoglobins in both the coelom and the vascular system *(Nephtys)* makes the adaptive significance of hemoglobin-containing cells in the annelids puzzling [Mangum, 1976]. The oxygen affinities of most terebellid and opheliid coelomic cell hemoglobins are higher than those of their respective extracellular hemoglobins; this finding has implied oxygen transfer from vascular to coelomic hemoglobin and presumably to tissue in contact with the coelomic fluid [Terwilliger, 1974; Mangum et al., 1975]. Although oxygen might be transferred via these coelomic cells to developing gametes, it also seems likely that some of the oxygen is used to maintain the high metabolic rate these cells exhibit and perhaps to enable them to carry out their multifunctional tasks.

PROBLEMS FOR FUTURE WORK

The diversity of invertebrate red cell morphology and respiratory proteins, as discussed in the three phyla above, suggests various sites of origin and patterns of differentiation and an array of functions for these cells as well as numerous problems for future research. For example, it is now thought that in mammals a pleuripotential stem cell gives rise to a series of progenitor cells, which in turn produce three main marrow lines [Hoffbrand and Pettit, 1980]. The site of red cell synthesis varies in the vertebrates from bone marrow in adult human to the kidney in amphibian and teleosts, the gonads of certain fish, the liver in turtles, and tissue around the heart in paddlefish and sturgeon [Beck, 1973]. The origin of many invertebrate red cells is not well known. In several sipunculans, including *T. dyscrita,* hemerythrin occurs in two apparently different cell populations, those in the coelomic cavity and those in the contractile vessels. Do these represent two distinct cell lines or just one at sequential stages of differentiation? Although the two cell populations have specific morphological differences, both types contain few organelles and resemble the nonmammalian vertebrate erythrocytes. This similarity in morphology is intriguing, especially since the respiratory proteins hemerythrin and hemoglobin have no known structural resemblance to one another. In contrast to the sipunculans, both the echiurans and the annelids synthesize hemoglobin; however, their cells are quite different morphologically from vertebrate erythrocytes. The cells of *U. caupo* and *P. pacifica* shown above appear to be more multifunctional, on the basis of general morphology, than the cells of sipunculans and vertebrates. A knowledge of the site of cell origin, the precise maturation process, and the question of pleuropotential properties of the invertebrate cells might shed light on the ancestry of some of the vertebrate erythrocytes.

A second area for future study involves the mode of hemoglobin and hemerythrin synthesis in these cells. Although both hemerythrin-and hemoglobin-containing cells are presumably involved in oxygen transport, it is not at all clear that there should be a priori similarities in synthesis of the two very different kinds of proteins. Studies in this area might elucidate some unique routes and modulation of hemoglobin synthesis and the as yet unstudied synthesis of hemerythrin, the iron-containing protein without a heme.

A third area of interest concerns the functional properties of these invertebrate cells. Although members of the Sipuncula, Echiura, and Annelida synthesize intracellular respiratory proteins, it is by no means clear that oxygen transport is the cells' sole function. The invertebrate intracellular hemoglobins and hemerythrins are noteworthy for their lack of heterotropic and homotropic interactions, features which usually confer adaptive oxygen transport abilities upon the molecule. It has been suggested, and it appears likely from the cells' complex morphology, that some of these cells are multifunctional, with properties similar to those of vertebrate leukocytes. If so, potentially interesting areas for study include cell recognition and selective active uptake of nutrients as well as the processing of phagocytosed compounds.

Finally, it is known that in mammalian erythrocytes ATP generated by glycolysis maintains cell volume, shape, and flexibility. Hemoglobin-containing cells of *G. dibranchiata* regulate their volumes in response to short- and long-term hyposmotic stress by reducing the intracellular free amino acid and K^+ content [Costa et al., 1980; Costa and Pierce, 1983] (see chapter by Pierce and Maugel, this volume). The red cells of the annelids contain mitochondria and are capable of oxidative respiration. Perhaps aspects of membrane permeability regulation, membrane structure, or cytoskeletal integrity utilize the elaborate array of organelles seen in some of these invertebrate red cells.

ACKNOWLEDGMENTS

This work was supported by National Science Foundation grant PCM 8207548.

REFERENCES

Addison A, Bruce R (1977): Chemistry of *Phascolosoma lurco* hemerythrin. Arch Biochem Biophys 183:328–332.

Addison A, Dougherty P (1982): The coelomic hemerythrin of *Siphonosoma cumanense*. Comp Biochem Physiol 72B:433–438.

Anderson RGW, Orci L, Brown MS, Garcia-Segura LM, Goldstein JL (1983): Ultrastructural analysis of crystalloid endoplasmic reticulum in UT-1 cells and its disappearance in response to cholesterol. J Cell Sci 63:1–20.

Antonini E, Chiancone E (1977): Assembly of multisubunit respiratory proteins. Annu Rev Biophys Bioeng 6:239–271.

Baumberger J, Michaelis L (1931): The blood pigments of *Urechis caupo.* Biol Bull 61:417–421.

Beck WS (1973): "Hematology." Cambridge: MIT Press, pp 1–484.

Block VH (1972): The development of smooth-surfaced endoplasmic reticulum in adrenal cortical cells of fetal guinea pigs. Am J Anat 135:381–418.

Bonaventura J, Kitto B (1973): Ligand linked dissociation of some invertebrate hemoglobins. In L Bolis K, Schmidt-Nielsen, Maddrell SHP (eds): "Comparative Physiology." Amsterdam North-Holland, pp 493–507.

Costa C, Pierce S (1983): Volume regulation in the red coelomocytes of *Glycera dibranchiata:* An interaction of amino acids and K^+ effluxes. J Comp Physiol 151:133–144.

Costa C, Pierce S, Warren M (1980): The intracellular mechanism of salinity tolerance in polychaetes: Volume regulation by isolated *Glycera dibranchiata* red coelomocytes. Biol Bull 159:626–638.

Cowden R (1966): A cytochemical study of the nucleated, hemoglobin-containing erythrocytes of *Glycera americana.* Trans Am Microsc Soc 85:45–53.

Dales R (1964): The coelomocytes of the terebellid polychaete *Amphitrite johnstoni.* Q J Microsc Sci 105:263–279.

Dales R, Dixon LRJ (1981): Polychaetes. In Ratcliffe N, Rowley A (eds): "Invertebrate Blood Cells." New York: Academic, pp 35–74.

Dehorne A (1949): Le probleme des corpuscules du sang vasculaire de *Magelona papillicornis* F. Mull. Arch Zool Exp Gén 86:41–49.

Ditadi A (1975): On the coelomic fluid of *Lissomyema exilii* (F. Müller, 1883) (Echiura). In Rice ME, Todorović M (eds): "Proc Int Symp Biol Sipuncula and Echiura." Belgrade: Naučno Delo, Vol 2, pp 191–196.

Dybas L (1975): Cell within a cell or a circulating pair. Nature 257:790–791.

Dybas L (1981): Sipunculans and echiuroids. In Ratcliffe NA, Rowley AF (eds): "Invertebrate Blood Cells." New York: Academic, Vol 1, pp 161–188.

Dybas L (1981): Sipunculans and echiuroids. In Ratcliffe NA, Rowley AF (eds): "Invertebrate Blood Cells." New York: Academic, Vol 1, pp 161–188.

Elam WT, Stern EA, McCallum JD, Sanders-Loehr J (1982): Structure of the binuclear iron center in hemerythrin by X-ray absorption spectroscopy. J Am Chem Soc 104:6369–6372.

Fox HM (1949): On chlorocruorin and haemoglobin. Proc R Soc B 136:378–388.

Fox HM, Vevers G (1960): "The Nature of Animal Colours." London: Sidgwick and Jackson.

Garey J, Davis B (1978): Modulation of hemoglobin from *Urechis caupo* by organic phosphates in response to low oxygen. Physiologist 21:42.

Garey J, Riggs A (1982): Structure and function of hemoglobin from *Urechis caupo.* Fed Proc 41:650.

Garey J, Riggs A (1983): Preparation of c-DNA from the m-RNA of *Urechis* red cells. Fed Proc 42:1971.

Garlick R, Riggs A (1982): The amino acid sequence of a major polypeptide chain of earthworm hemoglobin. J Biol Chem 257:9005–9015.

Garlick R, Terwilliger R (1974): Coelomic cell haemoglobin of the terebellid polychaete *Thelepus crispus* Johnson. Structure and oxygen equilibrium. Comp Biochem Physiol 47A:543–554.

Hall R, Terwilliger R, Terwilliger N (1981): Hemoglobins and myoglobin of the echiuran *Urechis caupo* (Fisher and MacGinitie). Comp Biochem Physiol 70B:353–357.

Harrington J, Suarez G, Borgese T, Nagel R (1978): Subunit interactions of *Glycera dibranchiata* hemoglobin. J Biol Chem 253:6820–6825.

Hendrickson WA, Co MS, Smith JA, Hodgson KO, Klippenstein GL (1982): X-ray absorption spectroscopy of the dimeric iron site in azidomethemerythrin from *Phascolopsis gouldii.* PNAS 79:6255–6259.

Hoffbrand A, Pettit J (1980): "Essential Haemotology." Oxford: Blackwell Scientific, pp 1–236.

Hoffman R, Mangum C (1970): The function of coelomic cell hemoglobin in the polychaete *Glycera dibranchiata.* Comp Biochem Physiol 36:211–228.

Horowitz N, Baumberger J (1941): Studies on the respiratory pigment of *Urechis* eggs. J Biol Chem 141:407–415.

Hyman L (1959): The protostomatous coelomates—phylum Sipunculida. In "The Invertebrates: Smaller Coelomate Groups." New York: McGraw-Hill, pp 610–690.

Klippenstein G (1980): Structural aspects of hemerythrin and myohemerythrin. Am Zool 20:39–51.

Klippenstein G, Holleman J, Klotz I (1968): The primary structure of *Golfingia gouldii* hemerythrin. Order of peptides in fragments produced by tryptic digestion of succinylated hemerythrin. Complete amino acid sequence. Biochemistry 7:3868–3878.

Klippenstein G, Van Ripper D, Oosterom E (1972): A comparative study of the oxygen transport proteins of *Dendrostomum pyroides.* Isolation and characterization of hemerythrins from muscle, the vascular system and the coelom. J Biol Chem 247:5959–5963.

Klippenstein G, Cote J, Ludlam S (1976): The primary structure of myohemerythrin. Biochemistry 15:1128–1138.

Klotz I, Klippenstein G, Hendrickson W (1976): Hemerythrin: Alternative oxygen carrier. Science 192:335–344.

Lankester ER (1881): On *Thalassema neptuni* Gaertner. Zool Anz 4:350–356.

Liberatore FA, Truby MF, Klippenstein GL (1974): The quaternary structure of *Phascolosoma agassizii* coelomic hemerythrin. Arch Biochem Biophys 160:223–229.

Loehr J, Loehr T (1979): Hemerythrin. A review of structural and spectroscopic properties. In Eichhorn J, Marzilli P (eds): "Advances in Inorganic Biochemistry." Amsterdam: Elsevier North-Holland, pp 235–253.

Loehr J, Lammers P, Brimhall B, Hermodson M (1978): Amino acid sequence of hemerythrin from *Themiste dyscritum.* J Biol Chem 253:5726–5731.

Mangum C (1976): Primitive respiratory adaptations. In Newell R (ed): "Adaptation to Environment." London: Butterworths, pp 191–278.

Mangum C, Carhart J (1972): Oxygen equilibrium of coelomic cell hemoglobin from the bloodworm *Glycera dibranchiata.* Comp Biochem Physiol 43A:949–958.

Mangum C, Kondon M (1975): The role of coelomic hemerythrin in the sipunculid worm *Phascolopsis gouldi.* Comp Biochem Physiol 50A:777–785.

Mangum C, Woodin B, Bonaventura C, Sullivan B, Bonaventura J (1975): The role of coelomic and vascular hemoglobin in the annelid family Terebellidae. Comp Biochem Physiol 51A:281–294.

Mangum C, Terwilliger R, Terwilliger N, Hall R (1983): Oxygen binding of intact coelomic cells and extracted hemoglobin of the echiuran *Urechis caupo.* Comp Biochem and Physiol 76A:253–257.

Manwell C (1960a): Histological specificity of respiratory pigments. 1. Comparisons of the coelom and muscle hemoglobins of the polychaete worm *Travisia pupa* and the echiuroid worm *Arhynchite pugettensis.* Comp Biochem Physiol 1:267–276.

Manwell C (1960b): Histological specificity of respiratory pigments. II. Oxygen transfer systems involving hemerythrins in sipunculid worms of different ecologies. Comp Biochem Physiol 1:277–285.

Manwell C (1963): Genetic control of hemerythrin specificity in a marine worm. Science 139:755–758.

Manwell C (1964): Chemistry, genetics, and function of invertebrate respiratory pigments—configurational changes and allosteric effects. In Dickens F, Neil E (eds): "Oxygen in the Animal Organism." New York: Macmillan, pp 49–119.

Manwell C (1977): Superoxide dismutase and NADH diaphorase in haemerythrocytes of sipunculans. Comp Biochem Physiol 58B:331–338.

Metalnikoff S (1900): *Sipunculus nudus.* Z Wissensch Zool 68.

Nemhauser I, Ornberg R, Cohen W (1980): Marginal bands in blood cells of invertebrates. J Ultrastruct Res 70:308–317.

Ochi O (1969): Blood pigments and erythrocytes found in some marine annelida. Mem Ehime Univ Sci Ser B 6:64–131.

Ochi O (1975): The erythrocyte and its pigment in echiurans *Urechis unicinctus* and *Ikedosoma gogoshimense.* In Rice M, Todorović M (eds): "Proc Int Symp Biol Sipuncula and Echiura." Belgrade: Naučno Delo, Vol 2, pp 197–204.

Ochi O, Ohnishi S (1971): Fine Structures of the Coelomic Cells in the Sipunculid, *Phascolosoma scolops.* 1. General Observations. Mem Ehime Univ Sci Ser B, 6:7–19.

Ohuye T (1937): On the coelomic corpuscles in the body fluid of some invertebrates. Sci Rep Tohoku Univ Biol 12:203–239.

Padlan E, Love W (1968): Structure of hemoglobin of the marine annelid worm *Glycera dibranchiata* at 5.5 Å resolution. Nature (London) 220:376–378.

Pritchard A, White F (1981): Metabolism and oxygen transport in the innkeeper *Urechis caupo.* Physiol Zool 54(1):44–54.

Redfield A, Florkin M (1931): The respiratory function of the blood of *Urechis caupo.* Biol Bull 61:185–210.

Rice ME (1975): In Rice ME, Todorović M (eds): "Proc Int Symp Biol Sipuncula and Echiura." Belgrade: Naučno Delo, Vol 2, p. 8.

Romieu M (1923): Recherches histophysiologiques sur le sang et sur le corps cardiaque des Annélides polychétes. Arch Morphol gén et exp 17:1–339.

Seamonds B, Schumacher H Jr (1972): Fine structure of erythrocytes of the common bloodworm *Glycera dibranchiata.* Cytologia 37:359–363.

Shafie S, Vinogradov S, Larson L, McCormick J (1976): RNA and protein synthesis in the nucleated erythrocytes of *Glycera dibranchiata.* Comp Biochem Physiol 53B:85–88.

Smith JA, Hendrickson WA, Addison AW (1983): Structure of trimeric haemerythrin. Nature 303:86–88.

Stenkamp R, Sieker L, Jensen L, Loehr J (1976): Structure of methemerythrin at 5 Å resolution. J Mol Biol 100:23–34.

Stenkamp R, Sieker L, Jensen L (1978): Crystallographic studies of azide, thiocyanate and perchlorate complexes of methemerythrin. J Mol Biol 126:457–466.

Svedberg T, Eriksson-Quensel IB (1934): The molecular weight of erythrocruorin. II. J Am Chem Soc 56:1700–1706.

Terwilliger R (1974): Oxygen equilibria of the vascular and coelomic hemoglobins of the terebellid polychaete *Pista pacifica.* Evidence for an oxygen transfer system. Comp Biochem Physiol 48A:745–755.

Terwilliger R (1980): Structures of invertebrate hemoglobins. Am Zool 20:53–67.

Terwilliger R, Garlick R (1978): Hemoglobins of *Glycera robusta:* Oxygen equilibrium properties of coelomic cell hemoglobin and body wall myoglobin. Comp Biochem Physiol 59A:359–362.

Terwilliger R, Koppenheffer T (1973): Coelomic cell hemoglobins of the polychaete annelid, *Pista pacifica* Berkeley. Comp Biochem Physiol 45B:557–566.

Terwilliger RC, Terwilliger NB (1983): Oxygen binding domains in invertebrate hemoglobins. In "Structure and Functions of Invertebrate Respiratory Proteins." Life Chem Rep Suppl 1:227–238. London: Harwood Acad Pub.

Terwilliger R, Terwilliger N, Roxby R (1975): Quaternary structure of *Pista pacifica* vascular hemoglobin. Comp Biochem Physiol 50B:225–232.

Terwilliger RC, Terwilliger NB, Schabtach E (1976): Comparison of chlorocruorin and annelid hemoglobin quaternary structures. Comp Biochem Physiol 55A:51–55.

Terwilliger R, Garlick R, Terwilliger N (1980): Characterization of the hemoglobins and myoglobin of *Travisia foetida*. Comp Biochem Physiol 66B:261–266.

Valembois P, Boiledieu D (1980): Fine structure and functions of haemerythrocytes and leucocytes of *Sipunculus nudus*. J Morphol 163:64–77.

Van Holde KE, Miller KI (1982): Haemocyanins. Q Rev Biophys 15:1–129.

Vinogradov SN, Kapp OH, Ohtsuki M (1982): The extracellular haemoglobins and chlorocruorins of annelids. In Harris JR (ed): "Electron Microscopy of Proteins." London: Academic Press, Vol. 3, pp 135–164.

Ward K, Hendrickson W, Klippenstein G (1975): Quaternary and tertiary structure of haemerythrin. Nature 257:818–821.

Weber RE (1973): Functional and molecular properties of corpuscular haemoglobin from the bloodworm *Glycera gigantea*. Neth J Sea Res 7:316–327.

Weber RE (1978): Respiratory pigments. In Mill P (ed): "Physiology of Annelids." New York: Academic, pp 393–446.

Weber RE (1980): Functions of invertebrate hemoglobins with special reference to adaptations to environmental hypoxia. Am Zool 20:79–101.

Weber RE, Magnum C, Steinman H, Bonaventura C, Sullivan B, Bonaventura J (1977): Hemoglobins of two terebellid polychaetes: *Enoplobranchus sanquineus* and *Amphitrite ornata*. Comp Biochem Physiol 56A:179–187.

Wells RMG (1982): Respiratory characteristics of the blood pigments of three worms from an intertidal mudflat. N Zealand J Zool 9:243–248.

Wells RMG, Dales RP (1974): Oxygenational properties of haemerythrin in the blood of *Magelona papillicornis* Müller (Polychaeta: Magelonidae). Comp Biochem Physiol 49A:57–64.

Wells R, Dales R (1975): Haemoglobin function in *Terebella lapidaria* L., an intertidal terebellid polychaete. J Mar Biol Assoc UK 55:211–220.

Blood Cells of Marine Invertebrates: Experimental Systems in Cell Biology and Comparative Physiology, pages 227–247

Chapter Eight
Molluscan Hemoglobins

Ronald L. Nagel

Division of Hematology, Albert Einstein College of Medicine, Bronx, New York 10461 and the Marine Biological Laboratory, Woods Hole, Massachusetts 02543

INTRODUCTION

Among the Metazoans, the Phylum Mollusca represents about 110,000 different living species, a number that is almost three times larger than the known species of vertebrates living today on the earth. This diversity attests to the great adaptative success of the molluscs, surpassed only by the awesome proliferation of the Phylum Arthropoda, whose members number more than 800,000 different living species [Russell-Hunter, 1968].

Most molluscs are characterized by a hard calcareous outer shell that protects them from predators (except when these are endowed with ingeniously constructed and specifically dedicated apparatus such as the claws of lobsters). In addition, they exhibit a sophisticated use of ciliary and mucous mechanisms for feeding, locomotion, and reproduction. Their ciliated gill, the *ctenidium* (which can contain hemoglobin), is an important organ for feeding and respiration and is the centerpiece of the mantle-cavity and semi-internal respiratory chamber.

The ctenidium has an elaborate system of particle-sizing surfaces that molluscs, particularly bivalves, can change to adapt to feeding conditions (this mechanism permits clams and oysters to concentrate the hepatitis virus and become a health hazard in contaminated waters). The ctenidia contain coelomic fluid, which in some bivalves contains hemoglobin-carrying erythrocytes. Hence, the surface of the organ is not only a particle-size discriminator but a respiratory organ. The coelomic fluid circulates inside the ctenidia by way of afferent and efferent blood vessels and is pumped by a rudimentary single-cavity heart.

In all molluscs the alimentary canal is ciliated and the typical gut is constructed to handle the finely chopped material generated by the filter mechanism of the bivalves or the characteristic rasping tongue (*radula*) of the grazing molluscs (snails and gastropods). The radula (which we will encounter again because it can contain hemoglobin) is a chitinous surface bristling with teeth that cover a tongue supported by an odontophore. This apparatus can be moved as a conveyor belt by buccal muscles and can rasp off material and transport it into the gut.

The major classes of Molluscs are Gastropods (snails), Bivalves (clams), and Cephalopods (octopus, squid). Minor classes of living Molluscs are a) Scaphopoda (elephant tusk-shells), which are intermediate between bivalves and gastropods, b) Aplacophora (worm-like with mantle and no shell), c) Polyplacophora (Chitons), and d) Monoplacophora, with only one living genus, *Neopilina* (an animal with limpet-like shell and sucker-like foot). The minor classes (a) and (c) were previously known as Amphineura.

EXPERIMENTAL STUDIES: ERYTHROCYTES OF EASTERN U.S. SPECIES

Anadara ovalis

In collaboration with Tom Borgese, Eugene F. Roth, and John Harrington, we have been studying in Woods Hole the hemoglobins found in the red cells of the "blood ark," *Anadara ovalis*. These cells, present in the hemolymph of this clam, are of great interest. Giemsa stain (Fig. 1A) shows that they are nucleated (as are red cells of nonmammalian vertebrates) but that, in addition, they have a number of cytoplasmic inclusions not observed in the red cells of vertebrates. The most striking inclusions are very dense granules that Eugene F. Roth has identified, by specific stain, to be iron containing aggregates (Fig. 1B). The significance of this finding requires further work, but it would not be surprising if these aggregates represent the iron stores necessary for hemoglobin synthesis. Vertebrate red cells also contain iron in the form of ferritin, but those are submicroscopic inclusions. Scanning electron microscopy of the *Anadara ovalis* red cells, fixed directly from the coelomic fluid, shows them to be relatively smooth-surfaced, with the nucleus apparently producing a bulge visible in some cells (Fig. 2). Images compatible with the presence of a marginal band of microtubules are also apparent (Fig. 2; see Chapter One by Cohen and Nemhauser).

The erythrocytes of *A. ovalis* contain two electrophoretically definable hemoglobins, a major component with a molecular weight of 56,200 (a tetramer) and a minor component of 30,000 molecular weight (a dimer) (Fig. 3).

Oxygen binding measurements demonstrate that at low hemoglobin concentration the p_{50} is 13.5 with an n value of 2.4, pH 7.0, 25°C. As the

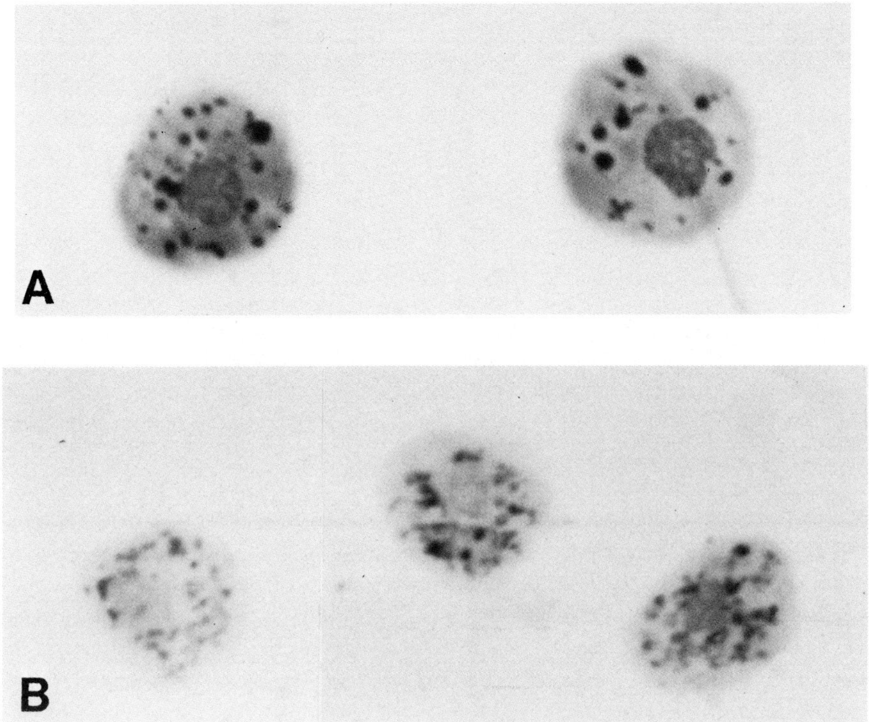

Fig. 1 A. Wright-stained *Anadara ovalis* red cells. B. Prussian blue stain of the same cells. Contrastained with Saphranin. Notice that the heavy intracellular aggregates are iron-containing. (Eugene F. Roth).

protein concentration is increased, the p_{50} also increases with a small elevation in the n value, suggesting ligand-dependent polymerization. No alkaline Bohr effect is present nor is an ATP or 2,3-DPG effect on oxygen affinity observed.

The minor component has a lower p_{50} of 6 mmHg, pH 7.0, 25°C and an n value of 1.4, with no alkaline Bohr effect. Red cell phosphate composition analysis demonstrates that *Anadara ovalis* red cells contain ATP (6 μm/gmHb) and GTP (2.5 μm/gmHb).

An interesting phenomenon observed with both components but particularly with the major component was its dissociation to monomers after methemoglobin conversion. Increased thermal denaturation (as compared to human Hb A) was observed with the major component. The minor component was only slightly more thermal-unstable than human Hb A.

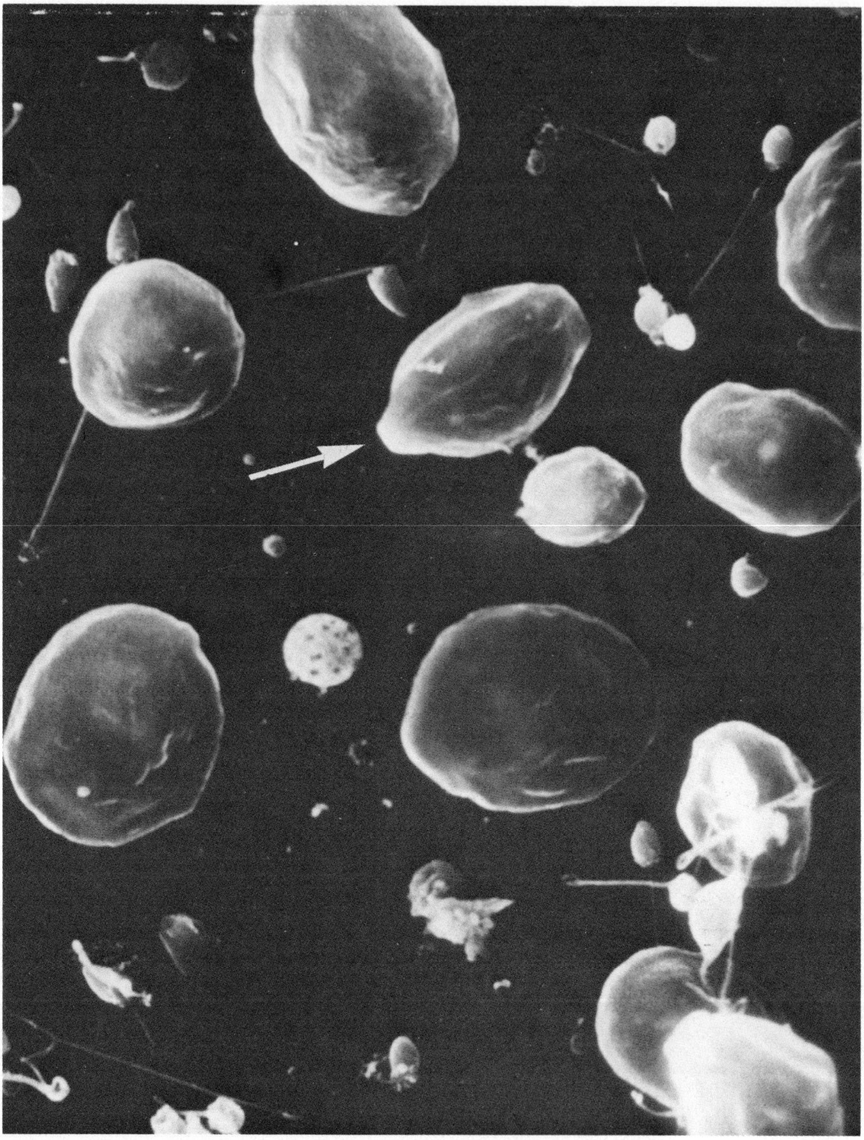

Fig. 2. Scanning electron microscopy of cells in coelomic fluid from *Andara ovalis*. Large cells are red cells. The arrow points to an image compatible with the presence of a marginal band underlining the cell membrane in the plane of flattening. Notice the nucleus bulging on the surface of other red cells. Sperm cells are also present in this sample. (Nagel and Raventos-Suarez).

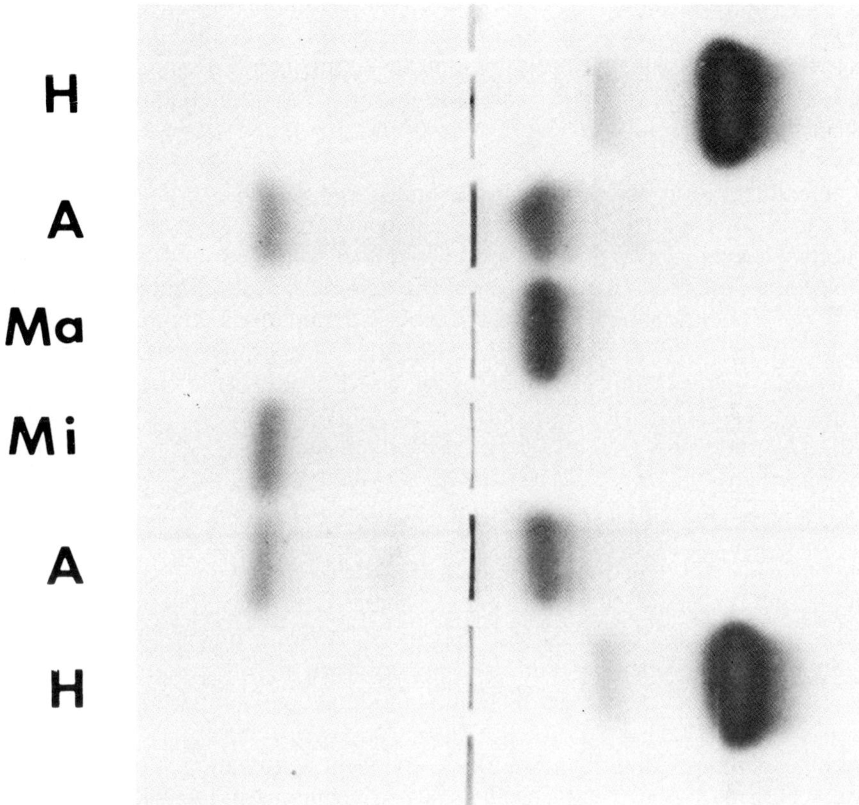

Fig. 3. Starch gel electrophoresis (pH 8.6). H. Human red cell hemolysate (Hb A, major component; Hb A_2, minor component). A. *Anadara ovalis* red cell hemolysate, exhibiting a major and a minor component, plus other components at very low concentrations. Ma. DEAE chromatography-purified major component from *Anadara* hemolysate. Mi. DEAE chromatography-purified minor component from *Anadara* hemolysate. (Borgese and Nagel)

The erythrocytes of the related species *Anadara transversa* also have major and minor Hb components, with different electrophoretic migration rates at pH 8.6 than the hemoglobins of *A. ovalis*. No functional or structural studies are yet available.

Noetia ponderosa

This arcid clam was first studied by Manwell [1963], who found red cells containing hemoglobin in the coelomic fluid. Two electrophoretically separable components were observed, which he estimated to have a molecular weight of about 30,000 daltons.

Freadman and Mangum [1976] confirmed that the molecular weight of the *Noetia* hemoglobin was 34,500 daltons, suggesting a dimeric molecule. The p_{50} of intact red cells was 5.3 mmHg at 10°C (pH 6.6–7.4) and 6.25 mmHg at 23°C. The curve had two phases, suggesting that each component had an intrinsically different p_{50}. The n value of the first phase was 1.81 and of the second phase, 1.23.

In collaboration with Dr. Richard San George we have further studied the properties of isolated hemoglobin components from this "ponderous ark." The two principal components are unevenly represented, and generally the Major component amounts to 80% of the hemolysate, the Minor component 20%, with occasional observations of other electrophoretically distinct hemoglobins at very low proportions. Interestingly, these proportions vary among individual clams and we do not know whether the variations are due to different developmental stages, environmental factors, or genetic polymorphism. The molecular weights of the two hemoglobin components, determined by light scattering, were 34,100 and 35,600 daltons.

The oxygen-binding properties of the principal hemoglobin components are as follows: The major hemoglobin has a p_{50} of 17.8 at 25°, pH 7.2 with an n value of 1.4. The minor component binds oxygen with a higher affinity, p_{50} = 8.7, at same pH and temperature, but with less cooperativity (n = 1.2). Under these circumstances, human Hb A has a p_{50} of 14.1 and an n value of 2.8. No alkaline Bohr effect is observed in either component. The temperature effect on oxygen binding is moderate and similar to mammalian hemoglobins. There is no protein-concentration dependence of oxygen affinity, strongly suggesting that no ligand-dependent aggregation is present. This was confirmed by light-scattering measurements. An intriguing and yet unexplained phenomenon is the slight biphasicity of the Hill plot of O_2 binding of the major component. Further work is needed to elucidate this phenomenon.

The subunit structure is of interest. The major component is a heterodimer composed of chains with different molecular weights as detected by SDS-polyacrylamide electrophoresis. The minor component exhibited one band in SDS gels and one band by HPLC globin separation, suggesting that it is a homodimer. This band migrates in HPLC with one of the chains found in the major component. Further work is needed to certify that it is indeed a homodimer and that both components have a common chain. A spectral characteristic of interest in these hemoglobins is a pronounced shoulder at 505 nm for the deoxy state, similar to that reported for *S. inaequivalvis* (see below).

Noetia's red cells are also nucleated with an approximate diameter of about 15–20μm. The hematocrit of the coelomic fluid is about 9%, with a hemoglobin concentration of 1.6 gm/dl. The intracellular hemoglobin concentration calculation has to consider the volume occupied by the nucleus.

Our best estimate is that the concentration of hemoglobin in the cytoplasm of these cells is over 40 gm/dl, somewhat higher than vertebrate red cells. We also find that the coelomic fluid pH is close to 7.0 and the osmolarity is about 730 mOsm.

HEMOGLOBINS IN OTHER MOLLUSCS: DISCUSSION

Of the classes of molluscs, the cephalopods are the most advanced and are considered the zenith of the evolution of invertebrates. The bivalves are probably the most primitive molluscs. In Table I we have summarized the available knowledge of the presence of hemoglobins among species that belong to the Phylum Mollusca. We will not discuss the hemoglobins (most properly myoglobins) found in radular or abductor muscle, but limit ourselves to more detailed description of intraerythrocytic and extracellular hemoglobins.

Red Cell Hemoglobins

In addition to those described above, the better-studied species with hemoglobin-containing red cells are the following.

Anadara broughtonii (inflata). Furuta and co-workers [1977] have reported that this clam has red cells containing 33% dimeric hemoglobin and 60% tetrameric hemoglobin. Yagi et al [1957] had previously crystalized and studied the tetrameric form of this clam hemoglobin.

The tetrameric hemoglobin is composed of two dissimilar chains (α and β) as determined by SDS-polyacrylamide gel electrophoresis and CM cellulose chromatography in 8 M urea. The dimeric hemoglobin showed a single band on two types of electrophoresis, but this chain (γ) was distinctly different from the two found as constituents of the tetrameric hemoglobin. Peptide mapping demonstrated considerable homology between α and β but both are very different from γ. The oxygen-binding properties of the two hemoglobins are very similar to those of *S. inaequivalvis* (see below). The tetramer shows high cooperativity (although Sumita et al. [1964] reported an $n = 1.7$ and Furuta et al [1975] reported an n of 2.8–3.0). The dimer has an $n = 1.8$. No alkaline Bohr effect nor 2,3-DPG effect was observed. Furuta et al. [1980] have demonstrated that both hemoglobins from *Anadara broughtonii* exhibit R-T transformation as detected by a) ligand dependency of the iodoacetamide reaction, b) ligand-dependent circular dichroism (CD) changes in the far ultraviolet (UV), and c) ligand-dependent binding of l-anilinonaphthalene-8-sulfonate. They have also demonstrated that the binding of –SH groups by p. hydroxi mercuribenzoate (PMB) increases oxygen affinity and decreases cooperativity in both hemoglobins, probably by displacing the equilibrium toward an increased stability of the oxy conformer.

Furuta and co-workers [1981] have also demonstrated that the tetrameric *A. broughtonii* hemoglobin, as in the case of *Scapharca*, polymerizes during

TABLE I. Molluscan Hemoglobins and Myoglobins

Approximate mol. wt.	Degree of aggregation	Class	Species	Site	Reference
16k	Monomer	Gastropod	*Aplysia limacina*	Radula	Rossi-Fanelli and Antonini [1957]
			Helisoma trivolvis	Radula	Terwilliger and Terwilliger [1977]
16k	Monomer	Bivalve	*Mercenaria mercenaria*	Abductor	Koppenheffer and Read [1969]
34k	Dimer	Gastropod	*Busycon canaliculatum*	Radula	Terwilliger and Read [1971]
			Nassa mutabilis	Radula	Geraci et al. [1977]
15k + 60k + Xk	Monomer + tetramers + polymers	Bivalve	*Phacoides pectinatus*	Ctenidia	Read [1965]
34k	2 Dimers	Bivalve	*Noetia ponderosa*[a]	Red cells	Manwell [1963]; San George, Nagel[c]
34k + 64k	Dimer + tetramer (polymers on deoxygenation)	Bivalve	*Scapharca inaequivalvis*[a]	Red cells	Chiancone et al. [1981]
			Anadara broughtonii (inflata)	Red cells	Furuta et al. [1977]
			A. ovalis (pexata)	Red cells	Borgese, Nagel, Harrington[c]
			A. transversa	Red cells	Borgese, Nagel, Harrington[c]
			A. trapezia	Red cells	Collett and O'Gower [1972]
			A. granosa	Red cells	
			A. maculosa	Red cells	
			A. satowi	Red cells	Ohnoki et al. [1973]
			A. senilis	Red cells	Djangmah et al. [1978]
64k	Tetramer	Bivalve	*Calyptogena magnifica*[b]	Red cells	Terwilliger et al. [1983]
64k + 430k	Tetramer + polymer	Bivalve	*Barbatia reeveana*[a]	Red cells	Grinich and Terwilliger [1980]
1,700k	Polymers	Gastropod	*Helisoma trivolvis*	Hemolymph	Terwilliger et al. [1976]
			Planorbis corneus		Wood and Mosby [1975]
			Biomphalaria glabrata		Figueiredo et al. [1973]
12,000k	Polymers	Bivalve	*Cardita borealis*[b]	Hemolymph	Terwilliger et al. [1978]

[a]Taxodont (arcid) clams.
[b]Heterodont clams.
[c]unpublished

deoxygenation. The largest aggregate observed is of a molecular weight of about 195,000 daltons, suggesting that it is constituted by three tetramers. They were also able to inhibit polymerization by blocking the reactive –SH group with p-chloromercuribenzoate. This finding should not necessarily be interpreted to mean that aggregation requires –SH groups, but that, alternatively, the conformational modification induced by the binding of PMB to this site (as demonstrated by oxygen binding changes) modifies the areas of contact needed for further aggregation.

Interesting information has been generated recently by the complete amino acid sequence determined on the polypeptide chain that constitutes the homodimer [Furuta and Kajita, 1983]. The globin chain has 146 amino acids with proline at the N terminus and leucine at the C terminus. Maximal homology is obtained with the β human chain if seven extra residues are added to the N terminal and four are deleted from the C terminal. Other deletions are present throughout the sequence. Homology with the human α chain is 21.9% at the amino acid sequence level, but with human α chains it is lower, amounting to about 15%. Interestingly, the homology with *Aplysia limacina* hemoglobin is 22.6%. Notably, there are only two histidines (proximal and distal heme-related) and one cysteine. The homology around the heme is very high when compared to horse hemoglobin (about 70%) but very low (5.6%) in the residues involved in the $\alpha_1\beta_2$ area of contact. This is not surprising, as this hemoglobin does not form tetramers. The $\alpha_1\beta_1$ contact area has a higher degree of homology (14.3%).

The C terminus is quite homologous with human β chain; within the 19 final residues, the homology is 60%. In terms of the spectral changes observed with clam hemoglobin, it is interesting that a two-residue addition is found in the FE loop (between the two heme-linked histidines). In addition, the entrance of the heme pocket flanked by Phe and Val in the human β chain are replaced in this clam hemoglobin by tyrosine and leucine. This change could have an effect on ligand affinity.

Scapharca inaequivalvis. This mollusc, found in the Mediterranean basin, specifically the Adriatic Sea, has erythrocytes circulating in its coelomic fluid. The cells contain two electrophoretically separable hemoglobins, one (Hb I), with a molecular weight of a dimer ($\approx$ 32,000 daltons) and the other (Hb II) of a tetramer ($\approx$ 64,000 daltons) [Chiancone et al., 1981].

In terms of the chain composition of these hemoglobins, there is good evidence that the tetrameric Hb II is composed by two distinct chains of slightly different molecular weight (16,400 and 16,800 daltons). With HB I, the results are less clear. In SDS-polyacrylamide gel electrophoresis, Hb I exhibits a single band. Of course, this might mean that the molecule is a homodimer, or that it is heterogeneous as to chain conformation but that the individual chains have the same molecular weight. The single peak in globin electrophoresis for apo-Hb I argues for a single chain but, again, does not entirely eliminate the possibility of two different polypeptide chains with small or no net pI differences. Another interesting structural feature is the presence of 1.5–SH groups per heme in Hb II and 1.0 per heme in Hb I. The result for Hb II could mean that one of the chains might have 2–SH and the other 1–SH. Also, Chiancone et al. [1981] find one heme per 17,000–18,000 gm of protein for both hemoglobins.

Spectroscopic properties of these two hemoglobins are of interest. The absorption spectra are different in two respects from human Hb A. There is a pronounced shoulder at 590 nm for the deoxy conformer, as seen in *Noetia ponderosa*. The UV spectrum is notable for the fact that the tryptophan peak at 290 nm does not disappear with oxygenation as in human Hb A.

The visible circular dichroism spectrum is different in the deoxy conformer from that of human Hb A. In the UV CD spectra, both deoxy clam hemoglobins have an additional negative band at 425 nm. Calculation of ellipticity from CD data shows that there is no change upon deoxygenation, unlike mammalian hemoglobins where the α-helical content increases by 8%.

The above results can be rationalized on the basis of potentially significant differences in the sequence of these hemoprotein chains as compared to the α and β chains of mammalian hemoglobins. These differences could explain the spectrophotometric results and are not unexpected, as globin chains in clam hemoglobin and human hemoglobin had a long time to diverge in evolutionary terms.

Another important feature of these hemoglobins is their oxygen-binding properties. Surprisingly, both components exhibit oxygen-binding cooperativity, as demonstrated by an n value of 2 for the tetramer (Hb II) and of 1.5 for the dimer form. This is particularly remarkable, as the dimer of mammalian hemoglobin has no cooperativity (in spite of initial confusion in the matter generated by the misinterpretation of the extent of dimerization induced by high concentrations of NaCl). This result alone separates clam hemoglobins from the functional behavior of mammalian hemoglobins.

No acid or alkaline Bohr effect is observed in the dimeric clam hemoglobin. While there is no alkaline Bohr effect in the tetrameric clam hemoglobin, an acid Bohr effect is observed below pH 6.5.

Another interesting property of the tetrameric clam hemoglobin is that its oxygen affinity decreases (and the n value increases) with increasing protein concentration. This result immediately suggested the presence of ligand-dependent hemoglobin polymerization. Chiancone et al [1981] confirmed this by sedimentation velocity measurement of deoxy tetrameric Hb, at different hemoglobin concentrations for different pH's as well as at different hemoglobin concentrations at the same pH. The result demonstrates that the tetramer polymerizes between pH 6 and pH 9.5, and depolymerizes outside these pH's. Between 3 and 8 mg/ml, the extent of polymerization increases until it reaches a plateau (at about an aggregation state of four tetramers). The polymerization is also deaggregated by high salt concentration. The pH and salt dependency of polymerization suggests that the *Scapharca* tetrameric hemoglobin polymerization is stabilized by electrostatic interaction. But the negative temperature coefficient of the reaction (less aggregation at low temperatures) suggests that hydrophobic interactions are also stabilizing forces in the polymer formation. The monomeric hemoglobin does not polymerize within the concentrations studied (1–20 mg/ml).

More recently, Ikeda-Saito et al [1982] have studied the thermodynamic properties of the oxygen binding of the two *Scapharca* hemoglobins. The calculation of Van't Hoff's heats of oxygenation are not uniform with respect to each oxygenation step, as observed for human Hb A. Nevertheless, as these hemoglobins do not have a Bohr effect, the heat or release of heterotropic ligands cannot be the explanation.

Anadara trapezia. This Australian arcid clam has two main electrophoretically distinct hemoglobins, one major and the other a minor component. *A. trapezia* hemoglobin is of considerable interest because it has an important and complex temperature dependency for oxygen binding [Collett and O'Gower, 1972]. Oxygen affinity decreases significantly above 20°C. Also, cooperativity of oxygen binding is highly temperature-dependent, with an n value of 2.1 at 20°C, 1.7 at 25°C, and 1.4 at 30°C. Caution should be exercised in the detailed interpretation of these data, until the two components in this hemolysate are studied separately. The n values of mixtures of hemoglobin can be misleading. Probably connected with this phenomenon is the fact that *A. trapezia* is polymorphic as to its hemoglobin composition [Nicol and O'Gower, 1967]. The minor component can be homozygous for the type Hb 2a or Hb 2b variants that are definable in a Cellogel strip electrophoresis (pH 9.5). Heterozygote individual clams for these hemoglobins have been described with both hemoglobins (Hb 2a and Hb 2b) simultaneously present. O'Gower and Nicol [1968] have calculated gene frequencies in clam beds harvested throughout the southeastern coast of Australia. Hb 2a frequency is highest at the northern tip and Hb 2b has its highest frequency in the south, with a continuous latitudinal cline between these two points with slight reversals of the trend at the extreme points. Of course, until we know more about the genomic structure of these clams, it cannot be ascertained if they differ in their genetic composition (globin genes) or if they express or activate differentially (as temperature varies, for example) different portions of their globin genome.

Similar temperature dependence of hemoglobins has been described by Collett and O'Gower [1972] on the other Australian clams, *Anadara granosa* and *Anadara maculosa*.

Anadara satowi. Ohnoki and co-workers [1973] have demonstrated that two major hemoglobin components can be purified from red cells of this Japanese arcid clam by DEAE-cellulose and CM-cellulose chromatography. The molecular weights are compatible with a dimer and a tetramer. In terms of oxygen-binding characteristics, again, as in other arcid clams, both components exhibited cooperativity (dimer has an n value of 1.5 and the tetramer an n value of 2.1). No alkaline Bohr effect is present although a small acid Bohr effect in the tetramer is detectable, and the affinity at 20°C, pH 7.3, and low concentration (60 μM heme) is lower than human hemoglobin.

Anadara senilis. This arcid clam inhabits the coast of West Africa and has been studied by Djangmah et al [1978]. The hemolymph contains red cells with two electrophoretically distinct hemoglobins. One has a molecular weight of 24,000–28,500 daltons (37%) and the other 54,500–55,500 daltons (63%). Hence this arcid clam has a dimer and a tetramer as major constituents in its erythrocytes. Interestingly, isoelectric focusing resolves the tetramer into two major bands (pI $\approx$ 6.0 and $\approx$ 5.3) and some minor components. The dimer exhibits a single band under these conditions. Subunit composition, as studied by SDS-polyacrylamide gel electrophoresis, resolved both hemoglobins into a single diffuse band with molecular weight of 12,000–14,000 daltons. Significant amino acid differences were observed between the two hemoglobins. The oxygen-binding curves of the tetrameric hemoglobin demonstrated a p_{50} of 8–13 mmHg, in the 6.5–7.5 pH range and an n value of 1.6–2.3. The dimeric hemoglobin had a p_{50} of 4.2–6.7 mmHg at the same pH range and an n value of 1.6–2.3. The scarcity of data points makes the presence or absence of a Bohr effect unreliable and further work is needed to define this heterotropic property.

Calyptogena magnifica. An extraordinarily interesting species is the thermal vent clam, studied by Terwilliger et al. [1983]. This heterodont bivalve mollusc, from the East Pacific ridge and the Galapagos Rift hydrothermal vent areas, also contains hemoglobins inside red cells. These clams are very large (26 cm long), have a white calcareous outer shell and red interior organs, and live at depths of 2.5 km. Temperature variations span 22°C (with 350 μM H_2S, pH 6.5, and very low pO_2 [vent water]) to 20°C (no H_2S, pH 7.5, and 0.110 μM O_2).

The hemoglobin harvested from red cells exhibited a molecular weight of 68,000 when studied by gel chromatography on Sephadex G 100 Bio Gel A-1.5M. A minor peak at 28,000 was also apparent but the sample contained methemoglobin and had been previously frozen. The major fraction, by dilution, dissociates into a molecular weight of 42,000. DEAE-cellulose column chromatography separated the major component into three fractions with different pI's. SDS gels on each fraction suggest the following structure: fraction I: $\alpha_2\beta_2$; fraction II: possibly $\alpha_2\beta_2$, $\beta_2\gamma_2$, $\alpha_2\gamma_2$, or only two of these;

and fraction III: γ_4. In this case, α and β had a molecular weight of 14,200, whereas γ was 13,400. The amino acid composition of α and β chains predict a homology of about 75% according to the method of Harris and Teller [1973]. On the other hand, little similarity in amino acid composition with other bivalve hemoglobins was found.

The oxygen affinity within cells is relatively high: the p_{50} was 7.6 $\pm$ 0.23, at pH 6.78 and 10.1°C with a Hill coefficient of 1.24. No temperature dependence of O_2 affinity was observed.

Of extraordinary potential significance is the fact that these clams might utilize chemoautotrophic sulphide-oxidizing bacteria to fix nitrogen. Hence, for these gigantic deep-sea bivalves, this hemoglobin could be playing the role that leghemoglobin plays in the root nodules of legumes.

Barbatia reeveana. This arcid clam studied by Grinich and Terwilliger [1980] contains a very unusual intracellular hemoglobin. The major component has a molecular weight of 430,000, which decomposes to a minimum molecular weight of 35,000 in SDS-urea plus reducing agents or 6 M guanidine. Subtilisin digestion produces both a 60,000-dalton and a 30,000-dalton species further dissociable by reducing SDS into 16,000-dalton polypeptides. Nevertheless, there is 1 heme per 16,000 gm of protein. Hence, the structure suggested by these findings is a dodecapolymer of a subunit of about 35,000 consisting of 2 heme-containing 35,000 domains, probably held together by covalent bonds.

The complete polymer has a very low affinity for O_2 with a p_{50} of 36 mmHg, at 20°C, no alkaline Bohr effect, and low cooperativity (n = 1.7). The subtilisin digestion product of 30,000 daltons binds O_2 reversibly with an affinity greater than that of the intact polymer but with no change in cooperativity.

These results suggest that the functional unit is a cooperative dimer covalently linked. The polymer structure seems to increase the oxygen affinity of the molecule, but not its cooperativity, suggesting that it affects its conformation in some other way, maybe changing the stereochemical restraints around the heme pocket of the O_2 binding domains.

A minor component of these red cells has a molecular weight of 64,000 with different chain constituents than the polymer, but no further data on this hemoglobin have been published.

The remarkable feature of the intraerythrocytic *Barbatia* hemoglobin is its molecular weight and unique polymeric structure similar to the type found in extracellular hemoglobins.

Myoglobins and Extracellular Hemoglobins

As shown in Table I, various species of molluscs contain extracellular hemoglobin in the hemolymph, or tissue myoglobins. These are of interest from a comparative perspective. The following are some of the better-studied examples of extracellular hemoglobins.

Phacoides pectinatus. Kenneth Read [1965] has studied the hemoglobins present in the ctenidia of this clam and has found three components identifiable by electrophoresis, gel filtration, and ion exchange chromatography: Hb 1, Hb 2, and Hb 3.

Hemoglobin 1 has a molecular weight of 14,581, computed on the basis of its amino acid composition. This monomer contains one heme group. Hemoglobin 2 is probably tetrameric at high concentration, as it co-elutes with mercaptalbumin (66,000 daltons) on Sephadex G 100. At lower concentrations, this hemoglobin elutes at a position that suggests a molecular weight of a dimer, and at even lower concentration the elution profile approaches that of a monomer ($\approx$ 17,000 daltons).

Interestingly, Hb 3 at high concentrations elutes in two peaks, one that can be assigned as a polymer (higher than a tetramer) and another fraction that elutes between 66,000-dalton and 25,000-dalton markers. Ultra centrifugation suggests an octamer and a tetramer for these fractions. At low concentration Hb 3 elutes from Sephadex G 100 in a way that is compatible with a molecular weight somewhat higher than that of a monomer.

Amino acid composition of Hb 1 demonstrates that it has only two histidines and one cysteine. The oxygen-binding properties and chain composition of these hemoglobins are not known.

Helisoma trivolvis. This planorbid snail has a hemoglobin (or myoglobin) localized in the radular muscle and, in addition, a high-molecular-weight extracellular hemoglobin. Interestingly, the two hemoglobins found might be closely related [Terwilliger et al., 1976].

The radular muscle intracellular hemoglobin is a monomer (molecular weight 15,400–17,800) and is present in the bright red odontophore complex. The extracellular hemoglobin found in the hemolymph of these snails has a molecular weight of 1,750,000 daltons, which according to the electron microscopy and ultracentrifugation data collected and interpreted by Terwilliger et al [1976] exists in circular arrangements of ten subunits of 175,000 daltons (dm: 200A°). It is intriguing, however, that the center of the circle does not appear empty in the micrographs published by Terwilliger et al [1976]; hence the possibility exists that there is an 11th subunit in the center of the disk (or alternatively extensions of the peripheral subunits). For many years, negatively stained cross sections of Hb S polymer were misinterpreted to be hollow, tubular structures when in reality they were solid rods. Limited subtilisin digestion breaks down this sununit into polypeptide fractions of 17,000–19,000 daltons that should be regarded as oxygen-binding domains. As there is one heme per 19,000 gm of protein, each 175,000-dalton subunit must comprise about 10 heme-containing domains [Terwilliger et al., 1977].

Again, this molecule could have been generated by the fusion of about 10 ancestral myoglobin genes.

Planorbis corneus. This snail, found on the coast of England, contains high-molecular-weight hemoglobin dissolved in the hemolymph. Wood and Mosby [1975] have determined by sedimentation velocity experiments and amino acid composition that this single hemoglobin component has a molecular weight of $1.65 \times 10^6 \pm 0.04 \times 10^6$. Electron microscopy of this protein revealed a ring arrangement of about six subunits with a diameter of 12.2 nm, half of the width observed in worm erythrocruorins. The center of the ring appeared empty in negatively stained electron micrographic materials, in contrast with the discoid arrangement from *Cardita* hemoglobin (see below). The heme content analysis suggested about 74 hemes per molecule. Each subunit member of the ring should have 9–12 hemes. The amino acid composition is significant for the low number of histidines and the possible absence or scarcity of cysteine. This separates this *Planorbis* hemoglobin and *Biomphalaria* hemoglobin (which are only similar in amino acid composition) from the erythrocruorin found in worms (*Arenicola*, *Lumbricus*, etc.), which is characterized by a higher number of histidines and cysteines.

The oxygen-binding curves of the *Planorbis* hemoglobin showed a relatively high oxygen affinity (p_{50} = 4–5 mmHg, pH 7.0–8.4) at temperatures between 16 and 25°C with an n value of 17–34. No alkaline Bohr effect was observed.

In terms of the molecular organization of this huge molecule, Wood and Mosby [1975] obtained, by heme content determination, a molecular weight of 22,300 daltons for the minimal, heme-containing unit or domains. This number is considerably higher than the 17,700-dalton heme-containing unit calculated by Figueiredo et al. [1973] for *Biomphalaria*. Again, dissociating and reducing agents did not generate a subunit of this size, suggesting that the structural subunit might be a multiple of the heme domain stabilized most likely by covalent bonds.

Biomphalaria glabrata. This Brazilian gastropod, the intermediate host of *Schistosoma mansoni*, contains hemoglobin dissolved in its hemolymph. Figueiredo et al [1973] have characterized the molecular weight of the single hemoglobin present as 1.69×10^6 daltons. The molecule contains one heme per 17,700 gm of protein, suggesting that it has 96 hemes per molecule. Low pH and high ionic strength dissociated the polymer into smaller subunits. The smaller subunit obtained by reduction of pH to 2.3, is 1/48 of the intact polymer, or a 92 heme-containing 34,000-dalton subunit. The p_{50} is slightly to the left of human hemoglobin at pH 7.05, and with an n value of 1.08, attesting to the almost entire absence of cooperativity.

More recently, further work on this hemoglobin has been reported by Almeida and Neves [1974] from Belo Horizonte, Brazil. These authors calculated a molecular weight of 1.75×10^6, somewhat higher than Figueiredo's determination. The amino composition reveals two histidines, a half-cysteine, eight arginines, and six isoleucines per heme-containing domain. All of these features are in contrast with human β-globin but are similar to the extracellular hemoglobin of other gastropods. Interestingly, Arrieta [1970] has reported the presence of carbohydrate in this hemoglobin, suggesting that it is really a low-sugar-containing glycoprotein.

Cardita borealis. This heterodont clam has an extracellular hemoglobin that is dissolved in the hemolymph of the pallial cavity and is characterized by a molecular weight of approximately 12×10^6 in the pH range of 5.7 to 8 and in the presence of Mg [Terwilliger et al., 1978]. The elution peak of *Cardita* hemoglobin in Sepharose 4B chromatography is broad and asymmetric, suggesting heterogeneity in molecular weights. At high pH (9.0–10.5) it is dissociated into a component with an apparent molecular weight of 1.4×10^6. SDS gel electrophoresis demonstrates that the smallest subunit is approximately 290×10^3 (but anomalous SDS behavior could render this result somewhat unreliable). *Cardita* hemoglobin apparently contains one heme per 22,000 gm of protein. These numbers suggest that the undissociated polymer is constituted by 40 subunits, each one containing about 13 hemes.

Spectral properties of O_2, CO, and cyanmet derivatives are similar to those of other hemoglobins. Electron microscopy of the large polymeric form discloses a rod-like supramolecular structure. Three morphological types are observed. Some molecules are cylinders (365 Å wide) with barely discernible substructure. The second type of molecule resembles parallel rows of repeating units, with a width of 210 Å and an apparent central cavity. The third category also are cylinders but with a very strongly stained central rod and poorly defined outer borders. The length of all these types is quite variable (from 365 Å to about 1,200 Å).

The amino acid composition reported by Terwilliger et al [1978] discloses a lack of similarity to other mollusc hemoglobins, except for the *Planorid* snails. Of interest is the fact demonstrated by Terwilliger and Terwilliger [1978] that gentle proteolysis cleaves the protein into heme-containing domains of molecular weight between 15,000 and 17,000 and multiples thereof. These domains, when isolated by gel chromatography, can bind oxygen reversibly. The amino acid composition of the isolated domain fractions are very similar and contain one heme per 17,000 gm of protein, suggesting a genome structure in which 13 duplicated copies of an original globin gene have been fused together. More intriguing is the fact that the functional properties of the complete molecule are no different from its individual domains (no cooperativity or Bohr effect), suggesting that the purpose of this elaborate construction is to reduce the number of particles or osmolarity; after all, this is an extracellular protein and the hemolymph has to be maintained at fixed oncotic pressure.

GENERAL OVERVIEW

Mollusc hemoglobin, an infrequent occurrence in this phylum, can be classified in three main types: a) the *intratissue hemoglobins* or myoglobins found in radular and abductor muscle, nerves, etc. of gastropods and amphineurans; b) the *intraerythrocytic hemoglobins* found up to now exclusively among bivalves; c) the *extracellular hemoglobins* found in the hemolymph of bivalves and gastropods. No hemoglobins have been found in cephalopods.

The interesting feature of these three groups is that their properties are quite different.

a. The myoglobins or intratissue hemoglobins found among molluscs can be single-chain hemoproteins, such as the vertebrate myoglobins. In addition, they can be dimeric and exhibit cooperativity. This feature, found among gastropods, for example, is a remarkable and striking departure from the structural-functional model "adopted" by the chordates.

b. The intraerythrocytic hemoglobins are of great interest as this is one of the first appearances of red cells in the phylogenetic tree. The only competition comes from the Phoronids (location of this Phylum in the evolutionary tree is controversial but Russell-Hunter [1968] believes that they belong in the arm that culminates in the chordates), which also have erythrocytes suspended in the coelomic fluid. The surprise is that hemoglobins can be exclusively dimeric (*Noetia ponderosa*), a mixture of dimers with tetramers (*Anadara spp*), only tetramers (*Calyptogena magnifica*) or even tetramers plus non-ligand-dependent polymers (*Barbatia reeveana*) (Table I). The most significant finding here is the presence of a dimer with cooperativity and a stable polymer, two circumstances not found in intraerythrocytic hemoglobins among chordates. In addition, the presence of homodimers that are cooperative denies the generalization espoused by Benesch and Benesch [1974] that two unlike subunits were essential for homotropic effects.

c. Extracellular hemoglobins among the molluscs are all characterized by high-molecular-weight constructions in which the minimal subunit is *not* a myoglobin-length globin ($\approx$ 17,000) but a larger covalently stabilized multiple of this protounit. The name *erythrocruorin* for these hemoglobins would be appropriate, but it has gained little favor among workers in the field, probably because of its cacophonicity. Polyhemoglobin or some other similar name might be necessary to use here, particularly when the application in the near future of molecular biology to this field identifies the gene location, size, and structure. It will of course be significantly different from the other globin genes.

The next question that needs answering is the exact position of molluscan hemoglobins in the evolutionary or phylogenetic tree. Do they represent an ancestral form of the chordate hemoglobins? If that is the case, why were some of the properties found in mollusc hemoglobins lost and others gained during their evolution towards the chordates? In effect, if one follows the phylogenetic views of Russell-Hunter [1968] and many others, the answer is that molluscs were not ancestors to chordates. In effect, after the protozoans (there is firm evidence for the presence of the globin gene in the form of a myoglobin-like molecule in *Paramecium*), the best-accepted phylogenia includes such minor phyla as the Cnidaria and Platyhelmynthes. After this point, three main branches are generated, each of which culminates in three major phyla: Chordata, Mollusca, and Arthropoda.

Hence, the design and characteristics of mollusc hemoglobin do not represent a development that was later incorporated in the evolution of the vertebrates, but a separate and distinct track that apparently was not very promising. Although it might represent a significant adaptation for the species exhibiting it, the most developed form of the molluscs, the cephalopods, have not been found to contain hemoglobins, but have opted for hemocyanins as the respiratory pigment.

What is the structural base that generates the unique characteristics of intraerythrocytic mollusc hemoglobins? If the *A. broughtonii* hemoglobin sequence is of general significance, the shift in the sequence (loss of residues in the N terminal and gains in the C terminal) might be an important clue. The low number of histidines (only two) explains the lack of Bohr effect and might play a significant role in the structural-functional relationships. In addition, the tetramers apparently have no organic phosphate-binding residues. This characteristic was added later, in the other evolutionary track, the one leading to the chordates. In this last track, thermostability also became a requirement that, interestingly, is already present in one of the two hemoglobins of *A. ovalis*.

The construction of hemoglobins for the extracellular compartment of molluscs is, of course, quite different, but this is not surprising. Some molluscs (bivalves and gastropods), and by the way also some arthropods, have gigantic molecules in diverse and complex arrays, with molecular weights from 1.7 million to 12 million daltons. The rules of the game are very different here. As mentioned, the minimal subunit is enormous (containing a large number of hemes), most probably the product of repetitive gene duplication and fusion, through several steps of unequal crossing-over events. The surprise is the low cooperativity among binding sites that, moreover, is restricted to low levels of aggregation. This situation suggests that these enormous constructions are not designed for complex regulation of O_2 delivery but respond to the need to conserve the number of particles suspended or dissolved in the hemolymph. Hence the larger the molecule, the larger the number of O_2-binding sites that can be accommodated without changing the osmotic or oncotic pressure.

Another point of interest is the physiological basis for the presence of multiple hemoglobins in each individual mollusc. In the case of *Anadara trapezia*, as commented before, the presence of polymorphism and a geographical gene frequency cline, in addition to significant and different temperature dependence for O_2 binding, strongly suggests that each hemoglobin has a distinct function in the individual and allows the carrier to adapt to diverse ecological needs.

It is of interest that most of the bivalves have at least two hemoglobins, one with higher O_2 affinity than the other. This situation might be particularly advantageous for intertidal clams, but firm data are not available. The function of *Calyptogena* hemoglobin might be as specific as its special habitat: It might be the leghemoglobin of the animal world.

In conclusion, molluscan hemoglobins offer the biochemist and physiologist the opportunity of studying a separate and distinct evolutionary pathway of the globin gene, guided by a very different set of selective pressures than the ones that have operated on the vertebrates.

ACKNOWLEDGMENTS

This work was possible because of the contributions of Eugene F. Roth, Thomas Borgese, Richard San George, and John Harrington. It was supported by NIH grant HL 21016.

REFERENCES

Almeida AP, Neves AGA (1974): The hemoglobin of *Biomphalaria glabrata*: Chemical composition and some physicochemical properties. Biochim Biophys Acta 371:140–146.

Arrieta MR (1970): Caracterization de la hemoglobines de la *Biomphalaria glabrata* como una glicoproteina. Thesis, Belo Horizonte, M.G. Brazil.

Benesch R, Benesch RE (1974): Homos and heteros among the hemos. Science 185:905–908.

Chiancone E, Vecchini P, Verzili D, Ascoli F, Antonini E (1981): Dimeric and tetrameric hemoglobins from the mollusc *Scapharca inaequivalvis*. J Mol Biol 152:577–592.

Collett LC, O'Gower AK (1972): Molluscan hemoglobins with unusual temperature-dependent characteristics. Comp Biochem Physiol 41A:843–850.

Djangmah JS, Gabbott PA, Wood EJ (1978): Physico-chemical characteristics and oxygen binding properties of the multiple haemoglobin of the West African blood clam, *Anadara senilis* (L). Comp Biochem Physiol 60B:245–250.

Figueiredo EA, Gomez MV, Heneine IF, Santos IO, Hargreaves FB (1973): Isolation and physico chemical properties of the hemoglobin *Biomphalaria glabrata* (Mollusca, Planorbid). Comp Biochem Physiol 44B:481–491.

Freadman MA, Mangum CP (1976): The function of hemoglobin in the arcid clam *Noetia ponderosa*. I. Oxygenation in vitro and in vivo. Comp Biochem Physiol 53A:173–179.

Furuta H, Kajita A (1983): Dimeric hemoglobin of the bivalve mollusc *Anadara broughtonii:* Complete amino acid sequence of the globin chain. Biochemistry 22:917–922.

Furuta H, Ohe M, Kajita A (1975): [in Japanese] Seikagaku 47:715.

Furuta H, Ohe M, Kajita A (1977): Subunit structure of hemoglobin from erythrocytes of the blood clam, *Anadara broughtonii*. J Biochem 82:1723–1730.

Furuta H, Ohe M, Kajita A (1980): Ligand-dependent allosteric transformation of hemoglobins from the clam, *Anadara broughtonii*. Biochim Biophys Acta 625:318–327.

Furuta H, Ohe M, Kajita A (1981): Ligand-dependent polymerization of tetrameric hemoglobin from the blood clam, *Anadara broughtonii*. Biochim Biophys Acta 668:448–455.

Geraci G, Sada A, Cirotto C (1977): Cooperative, low-molecular-weight dimeric myoglobins from the radular muscle of the gastropod mollusc *Nassa mutabilis L*. Eur J Biochem 77:555–560.

Grinich NP, Terwilliger RC (1980): The quaternary structure of an unusual high-molecular-weight intracellular hemoglobin from the bivalve mollusc *Barbatia reeveana*. Biochem J 189:1–8.

Harris C, Teller DJ (1973): Estimation of primary sequence homology from amino acid compositions of evolutionary related proteins. J Theor Biol 38:347–362.

Ikeda-Saito M, Yonetani T, Chiancone E, Ascoli F, Verzili D, Antonini E (1983): Thermodynamic properties of oxygen equilibria of dimeric and tetrameric hemoglobins from *Scapharca inaequivalvis*. J Mol Biol 170:1009–1018.

Koppenheffer TL, Read KRH (1969): The abductor muscle myoglobins of the bivalve mollusc *Mercenaria mercenaria L*. Comp Biochem Physiol 31:829–832.

Manwell C (1963): The chemistry and biology of hemoglobin in some marine clams. I. Distribution of the pigment and properties of the oxygen equilibria. Comp Biochem Physiol 8:209–218.

Nicol PI, O'Gower AK (1967): Haemoglobin variation in *Anadara trapezia*. Nature 216:684.

O'Gower AK, Nicol PI (1968): A latitudinal cline of haemoglobins in a bivalve mollusc. Heredity 23:485–491.

Ohnoki S, Mitomi Y, Hata R, Satake K (1973): Heterogeneity of hemoglobin from arca (*Anadara satowi*). Molecular weights and oxygen equilibria of arca HbI and HbII. J Biochem 73:717–725.

Read RHK (1965): The characterization of the hemoglobins of the bivalve mollusc *Phacoides pectinatus* (G melin). Comp Biochem Physiol 15:137–158.

Rossi-Fanelli A, Antonini E (1957): A new type of myoglobin isolated and crystalized from a muscle of Aplysiae. Biochimica 22:335–343.

Russell-Hunter WD (1968): "A Biology of Lower Invertebrates." London: McMillan.

Sumita N, Kajita A, Kaziro K (1964): Some properties of hemoglobin of *Anadara inflata*. J Biochem 55:148–153.

Terwilliger RC, Read KRH (1971): Oxygen equilibrium studies of the radular muscle myoglobin of the gastropod mollusc *Buccinum undatum L*. and *Busycon canaliculatum*. Int J Biochem 2:253–261.

Terwilliger RC, Terwilliger NB (1977): The hemoglobins of the mollusc *Helisoma trivolvis*: Comparison of the radular muscle myoglobin and vascular hemoglobin subunit structures. Comp Biochem Biophys 58B:283–289.

Terwilliger NB, Terwilliger RC (1978): Oxygen binding domains of a clam (*Cardita borealis*) extracellular hemoglobin. Biochim Biophys Acta 537:77–85.

Terwilliger NB, Terwilliger RC, Schabtach E (1976): The quaternary structure of a molluscan (*Helisoma trivolvis*) extracellular hemoglobin. Biochim Biophys Acta 453:101–110.

Terwilliger RC, Terwilliger NB, Bonaventura C, Bonaventura J (1977): Oxygen binding domains of *Helisoma trivolvis* hemoglobin. Biochim Biophys Acta 494:416–425.

Terwilliger RC, Terwilliger NB, Schabtach E (1978): Extracellular hemoglobin of a marine clam, *Cardita borealis:* An unusual hemoglobin quaternary structure. Comp Biochem Biophys 59B:9–14.

Terwilliger RC, Terwilliger NB, Arp A (1983): Thermal vent clam (*Calyptogena magnifica*) hemoglobin. Science 219:981–983.

Wood EJ, Mosby LJ (1975): Physicochemical properties of *Planorbis corneus* erythrocruorin. Biochem J 149:437–445.

Yagi Y, Mishima T, Tsujimura T, Sato K, Egami F (1957): Studies on the hemoglobin of *Anadara inflata* (Reeve). J Biochem 44:1–7.

NOTED ADDED IN PROOF

Of considerable interest are the recent, but unpublished, findings of William E. Royer and Warner E. Love at Johns Hopkins University. They have crystallized the hemoglobin dimer and tetramer of *Scapharca inaequivalvis* and determined their structure by X-ray crystallography. The two main findings are: a) the myoglobin fold, as we know it in vertebrate hemoglobins, is conserved in the individual subunits and b) the quaternary structure, that is, the way the subunits are arranged with respect to each other, is completely different from vertebrate hemoglobins. This last finding explains why the dissociation properties of mollusc hemoglobins are so unique and might explain the presence of stable dimers. It also lends support to the idea that the evolution of hemoglobins diverged after the definition of the myoglobin fold, with one track leading to mollusc hemoglobins and a separate and distinct one culminating in the mammalian hemoglobin structure and function.

A PRACTICAL GUIDE

Blood Cells of Marine Invertebrates: Experimental Systems in Cell Biology and Comparative Physiology, pages 251–279

Chapter Nine
Blood Cells of Marine Invertebrates: A Practical Guide

Chapter Contents

Species illustrations by Sarah R. Cohen.

INTRODUCTION

This chapter is a compilation of practical material on the animals and cells, contributed by many of the authors of this volume. It is intended to provide sufficient basic information for the novice to begin research on these cell types, as well as observations and suggestions of value to experienced workers. For each of the major experimental animals and blood cell types discussed in the previous chapters, we have attempted to answer the following questions: a) How are the animals maintained in the laboratory? b) How are the blood cells obtained? c) How are the cells washed and handled, and in what media? d) Where can one obtain the animals?

One problem common to many of these cell types (including some erythrocytes) is rapid loss of native cell shape upon removal of blood from the animals, presumably accompanied by intracellular physiological changes. In general, when beginning work on a given species, it is useful to fix a cell sample immediately upon withdrawal, or even to fix in situ if possible. This offers the best chance to determine native cell morphology and avoid confusion over the number of different kinds of cells present. Methods for preventing shape changes without fixation, and additional useful procedures applicable to each cell type, are presented in the sections that follow. Practical reference material, including a list of generally helpful reference works, several current sources of sea salts and refrigerated marine aquarium systems, and complete addresses of the suppliers of living animals cited in this chapter, is provided in the final section.

I. AMEBOCYTES OF THE AMERICAN "HORSESHOE CRAB," *LIMULUS POLYPHEMUS*

P.B. Armstrong

Department of Zoology, University of California, Davis, California 95616, and the Marine Biological Laboratory, Woods Hole, Massachusetts 02543

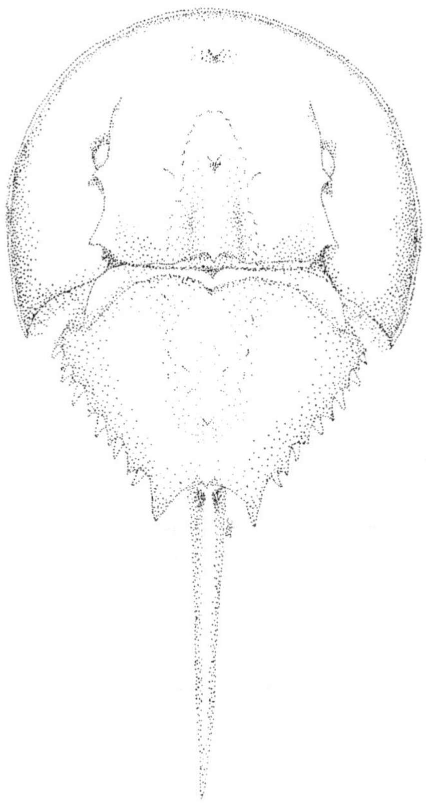

Fig. 1. The American "horseshoe crab," *Limulus polyphemus*.

Maintenance of Animals

L. polyphemus (Fig. 1) can be maintained for months in closed-system recirculating marine aquaria at 20°C. They should be fed weekly on crushed clams or pelleted dog chow, with reasonable attention to cleanliness.

Removal of Blood

Large quantities of blood can be obtained by cardiac puncture: Animals are removed from the aquarium and placed on a dry surface to allow excess seawater to drain from them. The cephalothorax and opisthosoma are bent at right angles at the cephalothorax-opisthosoma joint and the animal is held in this position with the left hand, with the thumb on the posterior end of the opisthosoma and the four fingers on the anterior rim of the cephalothorax. When numbers of animals are bled, wooden racks that hold the animal in a flexed position can be used (Fig. 2). The surface of the joint is carefully cleaned with 70% ethanol and a fresh, sterile 18-gauge needle is inserted into the heart by slipping the needle through the pliant tissue covering the joint into the cephalothorax. The point of insertion should be at the midline and the needle should be parallel to the dorsal line of the carapace of the cephalothorax [Levin and Bang, 1964; Hochstein et al., 1973; Jorgensen and Smith, 1973]. It is possible to collect 100 ml or more blood from a large animal. I know of no other readily obtainable invertebrate from which it is possible to collect so much blood so easily. A healthy animal has 2×10^7 to 6×10^7 cells per ml blood [Levin and Bang, 1968; Yeager and Tauber, 1935], and

1.4×10^7 cells contain 1 mg of protein [Levin and Bang, 1968]. In the interests of conservation, animals should be returned to the ocean as soon as possible after bleeding and should be protected from excessive stress (drying, overheating, etc.) in the interim (Fig. 2).

Preparation of Cells for Experimental Use

Two problems confront the investigator desiring to work with dispersed suspensions of amebocytes: cell aggregation and degranulation, and the formation of extracellular coagulum. The amebocyte is reactive to bacterial lipopolysaccharide (LPS). Amebocytes are stimulated to degranulate rapidly in the presence of 1–10 μg/ml LPS [Armstrong and Rickles, 1982], and the granule contents undergo gelation at picogram per milliliter concentrations of LPS [Levin et al., 1970]. Isolated cells readily become enmeshed in the extracellular gel so that gel formation must be avoided when it is important to maintain a suspension of isolated cells. This is accomplished by preventing contact of the cells with LPS. All glassware is autoclaved, then heated to 200°C for 2–4 hr. The saline that the cells are exposed to is the endotoxin-free 3% saline used in medical practice (Travenol Laboratories, Deerfield, IL, or Hyland, Costa Mesa, CA). When maintained in vitro, the amebocytes eventually degranulate spontaneously, even in the absence of lipopolysaccharide [Armstrong, 1980; Armstrong and Rickles, 1982], and the granule contents gelate spontaneously. The report that dimethylsulfoxide prevents the proteolytic cleavage necessary for conversion of the protein coagulogen into the form that can polymerize [Liang and Liu, 1982] suggests the possibility that gel formation can be suppressed by this agent. Amebocyte aggregation, degranulation, and coagulum formation can be prevented by treating freshly collected amebocytes with a warm solution of N-ethylmaleimide or formaldehyde. Cells treated in these ways are no longer viable. A variety of agents have been defined that are non-toxic but retard spontaneous and LPS-induced degranulation [Armstrong and Rickles, 1982]. These may prove useful in preparing viable, undegranulated cells. Degranulation can also be retarded by low temperatures: animals are chilled for 1–3 hr at 4°C, then bled into cold vessels [Levin and Bang, 1964; Pistole and Britko, 1978]. It is usually not possible to collect as much blood from chilled animals as from animals at room temperature, and the hemocrit is often lower.

I have found the following protocol useful for preparing viable, monodispersed suspensions of washed amebocytes. Prechilled animals are bled into virgin, prechilled 50-ml sterile screwcap plastic centrifuge tubes (Corning No. 25330-50) under endotoxin-free conditions. The blood cells are pelleted by a brief, low-speed centrifugation, preferably in a centrifuge equipped with a swinging bucket head. All centrifugation steps are as gentle as possible to avoid producing a cell pellet that is compact and difficult to resuspend, so

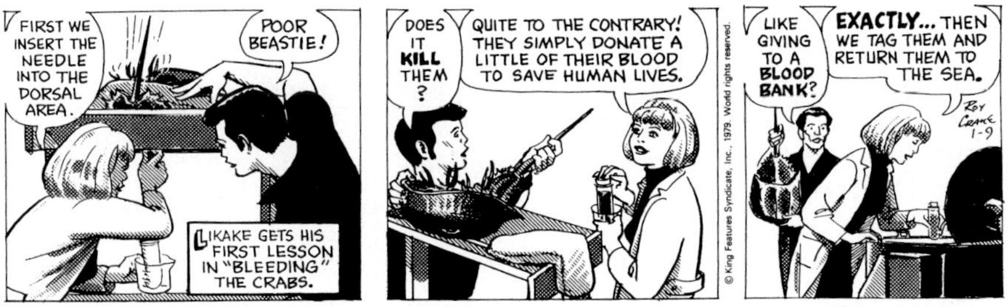
FIRST WE INSERT THE NEEDLE INTO THE DORSAL AREA.
POOR BEASTIE!
LIKAKE GETS HIS FIRST LESSON IN "BLEEDING" THE CRABS.
DOES IT KILL THEM?
QUITE TO THE CONTRARY! THEY SIMPLY DONATE A LITTLE OF THEIR BLOOD TO SAVE HUMAN LIVES.
© King Features Syndicate, Inc., 1979. World rights reserved.
LIKE GIVING TO A BLOOD BANK?
EXACTLY... THEN WE TAG THEM AND RETURN THEM TO THE SEA.
ROY CRANE 1-9

Fig. 2. Obtaining the blood of *Limulus*, as illustrated by Roy Crane in the Buz Sawyer comic strip. Reprinted with special permission of King Features. King Features Syndicate.

the speed and duration of centrifugation is kept just sufficient to pellet the cells. The plasma is removed by aspiration and the cells are resuspended in prechilled saline buffered to pH 4.6 with citrate and containing EDTA (to 500 ml of LPS-free 3% NaCl add: 9.0 gm dextrose (0.1 M), 4.5 gm sodium citrate dihydrate (0.03 M), 2.7 gm citric acid (0.026 M), and 1.9 gm disodium ethylenediamine tetraacetic acid (0.01 M), pH 4.6; [Soderhall and Smith, 1983]). Although the dry chemicals surely contain small amounts of LPS, the final amounts are not high enough to cause difficulty so long as the diluent is LPS-free. Any clumps of cells or masses of coagulum are removed with a sterile pipet and the cells are then pelleted and washed one or more times in prechilled LPS-free 3% NaCl. The final cell suspension remains monodispersive and viable for extended periods. The brief exposure to the anticoagulant appears to produce a cell suspension less prone to aggregation and degranulation. It has been found important to add Ca^{2+} (10 mM) when attempting to stimulate degranulation in cells prepared by this procedure.

Amebocytes undergo activation following removal from the animal, even under LPS-free conditions [Armstrong and Rickles, 1982]. Activation involves profound alteration in cell shape, protrusion of cell processes, and degranulation (see Armstrong, Chapter Three of this volume, Fig. 2). This has resulted in an overestimation of the number of different cell types in the blood when living extravasated cells were studied [Gregoire, 1955]. Activation of isolated cells can be prevented by bleeding into a fixative such as formaldehyde, glutaraldehyde, or N-ethylmaleimide [Armstrong, 1977]. For light microscopy, aldehyde-fixed cells can be attached to glass or plastic coverslips that have previously been derivatized with a polycation such as protamine sulfate or poly-L-lysine [Cohen et al., 1983]. Coverslips are exposed to a 1–10 mg/ml solution of poly-L-lysine [Mazia et al., 1975] or protamine sulfate [Vacquier, 1975] in distilled water for a few minutes and then are washed in distilled water. When glass coverslips are used, they must be completely free of grease or other hydrophobic material before derivatization. The cells should be washed in buffer before exposure to the derivatized coverglass. Cells can be fixed for plastic embedding, sectioning, and transmission electron microscopy in buffered glutaraldehyde [Dumont et al., 1966] or a fixative containing 1% glutaraldehyde, 3% paraformaldehyde, 3% NaCl, 3.5% sucrose, and 0.1 M phosphate buffer [Fahrenbach, 1970].

Observation of Cell Motility and Exocytosis

Amebocytes can be observed in situ in gill leaflets isolated from juvenile animals [Armstrong, 1979; Loeb, 1928]. The leaflets are sandwiched between a slide and a coverglass in 3% saline. The trauma of isolation induces a fraction of the cells to become motile in situ [Armstrong, 1979]. Amebocytes can also be observed in the abdominal spines of juvenile animals [Bang, 1979].

Motility of the cells can be studied either by allowing freshly collected cells diluted in 3% NaCl to attach directly to coverglasses that then are mounted on slides for viewing [Armstrong and Rickles, 1982] or by collecting 4–6 ml of blood into an embryo watchglass and allowing the cells to settle to the bottom of the dish and cohere into a tissue-like layer ("amebocyte tissue" [Loeb, 1920]). Small pieces of amebocyte tissue are removed and placed in contact with a coverglass in a suitable observation chamber. Within half an hour to 1 hr, numbers of amebocytes migrate from the explant over the surface of the coverglass, where they can be observed and studied [Armstrong, 1977]. Although the second procedure is more tedious, it is recommended for observation of cells showing the unflattened, contracted state. Cells prepared by the first method tend to flatten shortly after they contact the glass, but if the number of cells is large enough to generate a multilayer, the cells not in contact with the glass remain in the unflattened, contracted state.

The *Limulus* amebocyte is a useful cell for studying the process of exocytosis. A system for visual study of the process has been developed by Armstrong and Rickles [1982]. Four to ten drops of blood are diluted in 15 ml 3% NaCl contained in a 100-mm petri dish. Several 22-mm × 22-mm, No. 1½ coverglasses are placed on the bottom of the dish prior to bleeding. After 2–10 min, coverglasses are removed from the dish and are placed with the attached cells down over a few drops of 3% NaCl in a perfusion chamber constructed by supporting the coverglass above a 1 × 3-in microscope slide with fragments of No. 1½ coverglasses at the four corners. Two coverslips are placed on each slide, one to serve as the experimental, the other to serve as the principal control. The coverglasses are sealed to the slide with molten 1:3 vaseline:paraffin along the long edges of the slide, leaving the other two edges of the coverglass unsealed. Perfusion of the chamber is performed by introducing saline at one free edge with a Pasteur pipet and removing solution with absorbant tissue at the opposite free edge. The contents of the perfusion chamber can be exchanged in a few seconds, keeping the same cells in the field of view throughout the procedure. The cytoplasmic granules can be observed and the degree of degranulation scored visually.

Sources of This Species (complete addresses at end of chapter)

Limulus polyphemus occurs along the Atlantic Coast of North America from Maine to Yucatan [Shuster, 1979, 1982]. Mature and juvenile animals are collected along the shores of protected bays and estuaries, or dredged from the continental shelf. They can be purchased from the MBL Department of Marine Resources, from the Gulf Specimen Co., and from Maritech.

References

Armstrong PB (1977): Interaction of the motile blood cells of the horseshoe crab *Limulus*. Studies on contact paralysis of pseudopodial activity and cellular overlapping *in vitro*. Exp Cell Res 107:127–138.

Armstrong PB (1979): Motility of the *Limulus* blood cell. J Cell Sci 37:169–180.

Armstrong PB (1980): Adhesion and spreading of *Limulus* blood cells on artificial surfaces. J Cell Sci 44:243–262.

Armstrong PB, Rickles FR (1982): Endotoxin-induced degranulation of the *Limulus* amebocyte. Exp Cell Res 140:15–24.

Bang FB (1979): Ontogeny and phylogeny of response to gram-negative endotoxins among the marine invertebrates. Cohen E (ed): "Biomedical Applications of the Horseshoe Crab (Limulidae)." New York: Alan R. Liss, pp 109–123.

Cohen WD, Nemhauser I, Cohen MF (1983): Marginal bands of lobster blood cells: Disappearance associated with changes in cell morphology. Biol Bull (Woods Hole) 164:50–61.

Dumont JN, Anderson E, Winner G (1966): Some cytologic characteristics of the hemocytes of *Limulus* during clotting. J Morphol 119:181–208.

Fahrenbach WH (1970): The cyanoblast: Hemocyanin formation in *Limulus polyphemus*. J Cell Biol 44:445–453.

Gregoire C (1955): Blood coagulation in arthropods. IV. A study of phase contrast microscopy of blood reactions *in vitro* in Onychophora and in various groups of arthropods. Arch Biol (Liege) 66:489–508.

Hochstein HD, Elfin JF, Cooper JF, Seligmann EB, Wolfe SM (1973): Further developments of *Limulus* amebocyte lysate test. Bull Parenteral Drug Assoc 27:139–148.

Jorgensen JH, Smith RF (1973): Preparation, sensitivity, and specificity of *Limulus* lysate for endotoxin assay. Appl Microbiol 26:43–48.

Levin J, Bang FB (1964): The role of endotoxin in the extracellular coagulation of *Limulus* blood. Bull Johns Hopkins Hosp 115:265–274.

Levin J, Bang FB (1968): Clottable protein in *Limulus*: Its localization and kinetics of its coagulation by endotoxin. Thromb Diath Haemorrh 19:186–197.

Levin J, Tomasulo PA, Oper RS (1970): Detection of endotoxin in human blood and demonstration of an inhibitor. J Lab Clin Med 75:903–911.

Liang S-M, Liu T-Y (1982): Studies on the *Limulus* coagulation system: Inhibition of activation of the proclotting enzyme by dimethylsulfoxide. Biochem Biophys Res Commun 105:553–559.

Loeb L (1920): The movements of the amoebocytes and the experimental production of amoebocyte (cell fibrin) tissue. Washington Univ Studies 8:3–79, 1920.

Loeb L (1928): Amoebocyte tissue and ameboid movement. Protoplasm 4:596–625.

Mazia D, Schatten G, Sale W (1975): Adhesion of cells to surface coated with polylysine. Applications to electron microscopy. J Cell Biol 66:198–200.

Pistole TG, Britko JL (1978): Bactericidal activity of amebocytes from the horseshoe crab, *Limulus polyphemus*. J Invertebr Pathol 31:376–382.

Shuster CN (1979): Distribution of the American horseshoe "crab," *Limulus polyphemus* (L.). In Cohen E (ed): "Biomedical Applications of the Horseshoe Crab (Limulidae)." New York: Alan R. Liss, pp 3–26.

Shuster CN (1982): A pictorial review of the natural history and ecology of the horseshoe crab *Limulus polyphemus*, with reference to other Limulidae. In "Physiology and Biology of Horseshoe Crabs: Studies on Normal and Environmentally Stressed Animals." New York: Alan R. Liss, pp 1–52.

Soderhall K, Smith VJ (1983): Separation of the haemocyte populations of *Carcinus maenas* and other marine decapods, and prophenoloxidase distribution. Dev Comp Immunol 7:229–239.

Vacquier VD (1975): The isolation of intact cortical granules from sea urchin eggs: Calcium ions trigger granule discharge. Dev Biol 43:62–74.

Yeager JF, Tauber OE (1935): On the hemolymph cell counts of some marine invertebrates. Biol Bull (Woods Hole) 69:66–70.

II. AMEBOCYTES OF THE "HORSESHOE CRAB," *LIMULUS POLYPHEMUS*: ADDITIONAL NOTES

J. Levin and R.L. Ornberg

Departments of Laboratory Medicine and Medicine, University of California School of Medicine, San Francisco, California 94143 (J.L.); Laboratory of Cell Biology and Genetics, National Institute of Arthritis, Diabetes, Digestive, and Kidney Diseases, National Institutes of Health, Bethesda, Maryland 20205 (R.L.O.); and the Marine Biological Laboratory, Woods Hole, Massachusetts 02543 (J.L., R.L.O.)

Maintenance of Animals

L. polyphemus can be maintained for 3–6 months in closed-system circulating tanks of artificial sea water at 10–12°C. At this relatively low temperature feeding is not critical; if desired, the animal will feed if it is turned on its back and food is placed in the mouth. At higher temperatures (~20°C) the animals will also survive without feeding. However, it is best to feed them weekly, crushed shellfish being a good food source. The MBL Department of Marine Resources also recommends small worms and pieces of raw meat, and suggests use of a separate feeding tank to maintain cleanliness and viable conditions in the primary tank. The animals are kept in the feeding tank for only 1 day at a time. *Limulus* is also readily maintained in tanks in the running seawater available at a marine station.

Removal of Blood and Preparation of Cells for Experimental Use

Blood can be removed via syringe by puncturing the leg joints or by cardiac puncture. In either case the surface is first wiped with a 70% ethanol swab. A 1-in or 1.5-inch, 20-gauge needle is satisfactory, but a short (approx. ½–1 inch) large-bore needle (12–16 gauge) is most useful for rapidly obtaining large volumes of blood from the heart. For cardiac puncture, flex the cephalothorax and abdominal segments; using 70% ethanol, clean the muscle that covers the heart in the midline. Collect blood into sterile *and* pyrogen-free containers using a similarly prepared needle. This results in blood from which one can prepare unaggregated amebocytes if N-ethyl maleimide (NEM) is present. Dilution of blood with a solution of 5mM NEM in sterile, pyrogen-free 3% saline is helpful in obtaining a good yield of intact, unaggregated cells. It should be noted that NEM is useful in preparing cells for biochemical work but not for physiological studies of living cells.

Maintenance of sterile, pyrogen-free conditions is critical for preventing cell aggregation and degranulation. Blood should be continuously mixed with the NEM solution as it is obtained to prevent cell aggregation. Warming the initial solution of NEM to approximately 40°C further enhances the inhibition of aggregation, but is not needed for subsequent washing of cells. For biochemical work, the cells can be washed and maintained in 3% saline containing 5 mM NEM and stored at room temperature. However, after approximately 4 hr some cell aggregation will begin to occur, and subsequently the degree of aggregation increases. At 4°C the tendency for aggregation is increased; to minimize this, cells are handled at room temperature throughout.

For physiological studies of living cells, NEM should be avoided and a Ringer's solution used. A compatible Ringer's solution for *Limulus* amebocytes is the following: 454 mM NaCl, 10 mM KCl, 10 mM $CaCl_2$, 32 mM $MgCl_2$, 14 mM $MgSO_4$, 20 mM HEPES (N-2-hydroxyethyl-piperazine-N-2 ethane sulfonic acid), pH 7.8. In preparing this solution, all salts and glassware were baked at 200°C for 4 hr to destroy endotoxin potentially present. HEPES buffer, diluted from 0.5 M concentrated stock, was clarified with 0.22 μm Millipore filters after autoclaving. After baking $MgCl_2$ it decomposes to $MgOH_2$, which is redissolved with HCl. After the salts have been redissolved the buffer is added. Use of baking in combination with Millipore filtration prevents degranulation of the cells in the medium as observed by light microscopy. One can evaluate the potential presence of residual endotoxin in solutions by using the *Limulus* Amebocyte Lysate (LAL) test [Watson et al, 1982]. The exquisite sensitivity of the test easily permits detection of levels of endotoxin lower than that required to activate the cells.

Low temperature helps prevent cell shape change and secretion. Propranolol (1 mM) helps prevent aggregation, shape change, and secretion. Cytochalasin D at final concentrations in the range of 1–10 mg/ml prevents the shape change but does not prevent secretion. The effects of both propranolol and cytochalasin are reversible, and they can be washed out within 15–20 min. To obtain low-temperature cells, the animals can be put in seawater (or artificial seawater) containing bags of ice; a cold room is not necessary. Drugs can be added to cells using cell-free plasma as a medium. Whole blood is withdrawn and centrifuged, and the plasma supernate saved. Drugs are added to this plasma at twice the desired final concentration. The syringe is pre-loaded with one volume of the drug-plasma mixture, and blood is drawn directly from the animal into this syringe until an appropriate or equal volume is reached. This procedure ensures very rapid exposure of cells to drugs under nearly physiological conditions [Ornberg and Reese, 1981].

References and Additional Information

Cohen E, Bang FB, Levin J, et al, eds (1979): "Biomedical Applications of the Horseshoe Crab." New York: Alan R. Liss, Inc.

Levin J, Bang FB (1968): Clottable protein in *Limulus*: Its localization and kinetics of its coagulation by endotoxin. Thromb Diath Haemorrh 19:186–197.

Ornberg RL, Reese TS (1981): Beginning of exocytosis captured by rapid-freezing of *Limulus* amebocytes. J Cell Biol 90:40–54.

Watson SW, Levin J, Novitsky TJ, eds (1982): Endotoxins and their detection with the *Limulus* Amebocyte Lysate test. New York: Alan R. Liss, Inc.

III. HEMOCYTES OF THE AMERICAN LOBSTER, *HOMARUS AMERICANUS*

W.D. Cohen and I. Nemhauser

Department of Biological Sciences, Hunter College of the City University of New York, New York, New York 10021, and the Marine Biological Laboratory, Woods Hole, Massachusetts 02543

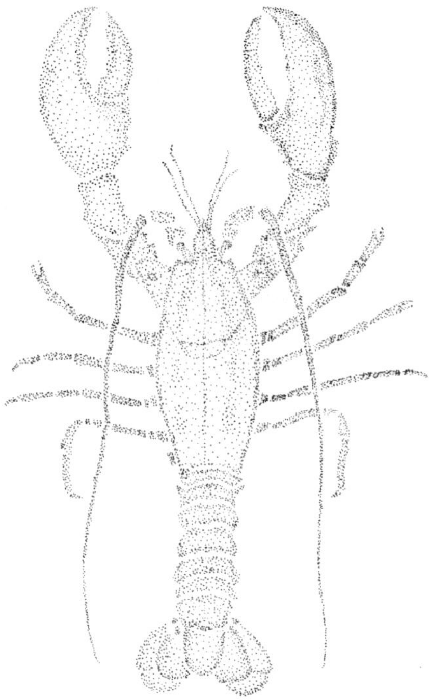

Fig. 3. The American lobster, *Homarus americanus*.

Maintenance of Animals

Homarus americanus (Fig. 3) is readily maintained in the laboratory (as in the market!) in closed-system circulating artificial seawater tanks at 10–15°C. They can be fed fish, clams, shrimp, or worms, but can also be maintained for long periods without feeding. A refrigerated 50-gallon or larger tank containing "Instant Ocean" (Aquarium Systems, Mentor, OH 44060) or other artificial seawater (for example, that of the Ruet Co., Saddle Brook, NJ 07662) is adequate. The claws should be held closed by wooden pegs or by heavy rubber bands. This not only protects the researcher, but also keeps the larger lobsters from snipping the claws off the smaller ones, something at which they are remarkably adept.

Other marine crustacea can be similarly maintained and fed at about 15°C. Shrimp, clams, and worms are recommended as food for various crustacea by the Committee on Marine Invertebrates of the National Research Council (U.S.) [CMI, 1981]. Their publication, entitled "Laboratory Animal Management, Marine Invertebrates," is a generally useful manual on maintenance and culture of many marine species.

Removal of Coelomic Fluid

Small blood samples (0.1–1 ml) are conveniently obtained from lobsters or crabs by snipping off the tip of a walking leg with heavy scissors. A simple way to handle the animals is to trap them within a strong net with fairly large holes. The body of the animal within the net can be held under a heavy cloth or with a thick glove. Usually one or more walking legs will protrude and can be grasped by hand for snipping. The fluid will quickly begin to drip out, or it can be drawn off by pipette immediately for fixation or other experimental treatment. Alternatively, larger samples can be withdrawn from the animal by syringe (i.e., without snipping).

Preparation of Cells for Experimental Use

Most of the cells in lobster blood undergo rapid activation, changing shape and initiating exocytosis ("explosive degranulation") shortly after removal from the animal. It is therefore imperative to work as quickly as possible and/or to use inhibitors if native shape or unactivated physiology are important. The same problem is likely to occur with all invertebrate clotting cells of this type. The method recommended by R. Ornberg for *Limulus* amebocytes, in which the time available for activation is minimized by drawing cells directly from the animal into a syringe containing experimental media, would appear to be useful with *Homarus* and other crustacean hemocytes as well. The coelomic fluid of the species, prepared in advance and from which cells have been removed by centrifugation, can be used as the base of such media (see previous section of this chapter). We have also found marine crustacean Ringer's solution at pH 7.0 (30.65 gm/liter NaCl, 0.99 gm/liter KCl, 1.82 gm/liter $CaCl_2 \cdot 2\,H_2O$, 5.04 gm/liter $MgCl_2 \cdot 6\,H_2O$, $NaHCO_3$ to pH 7.0 [Cavanaugh, 1975]) to be a useful blood diluent for lobster hemocytes.

Classification of Cell Types in Lobster Hemolymph

One of the difficulties which a researcher initially encounters in working with "blood" of *Homarus* and other crustacea is that of identifying cell types. Therefore we include here a synopsis of pertinent literature, pointing out some of the problems in this area in the hope that improved classification methods and data may result.

Toney [1958] described four cell types in fresh lobster blood (*H. americanus*) on the basis of size, morphology, and behavior, as observed in phase contrast: "lymphoid cells," "monocytes," and larger "explosive refractile granulocytes" containing either small (0.25 μm) or large (1 μm) granules. The "explosive refractile granulocytes" were identified as clotting cells, those containing large granules constituting 90–95% of the total blood cell population. Most of the blood cells were initially discoid or ellipsoid, subsequently undergoing drastic changes in morphology.

Hearing and Vernick [1967] fixed blood samples of *H. americanus* immediately after removal from animals and examined the cells by light and electron microscopy. They identified three cell types on the basis of staining and morphology: "eosinophils" (20% of population), "ovoid basophils" (20%), and "spindular basophils" (60%). Granules of various sizes were present in all of the cells, the largest occurring in the "spindular basophils." Thus there is a discrepancy with the classification of Toney [1958] in which one cell type, the explosive refractile granulocyte containing large granules, constitutes > 90% of lobster blood cells. However, since cell type was determined primarily by examination of cells in sections, it is possible that the "spindular basophils" and "ovoid basophils" were the same flattened, oval cells cut at various angles. This cell type, containing the larger granules, would then account for approximately 80% of the population.

In a more recent classification of *H. americanus* hemocytes based upon morphological, staining, and optical characteristics, Cornick and Stewart [1978] described four cell types: prohyalocytes (about 2% of the population), hyalocytes (64%), eosinophilic granulocytes (12%), and chromophobic granulocytes (22%). Observations were made on both stained and unstained films of cells fixed immediately after removal from the animal. Cells in the last three categories, constituting most of the population, were observed to contain granules of various sizes and staining properties. It is not clear just which of these cells correspond to the "explosive granulocytes" of Toney [1958], but on the basis of numbers, one can presume that it must be at least the "hyalocytes" and a majority of the others.

Classification of blood cell types in the lobster and in many other invertebrates is obviously a difficult task. There are several major factors that contribute to this difficulty, including a) the triggering of morphological changes in the native cells by the act of hemolymph removal (wounding, etc.), b) morphological changes induced by subsequent contact with glass slides or other experimental surfaces, c) possible variation in the health and physiological state of the animals, d) possible presence of cells in intermediate stages of differentiation, and e) sparsity of previous literature on the behavior and function of the cells. As noted above, precautions can be taken so as to minimize morphological changes of the a) and b) variety, reducing or eliminating the occurrence of activation stages. Once this is achieved, cell types can be characterized by morphological, behavioral, and biochemical criteria and perhaps separated by density gradient centrifugation or other means.

Other Crustacea

A good example of the application of such precautions and of separation methods to crustacean hemocytes is provided by the recent work of Soderhall and Smith [1983] on *Carcinus maenas* and several other species. Since such an approach is likely to be of general value, we include here some of the details. Animals were prechilled to 7°C for 2 hr prior to bleeding. Hemolymph was drawn directly into a syringe containing an anticoagulant solution (citrate/EDTA buffer = 0.45 M NaCl, 0.1 M glucose, 30 mM trisodium citrate, 26 mM citric acid, 10 mM EDTA, pH 4.6 at 7°C) using 1:1 or 1:2 hemolymph/anticoagulant volume ratios. This medium was reported to maintain cell integrity and viability during subsequent steps. Samples (1 ml) were layered onto continuous 10-ml Percoll gradients, pre-formed in polycarbonate tubes by centrifugation of 60% Percoll (Pharmacia Inc., Uppsala, Sweden) in 3.2% NaCl at 25,000 g for 20 min at 7°C. Before use, centrifuge tubes were washed in 6 M urea, pH 2.0, rinsed in distilled water, and coated

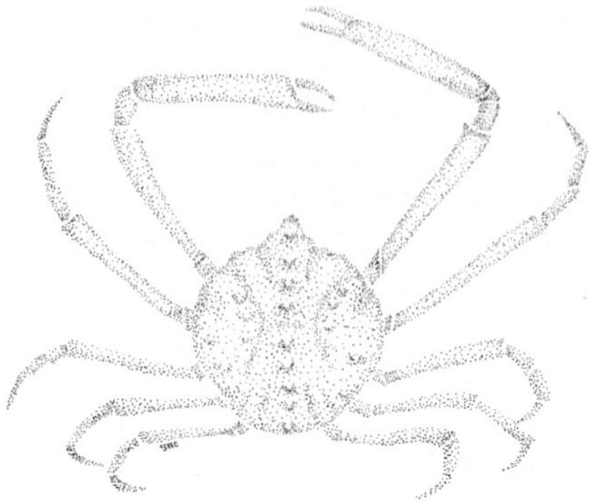

Fig. 4. The "spider crab," *Libinia emarginata*.

with dichlorosilane, to minimize attachment of cells to tube walls. Gradient tubes were centrifuged in a swing-out rotor at 2,900 g for 10 min at 7°C, and 0.5-ml fractions collected from the bottom of the tubes. For *C. maenas*, three major cell bands were observed and collected: the uppermost band at the sample-gradient interface, containing some small hyaline cells; a band about halfway down the tube containing many hyaline cells; and a band near the bottom containing only granular cells. Granular cell bands in the same location were also obtained with other species, though there was some variation in number and location of other bands. The distribution of prophenoloxidase in different cell fractions was found to be restricted to the granular cells, correlating well with the fact that the granular cells of *C. maenas* are believed to function in clotting and agglutinin release, whereas the hyaline cells of this species are responsible for phagocytosis in vitro [Smith and Ratcliffe, 1978]. Cell separation methods thus provide an excellent approach to hemocyte characterization and classification.

Our primary interest has been in the cytoskeleton of crustacean hemocytes, particularly marginal bands of microtubules [Cohen et al, 1983]. We have found obvious marginal bands not only in lobster hemocytes but also in similar cells of several species of marine crabs, including *Libinia emarginata* ("spider crab"; Fig. 4) and *Cancer borealis* ("Jonah rock crab"). We do not yet know whether these are all clotting cells, however. Thus it remains to be determined whether marginal bands are a diagnostic feature of clotting cells in marine Crustacea; if so, they may help considerably in cell classification schemes.

Sources of These Species and Usable Relatives (complete addresses at end of chapter)

Living specimens of *H. americanus* are readily available commercially in the United States in fish markets and supermarkets. Many species of crabs can be obtained at or from the MBL Department of Marine Resources, from Pacific Biomarine Inc., and from Gulf Specimen Co. *Callinectes sapidus* (the blue crab) is also available live in Northeastern U.S. fish markets at certain times of the year. These are usually shipped in baskets without water, but they are active for at least several weeks when restored to a seawater tank. Various crustaceans can of course be collected as permitted in shallow coastal waters.

References

Cavanaugh GM, ed (1975): "Formulae and Methods VI of the Marine Biological Laboratory." Woods Hole, Massachusetts: MBL (available from MBL).

CMI (Committee on Marine Invertebrates) (1981): "Laboratory Animal Management, Marine Invertebrates." Washington, DC: National Academy Press.

Cohen WD, Nemhauser I, Cohen MF (1983): Marginal bands of lobster blood cells: Disappearance associated with changes in cell morphology. Biol Bull 164:50–61.

Cornick JW, Stewart JE (1978): Lobster (*Homarus americanus*) hemocytes: Classification, differential counts, and associated agglutinin activity. J Invert Pathol 31:194–203.

Hearing V, Vernick SH (1967): Fine structure of the blood cells of the lobster, *Homarus americanus*. Chesapeake Sci 8:170–186.

Smith VJ, Ratcliffe NA (1978): Host defence reactions of the shore crab, *Carcinus maenas* in vitro. J Mar Biol Assoc UK 58:367.

Soderhall K, Smith VJ (1983): Separation of the haemocyte populations of *Carcinus maenas* and other marine decapods, and prophenoloxidase distribution. Dev Comp Immunol 7:229–239.

Toney ME Jr (1958): Morphology of the blood cells of some Crustacea. Growth 22:35–50.

IV. PETALOID/FILOPODIAL COELOMOCYTES OF THE GREEN SEA URCHIN, *STRONGYLOCENTROTUS DROEBACHIENSIS*

K.T. Edds

Department of Anatomical Sciences, School of Medicine, State University at Buffalo, Buffalo, New York 14214 and the Marine Biological Laboratory, Woods Hole, Massachusetts 02543

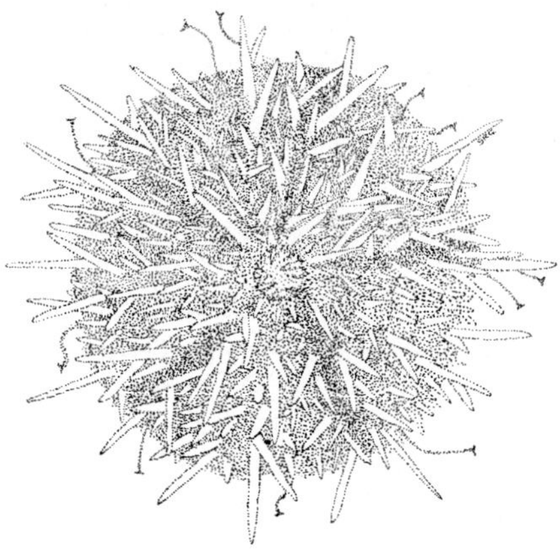

Fig. 5. The green sea urchin, *Strongylocentrotus droebachiensis*.

Maintenance of Animals

S. droebachiensis (Fig. 5) can be maintained easily in the laboratory in any sort of refrigerated aquarium that has seawater circulating through a sand/gravel bed in the bottom of the tank. Supplemental filters containing activated charcoal and mounted on the sides may be necessary if large numbers of animals are to be kept. We routinely keep 100 animals in a 135-gallon aquarium with only a "well seasoned" sub-gravel filter. Problem situations can usually be remedied by reducing the biological load on the aquarium system; see Spotte [1979] for techniques on invertebrate culture in closed systems. The animals do well in "Instant Ocean" artificial seawater (Aquarium Systems, Mentor, OH 44060) adjusted to specific gravity 1.025 in accordance with directions. *S. droebachiensis* lives in relatively cold Northeastern U.S. waters, and a laboratory temperature range of 10–15°C is usual. We try to match what the animals were experiencing at the time of collection. They are normally fed *Laminaria* (kelp), but can survive quite well without feeding for as long as 1 year, during which time internal organs diminish in size but coelomic fluid is maintained in experimentally useful volumes. Other species of sea urchins can also be used as a source of petaloid/filopodial cells (see below); maintenance temperature varies with species. The volume "Laboratory Animal Management—Marine Invertebrates" [CMI, 1981] contains a useful table on maintenance temperatures and feeding of many commonly studied animals including various urchin species.

Removal of Coelomic Fluid

After easing the animal from the side of the aquarium and draining most of the seawater from the outside, the animal is held oral side up such that the five white "teeth" of "Aristotle's Lantern" are visible. With a pair of sharp dissecting scissors or the equivalent, one cuts through the soft tissue immediately surrounding the lantern and then plucks it out with the scissors tips. With the coelomic cavity and its contents now accessible, one merely pours the fluid (2–30 ml depending on season, health, and unknown factors) out and into a beaker containing anticoagulant. The anticoagulant we use is a 50/50 mixture of 1 M EGTA, pH 7.5, and 1 M Tris-HCl (pH 7.5). We generally use 6 ml of each solution in a beaker and add coelomic fluid from two or more animals to a final volume of 60 ml; the final concentration of each component is therefore 0.1 M. This procedure prevents clotting and allows for separation of cell types by a sucrose step gradient [Edds, 1977].

Preparation of Cells for Experimental Use

The unclotted cell suspension is layered onto a solution consisting of 0.8 M sucrose made in 0.5 M NaCl and 20 mM Tris-HCl (pH 7.5) in 15-ml centrifuge-worthy test tubes. The tubes are spun at 5,000g for 5 min in a swinging-bucket rotor; a table-top centrifuge can be used but a larger, refrigerated machine is preferable. The petaloid/filopodial cells are collected from the sucrose-coelomic fluid interface and washed in 0.5 M NaCl, 20 mM Tris-HCl, pH 7.5. The cells can be concentrated by gentle centrifugation (650g for 3 min) or used as a suspension. Transformation to the filopodial morphology can be elicited by diluting the 0.5 M salt buffer to 0.3 M with 20 mM Tris-HCl, pH 7.5.

Interestingly, if the cells are allowed to remain in the anticoagulant/coelomic fluid solution they display motility that is not observed in the washed cells [Edds et al., 1983]. The nature of the factors present in the coelomic fluid that promote motility are not known but they can be added back, as cell-free fluid, to washed cells with similar effects on motility.

Sources of This Species and Usable Relatives (complete addresses at end of chapter)

Strongylocentrotus droebachiensis can be obtained from the MBL Department of Marine Resources, and from Mr. Donald A. Bryant, Bath, ME.

Strongylocentrotus purpuratus is also a good source of material and is available from Pacific Biomarine Inc., from Marinus Inc., and from Intertidal Marine Biologicals.

Any large urchin, such as *Lytechinus variegatus*, will be useful as a source of cells. Smaller animals, e.g., *Arbacia punctulata* or *Lytechinus pictus*, can also be used but the amount of fluid is correspondingly less. *Arbacia* can be obtained from the MBL Department of Marine Resources, from Gulf Specimen Co., from H.M. Terry Co., Inc., and from Maritech; *L. variegatus* from Gulf Specimen Co.; and *L. pictus* from Pacific Biomarine.

References

CMI (Committee on Marine Invertebrates) (1981): "Laboratory Animal Management, Marine Invertebrates." Washington, DC: National Academy Press.

Edds KT (1977): Dynamic aspects of filopodial formation by reorganization of microfilaments. J Cell Biol 73(2):479–491.

Edds KT, Chambers C, Allen RD (1983): Coelomocyte motility. Cell Motil 3(2):113–121.

Spotte S (1979): "Fish and Invertebrate Culture: Water Management in Closed Systems." New York: Wiley (Interscience).

V. ERYTHROCYTES OF THE SIPUNCULAN WORMS *PHASCOLOPSIS GOULDII* AND *THEMISTE DYSCRITA*

W.D. Cohen, I. Nemhauser, N.B. Terwilliger, and R.C. Terwilliger

Department of Biological Sciences, Hunter College of the City University of New York, New York, New York 10021 (W.D.C., I.N.), the Marine Biological Laboratory, Woods Hole, Massachusetts 02543 (W.C., I.N.), and the Oregon Institute of Marine Biology, University of Oregon, Charleston, Oregon 97420 (N.B.T., R.C.T.)

Maintenance of Animals

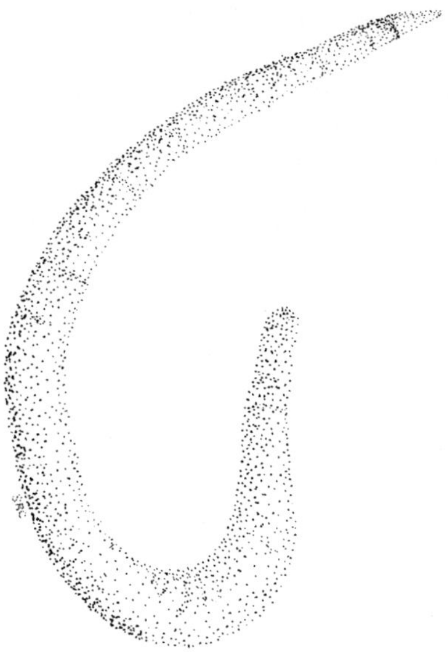

Fig. 6. The "peanut worm," *Phascolopsis gouldii*.

P. gouldii (formerly classified as *Phascolosoma gouldii* and *Golfingia gouldii*; Fig. 6) is readily maintained for long periods in the unfiltered running seawater available at a marine station. The animals will also survive for months in closed-system circulating tanks of artificial seawater at about 15°C. We have used 30-gallon tanks containing "Instant Ocean" artificial seawater (Aquarium Systems, Inc., Eastlake, OH) supplemented with trace elements (Hawaiian Marine Imports, Inc., Houston, TX), with feeding of "Marine Invertebrate Diet" (Hawaiian Marine Imports). Fine sand should be provided so that the animals can burrow under.

T. dyscrita can be maintained in the laboratory for months in unfiltered, running seawater at 15°C. Running seawater is preferable but not necessary. The animals are hardy and will survive for weeks under adverse conditions, such as in closed ziplock bags containing seawater.

Removal of Coelomic Fluid

Coelomic fluid can be drawn from the body cavity by syringe, or can be obtained by slitting the animal longitudinally with a scalpel or razor blade. In the latter case the fluid gushes out, and one must be prepared to catch it in a receptacle (slitting the animal in a petri dish is convenient). Additional squeezing of the slit animal will yield the maximum volume.

Removal of fluid from the contractile vessel of *Themiste* requires slitting the animal open, removing the pink fluid-filled diverticulae of the contractile vessel, and collecting the fluid.

Preparation of Cells for Experimental Use

The hemerythrin-containing erythrocytes of *P. gouldii* appear to be morphologically stable at room temperature in their native coelomic fluid. The coelomic fluid does not clot, though it is reported to do so in some other Sipunculan species [Hyman, 1959]. Amebocytes and gametes are typically present in addition to the erythrocytes. If the worm is female, the eggs can be centrifuged out, or will settle out if the fluid is left standing. Most sperm can be removed by gently sedimenting the erythrocytes and discarding the supernate, but they are difficult to remove completely. When pure suspensions of erythrocytes are required, it is best to examine the coelomic fluid of animals separately and discard those containing sperm (milky pink).

The coelomic hemerythrin-containing cells of *T. dyscrita* undergo shape changes shortly upon removal from the animal, the surface becoming increasingly indented and wrinkled. Neither low temperature nor dilution into filtered seawater appear to alter the course of shape transformation, whereas salinity extremes accentuate the changes in morphology. The hemerythrin-containing cells found within the contractile vessels of this species also change morphology upon removal, becoming cup-shaped. Neither of the cell types appears to aggregate upon removal from the animal.

Sources of These Species and Usable Relatives (complete addresses at end of chapter)

Phascolopsis gouldii can be obtained from the MBL Department of Marine Resources. *Themiste dyscrita* is not available commercially, but *Themiste zostericola* can be obtained from Pacific Biomarine, Inc. *Phascolosoma agassizii* is available from Pacific Biomarine and Sea Life Supply.

One should be sure to check the genus and species of the animals, using references such as Light's manual [Smith and Carleton, 1975]. Incorrect identification of peanut worms has led to confusion in the past.

References and Additional Information

Adolph EE (1936): Differential permeability to water and osmotic changes in the marine worm *Phascolosoma*. J Cell Comp Physiol 9:117–135.

Dybas L (1981): Sipunculans and echiuroids. In Ratcliffe NA, and Rowley AF (eds): "Invertebrate Blood Cells." London: Academic Press, pp 161–188.

Gibbs PE (1977): "British Sipunculans." New York, London: Academic Press.

Hyman LH (1959): "The Invertebrates. V. Smaller Coelomate Groups (Sipunculida)." New York, London, Toronto: McGraw-Hill, pp 610–696.

Meglitsch PA (1967): "Invertebrate Zoology." New York: Oxford University Press.

Morris RH, Abbot DP, Hoderlie EC (1980): "Intertidal Invertebrates of California." Stanford, California: Stanford University Press.

Smith RI, Carleton JT, eds (1975): Light's Manual: Intertidal Invertebrates of the Central California Coast. 3rd Ed. Berkeley, California: University of California Press.

VI. ERYTHROCYTES OF THE POLYCHAETE WORMS *GLYCERA DIBRANCHIATA* AND *PISTA PACIFICA*, AND OF THE ECHIURAN *URECHIS CAUPO*.

S.K. Pierce, N.B. Terwilliger, and R.C. Terwilliger

Department of Zoology, University of Maryland, College Park, Maryland 20742 (S.K.P.), the Marine Biological Laboratory, Woods Hole, Massachusetts 02543 (S.K.P.), and the Oregon Institute of Marine Biology, University of Oregon, Charleston, Oregon 97420 (N.B.T., R.C.T.).

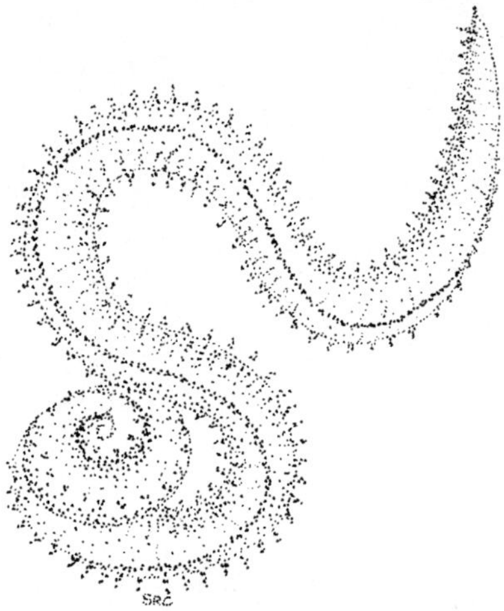

Fig. 7. The "blood worm," *Glycera dibranchiata*.

Maintenance of Animals

G. dibranchiata, the "blood worm" (Fig. 7), can be maintained without feeding for several weeks in closed-system circulating seawater tanks ("Instant Ocean" artificial seawater, salinity 920 mOsm) at 10°C or less. One should probably not use worms held more than 3 weeks, however. For some reason they keep much better if left in the dark. They can also be kept in cold running natural seawater at a marine station in floating containers or allowed to burrow into sand.

P. pacifica can be maintained for several weeks at 15°C in the running unfiltered seawater available at a marine station. *P. pacifica* is a tube-dwelling polychaete; it survives best in its own tube (about 2–3 feet long) or in a tank containing sufficient sand for new tube formation.

U. caupo, the "fat innkeeper worm" (Fig. 8), survives for months at 15°C in the running unfiltered seawater at a marine station. The animal lives in U-shaped burrows in mudflats, and does best if allowed to burrow into plastic tubing or a mud-filled aquarium.

Removal of Blood or Coelomic Fluid and Preparation of Cells for Experimental Use

The body wall of *Glycera* is cut with scissors and coelomic fluid is allowed to drain out. Care is taken not to cut into the gut. Alternatively, the proboscis can be cut open after it is extruded. The fluid does not clot. The hemoglobin-containing cells, which are spherical, are washed with a MOPS-buffered artificial seawater, pH 7.5 (460 mM NaCl, 10 mM KCl, 10 mM $CaCl_2$, 25 mM $MgCl_2 \cdot 6H_2O$, 27 mM $MgSO_4$, 2.3 mM $NaHCO_3$, 5 mM MOPS [Costa and Pierce, 1983]) and are usually kept on ice. Contaminating ameboid cells are easily separated by low-speed centrifugation.

Both the extracellular hemoglobin-containing vascular fluid and the erythrocytes (hemoglobin-containing coelomic cells) of *Pista* can be removed via syringe or by longitudinal incision. The color of the coelomic fluid can vary from red to black. Clotting is not observed, and the erythrocytes settle rapidly. They can be separated from extracellular hemoglobin by repeated washing and gentle centrifugation in filtered seawater. Variable hematocrit values have been observed, ranging from approximately 5% to 75%. This variation did not appear to correspond to animal size or blood color. The spherical cells do not undergo marked shape change after removal from the animal. While they show some volume responses to salinity extremes, the cells are relatively hardy and swell or shrink uniformly.

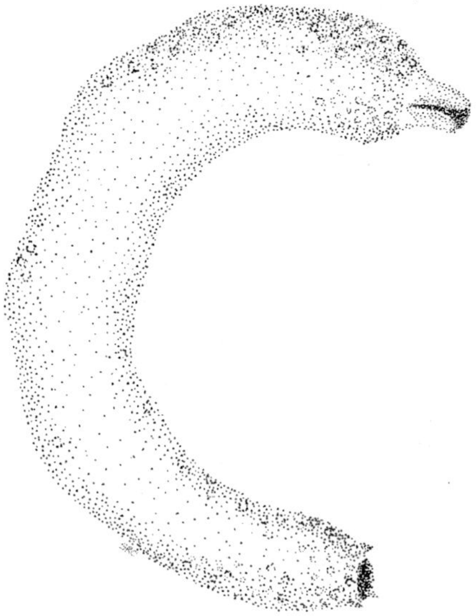

Fig. 8. The "innkeeper worm," *Urechis caupo*.

The coelomic fluid of *Urechis* with its hemoglobin-containing cells is removed by needle and syringe, or by longitudinal incision. The fluid varies in color from bright red to brown-black. The cells do not aggregate and the fluid does not clot. The cells, which are spherical, occupy 18–40% of the coelomic fluid volume and are relatively stable in either coelomic fluid or filtered seawater.

Sources of These Species (complete addresses at end of chapter)

Glycera dibranchiata can be obtained from the Maine Bait Co. and from the MBL Department of Marine Resources. *Pista pacifica* is not available commercially. It is found from British Columbia to Southern California, inhabiting sandy mudflats at approximately the 0.0 ft tide level. The animal lives in a tube about 1 meter deep in mud (see Morris et al. [1980] for further information).

Urechis caupo is available from Pacific Biomarine, from Sea Life Supply, and, upon inquiry, may also be obtainable from Intertidal Marine Biologicals.

References

Costa CJ, Pierce SK (1983): Volume regulation in the red coelomocytes of *Glycera dibranchiata*: An interaction of amino acid and K^+ effluxes. J Comp Physiol 151:133–144.

Morris RH, Abbot DP, Hoderlie EC (1980): "Intertidal Invertebrates of California." Stanford, CA: Stanford University Press.

VII. ERYTHROCYTES OF THE "BLOOD CLAMS" *NOETIA PONDEROSA*, *ANADARA OVALIS*, AND *ANADARA TRANSVERSA*

W.D. Cohen, I. Nemhauser, and S.K. Pierce

Department of Biological Sciences, Hunter College of the City University of New York, New York, New York 10021 (W.D.C., I.N.), Department of Zoology, University of Maryland, College Park, Maryland 20742 (S.K.P.), and the Marine Biological Laboratory, Woods Hole, Massachusetts 02543 (W.D.C., I.N., S.K.P.)

Maintenance of Animals

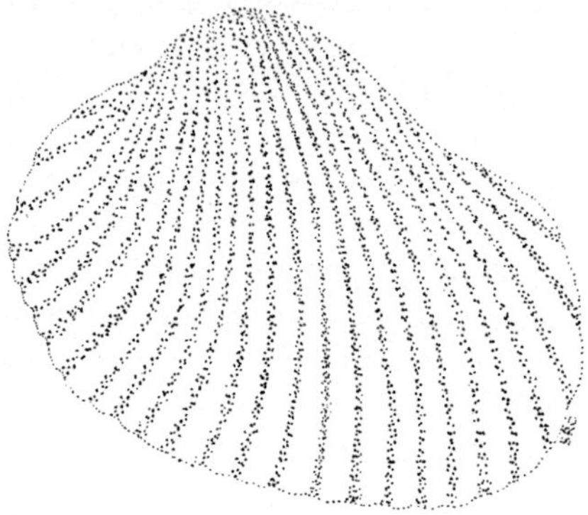

Fig. 9. The "blood ark," *Anadara ovalis*.

N. ponderosa (the "ponderous ark"), *A. ovalis* (the "blood ark," Fig. 9), and *A. transversa* (the "transverse ark") are all readily maintained for long periods in the running, unfiltered seawater at a marine station (15–20°C). *N. ponderosa* can be maintained for months in closed-system tanks of circulating, aerated artificial seawater ("Instant Ocean," Aquarium Systems, Inc.) at about 10°C without feeding, and at 18°C with feeding of "Marine Invertebrate Diet" (Hawaiian Marine Imports, Inc., Houston, TX). *A. ovalis* and *A. transversa* from Northeast US waters have been similarly maintained at 15°C, and *A. ovalis* from the Gulf of Mexico at 18°C.

Removal of Blood

If the animals cannot be caught by surprise with the valves (shells) open, they must first be wedged open. Various tools such as clam knife, spatula, metal probe or screwdriver are useful here. One reliable procedure is to file the edges of the shells where they meet, using a triangular file, until a small opening is produced. A probe is then inserted and used to pry open the shells sufficiently to insert a clam knife. The seawater can then be drained. Care must be taken so that the mantle is not punctured prematurely by inserting the probe or knife too deeply. The clam knife can be rotated to separate the shells further. Blood can be obtained quickly by slashing the adductor muscles and mantle with a razor blade. The blood is drained from the cut surfaces into a beaker. Alternatively, the shells can be pulled apart until the animal is unable to close them, exposing the reddish mantle surfaces that line them, under which much of the blood is pooled. These are then punctured by the tip of a Pasteur pipette, and the blood is pipetted or drained off. It is also possible to remove small volumes of blood without opening the animal by inserting a fine pipette or needle through a small hole in the shells into the mantle surface. *A. ovalis* is a bit more difficult than the other species to open

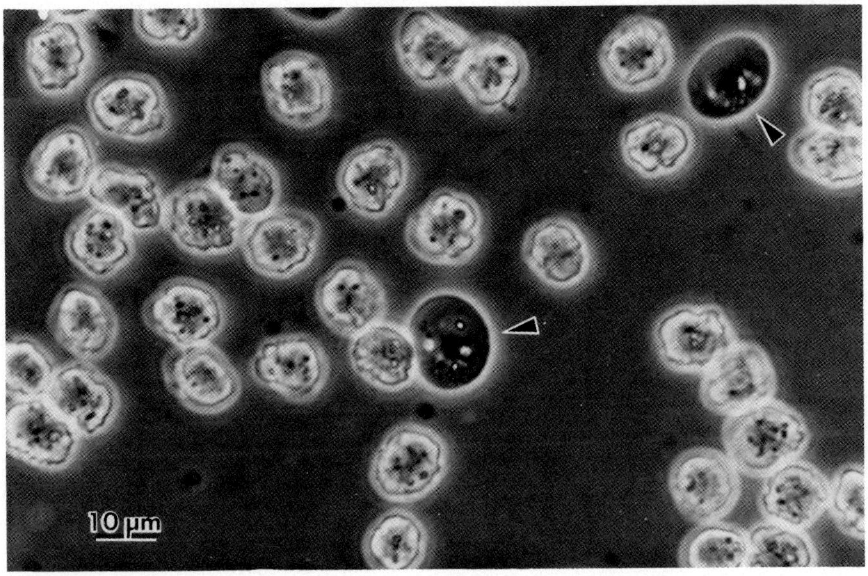

Fig. 10. Erythrocytes of *A. ovalis* in native fluid, shortly after removal from the animal. A few cells still have normal smooth, flattened morphology (arrowheads), but the rest have become lumpy and amorphous (phase contrast).

neatly; its shell is quite fragile, and small pieces will break off easily when stressed by the clam knife or probe.

The normal hematocrit for these hemoglobin-containing cells will be about 6–7%. In our experience, only bright red blood should be used. In some animals the blood is brown, and the cells have abnormal shapes.

Preparation of Cells for Experimental Use

While stringy material occasionally appears upon storage at room temperature, the blood does not clot. When kept in their native fluid at room temperature, most of the erythrocytes of *Anadara ovalis* and *Anadara transversa* undergo a shape change within minutes of removal of the animal. This can also occur within the erythrocytes of *Noetia ponderosa*, but it is far less frequent. The cells are initially flattened and elliptical, but after 5–10 min nearly all have become lumpy and amorphous ("potato-shaped"; Fig. 10). The phenomenon presents a problem for structural studies and for experiments in which native morphology is important to the function under investigation. There are several ways to avoid the problem, such as by working with *Noetia* as much as possible. Immediate dilution of the blood approximately 1:10–1:20 into marine molluscan Ringer's solution or other suitable diluents (see below) pre-chilled to 0°C prevents the shape change, but the conditions are not appropriate for certain kinds of experiments. The most useful procedure that we have discovered for obtaining normal cells at room temperature is immediate dilution of the blood into large volumes of diluent (approximately 1:200). This is usually, but not always, effective. A beaker containing the diluent at room temperature is set up in advance with continuous magnetic stirring. The blood is added continuously as it is being obtained, and the erythrocytes are then sedimented by relatively low speed centrifugation (for example, approx. 2,000 rpm for 2 min in the International HN centrifuge). As a general guide, animals of 2–3 cm (shell long dimension) yield about 1 ml blood; animals of 4–6 cm yield about 2 ml, etc. The appropriate volume of diluent for a 1:200 dilution can thus be estimated in advance.

We have found several media suitable for dilution of the blood and washing the cells. These include marine molluscan Ringer's solution, which consists of NaCl 30.97 gm/liter, KCl 0.8 gm/liter, $CaCl_2 \cdot 2H_2O$ 1.91 gm/liter buffered with phosphate at pH 7.2 (we use $NaH_2PO_4 \cdot H_2O$ 0.07 gm/liter) [Cavanaugh, 1975]; artificial seawater ("MBL formula": NaCl 24.72 gm/liter, KCl 0.67 gm/liter, $CaCl_2 \cdot 2\ H_2O$ 1.36 gm/liter, $MgCl_2 \cdot 6\ H_2O$ 4.66 gm/liter, $MgSO_4 \cdot 7\ H_2O$ 6.29 gm/liter, $NaHCO_3$ 0.18 gm/liter [Cavanaugh, 1975]); and MOPS-buffered artificial seawater [Costa and Pierce, 1983] (see preceding section of this chapter for recipe). The blood contains amebocytes and sometimes gametes in addition to erythrocytes, both of which are removed by several cycles of gentle centrifugation and resuspension. Amebocytes tend to clump and form a whitish layer overlying the erythrocyte pellet. This layer, containing trapped erythrocytes as well, can be dislodged in a single sheet by gentle squirts of fresh wash medium from a Pasteur pipette. The layer is then removed and discarded.

The rapid loss of normal erythrocyte shape in these species can be viewed as an experimental annoyance, but it is also an interesting problem, presumably involving changes in the cytoskeleton. Although we know little about the mechanism, it appears to be triggered by a factor in the extracellular fluid. If cells of normal shape, obtained by the dilution method described above, are added to extracellular fluid (from which the amorphous erythrocytes have been removed by centrifugation), they rapidly lose their shape. The activity of the fluid is not heat-labile, nor is it inhibited by protease inhibitors or EGTA (Joseph-Silverstein and Cohen, unpublished observations). The effect also cannot be mimicked by hyperosmotic Ringer's. Presumably it is the rapid dilution of this extracellular factor that prevents cell shape change in the method described above.

Observation of Native Cell and Cytoskeletal Morphology; Preparation of Anucleate Ghosts

A convenient way to see native cell shape in these or any other cell types in which morphological change is possible is to dilute blood immediately approximately 1:10 into Ringer's containing 1% or 0.1% glutaraldehyde. For observation of the cytoskeleton, it is necessary to clear hemoglobin from the cell. The hemoglobin is dense enough to obscure structures in phase contrast (or other types of light microscopy), and its electron density due to iron content is a problem in electron microscopy. One simple method is to dilute a drop of blood (approx 0.05 ml) into 0.5 ml of lysing medium consisting of 1 mM $MgCl_2$, 5 mM EGTA, 0.4% Triton X-100, 100 mM PIPES buffer, pH 6.8, containing 10 mM TAME and 0.1 mM PMSF or other protease inhibitors, and observe in phase contrast under oil immersion using a minimum volume sample flattened under the coverslip. The Triton clears the hemoglobin immediately, and both the nucleus and the marginal band of microtubules with its associated pair of centrioles are easily seen. Another useful technique is to lyse and fix the cells simultaneously. This is achieved by including Triton in a glutaraldehyde fixative. Typically, many of the cells are cleared of hemoglobin before the glutaraldehyde begins to take effect. In some cells the hemoglobin may not escape or be diluted sufficiently, and fuzzy material of moderate electron density will be present within the cell. Even in these cases, structural features are rendered much more visible than without the detergent.

To prepare *anucleate* ghosts, one can dilute fresh blood or washed cells into 50 mM PIPES, 0.5 mM $MgCl_2$, 2.5 mM EGTA, plus protease inhibitors, pH 6.8, and flux three times (i.e., in and out equals one time) through a 22-gauge needle on a syringe. Nuclei are released intact from the osmotically lysed cells, leaving behind nearly phase-transparent ghosts containing some smaller organelles. Appropriate centrifugation will sediment everything but the anucleate ghosts, which are less dense than nuclei or nucleated ghosts. The anucleate ghosts are subsequently collected from the supernate. Although the procedure seems to result in loss of tubulin, the anucleate ghosts are very useful for studying components of the membrane and cell surface-associated cytoskeleton (actin and spectrin-like proteins).

Sources of These Species and Usable Relatives (complete addresses at end of chapter)

A. ovalis and *A. transversa* can be obtained in small numbers from the MBL Department of Marine Resources. *N. ponderosa* and sometimes *A. ovalis* and related species such as *A. lienosa floridana* ("cut-ribbed ark") and *A. braziliana* ("incongruous ark") are available from the Gulf Specimen Co., Inc. Full-grown *A. lienosa floridana* are by far the largest blood clams we have encountered (up to 12 cm in length). *N. ponderosa* are also supplied by H.M. Terry Co., Inc.

Useful reference works for identifying various species of U.S. blood clams are "Guide to Identification of Marine and Estuarine Invertebrates" [Gosner,

1971], "Seashells of North America" [Abbott, 1968], and "American Seashells" [Abbott, 1974]. The major distinguishing features of *N. ponderosa*, *A. ovalis*, and *A. transversa* shells are illustrated on pages 422–425 of Abbott [1974].

Marine bivalves with hemoglobin-containing erythrocytes, closely related to the species described here, are found worldwide. There are representatives in Japan [Ochi, 1972], West Africa [Yoloye, 1975], and Australia [Sullivan, 1961], for example.

References

Abbott RT (1968): "Seashells of North America." New York: Golden Press, Racine, Wisconsin: Western Publishing Co.

Abbott RT (1974): "American Seashells," 2nd Ed. New York, Toronto, London, Melbourne: Van Nostrand Reinhold.

Cavanaugh GM, Ed (1975): "Formulae and Methods IV of the Marine Biological Laboratory." Woods Hole, Massachusetts: Marine Biological Laboratory.

Costa CJ, Pierce SK (1983): Volume regulation in the red coelomocytes of *Glycera dibranchiata*: "An interaction of amino acid and K^+ effluxes. J Comp Physiol 151:133–144.

Gosner KL (1971): "Guide to Identification of Marine and Estuarine Invertebrates. Cape Hatteras to the Bay of Fundy." New York: Wiley.

Ochi O (1972): Fine structures of the erythrocytes in a marine bivalve, *Barbatia virescens*. Mem Ehime Univ Sci Ser B (Biol) 7:14–20.

Sullivan GE (1961): Functional morphology, microanatomy, and histology of the "Sydney cockle," *Anadara trapezia* (Deshayes) (Lamellibranchia: Arcidae). Aust J Zool 9:219–257.

Yoloye V (1975): The habits and functional anatomy of the West African bloody cockle, *Anadara senilis* (L.). Proc Malac Soc Lond 41:277–299.

VIII. PRACTICAL REFERENCE MATERIAL

Reference works that the authors have found particularly useful are presented; a comprehensive listing has not been attempted. Sources of sea salts, refrigerated marine tanks, and living animals are also given below, with addresses and telephone numbers current as of 1984.

A. REFERENCE WORKS

Invertebrate Blood Cells and Comparative Physiology

Andrew W (1965): "Comparative Hematology." New York: Grune and Stratton.

Prosser CL, Brown FA Jr (1961): "Comparative Animal Physiology." 2nd Ed. Philadelphia, London: W.B. Saunders.

Ratcliffe NA, Rowley AF, eds (1981): "Invertebrate Blood Cells." General aspects, animals without true circulatory systems to cephalopods. London: Academic Press, Vol 1.

Ratcliffe NA, Rowley AF, eds (1981): "Invertebrate Blood Cells." Arthropods to urochordates, invertebrates and vertebrates compared. London: Academic Press, Vol 2.

Identification of Species

Abbott RT (1974): "American Seashells," 2nd Ed. New York, Cincinnati, Toronto, London, Melbourne: Van Nostrand Reinhold.

Gosner KL (1971): "Guide to Identification of Marine and Estuarine Invertebrates. Cape Hatteras to the Bay of Fundy." New York: Wiley.

Morris RH, Abbot DP, Hoderlie EC (1980): "Intertidal Invertebrates of California." Stanford, California: Stanford University Press.

Smith RI, ed (1964): "Keys to Marine Invertebrates of the Woods Hole Region." Contribution No. 11 of the Systematics-Ecology Program. Woods Hole, Massachusetts: Marine Biological Laboratory.

Smith RI, Carleton JT, eds (1975): "Light's Manual: Intertidal Invertebrates of the Central California Coast." 3rd Ed. Berkeley, California: University of California Press.

Maintenance of Marine Invertebrates in the Laboratory

Berg CJ Jr (1983): "Culture of Marine Invertebrates, Selected Readings." Stroudsburg, Pennsylvania: Hutchinson Ross.

Committee on Marine Invertebrates (1981): "Laboratory Animal Management, Marine Invertebrates." Washington, DC: National Academy Press.

deGraaf F (1973): "Marine Aquarium Guide." Pet Library, Ltd., Harrison, New Jersey: Sternco Industries.

Needham JG, Galtsoff PS, Lutz FE, Welch PS (1959): "Culture Methods for Invertebrate Animals." New York: Dover.

Smith WL, Chanley MH, eds (1975): "Culture of Marine Invertebrate Animals." New York, London: Plenum.

Spotte S (1979): "Fish and Invertebrate Culture: Water Management in Closed Systems." New York: Wiley (Interscience).

B. ANIMALS, EQUIPMENT, AND SUPPLIES

Sources of Sea Salts and Refrigerated Marine Aquarium Systems

Sea salts and other marine aquarium supplies are generally available in pet shops. For laboratory maintenance of invertebrates in seawater below room temperature, tanks can be kept in a coldroom, or else temperature-controlled systems must be used. The following U.S. suppliers provide sea salts in bulk amounts and/or refrigerated sea water systems.

Aquarium Systems, 8141 Tyler Blvd, Mentor, OH 44060; tel: (216) 255-1997 ("Instant Ocean" sea salts; other supplies).

Frigid Units, Inc., 3214 Sylvania Avenue, Toledo, OH 43613; tel: (419) 474-6971 (refrigerated tanks).

Marinus, Inc., P.O. Box 83098, Westchester, CA 90083; tel: (213) 670–8009 (refrigerated tanks, sea salts).

Pacific Biomarine Laboratories, Inc., P.O. Box 536, Venice, CA 90291; tel: (213) 822-5757 (refrigerated tanks, sea salts).

The Ruet Co., Inc., 441 Market Street, Saddle Brook, NJ 07662; tel: (201) 843-0844 (refrigerated tanks, sea salts).

Sources of Living Marine Invertebrates Cited in This Chapter

Donald A. Bryant, P.O. Box 461, Bath, ME 04530; tel: (207) 442-7521 (*Strongylocentrotus droebachiensis*).

Gulf Specimen Co., Panacea, FL 32346; tel: (904) 984-5297 (*Limulus polyphemus*, *Arbacia punctulata*, *Noetia ponderosa*, *Anadara ovalis*; various crustacea and many other invertebrate species).

Intertidal Marine Biologicals, 33 Cross Street, Shrewsbury, MA 01545; tel: (617) 842-2306 (*Strongylocentrotus purpuratus*).

Maine Bait Co., P.O. Box 204, New Castle, ME 04533; tel: (207) 563-3000 (*Glycera dibranchiata*).

Marine Biological Laboratory, Department of Marine Resources, Woods Hole, MA 02543; tel: (617) 548-3705 ext. 325 (*Limulus polyphemus*, *Libinia emarginata* and other crustacea, *Strongylocentrotus droebachiensis*, *Arbacia punctulata*, *Phascolopsis gouldii*, *Glycera dibranchiata*, *Anarada ovalis*, *Anarada transversa*, many other invertebrate species).

Marinus, Inc., P.O. Box 83098, Westchester, CA 90083; tel: (213) 670-8009 (*Strongylocentrotus purpuratus*, other invertebrate species).

Maritech, P.O. Box 129, Miami, FL 33145 (*Limulus polyphemus*, *Arbacia punctulata*).

Pacific Biomarine Laboratories, Inc., PO Box 536, Venice, CA 90291; tel: (213) 822-5757 (*Strongylocentrotus purpuratus*, *Lytechinus pictus*, *Themiste zostericola*, *Phascolosoma agassizii*, *Urechis caupo*, various crustacea, and many other invertebrate species).

Sea Life Supply, 740 Tioga Avenue, Sand City, CA 93955; tel: (408) 394-0828 (*Phascolosoma agassizii*, *Urechis caupo*, many other invertebrate species).

H.M. Terry Co. Inc., Willis Wharf, VA 23486; tel: (804) 442-6251 (*Noetia ponderosa, Arbacia punctulata*).

ACKNOWLEDGMENTS

We are indebted to Jacquelyn Joseph-Silverstein (Hunter College), Dr. Louis Leibovitz (MBL), Dr. Ronald Nagel (Albert Einstein College of Medicine), and Dr. Greenfield Sluder (Worcester Foundation) for additional contributions and/or consultations during preparation of this chapter.

Index